# Liver Cancers

Tim Cross • Daniel H. Palmer
Editors

# Liver Cancers

## From Mechanisms to Management

Springer

*Editors*
Tim Cross
Royal Liverpool University Hospital
Liverpool
Merseyside
UK

Daniel H. Palmer
University of Liverpool
Liverpool Early Drug Development Unit
Liverpool
UK

ISBN 978-3-319-92215-7 ISBN 978-3-319-92216-4 (eBook)
https://doi.org/10.1007/978-3-319-92216-4

Library of Congress Control Number: 2018957857



This Springer imprint is published by the registered company Springer Nature Switzerland AG
The registered company address is: Gewerbestrasse 11, 6330 Cham, Switzerland

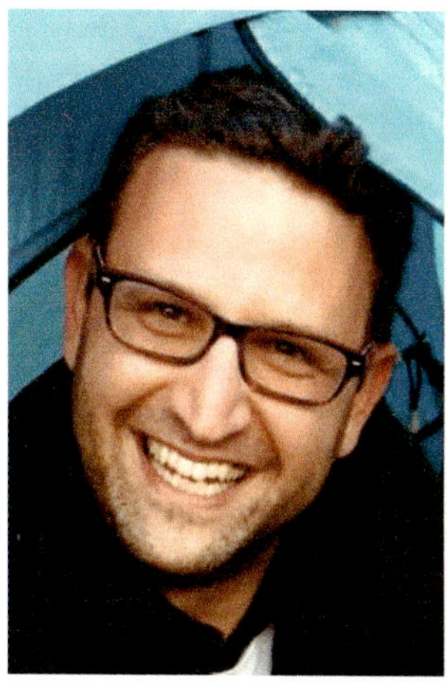

*Dedicated to the Memory of Dr. CG 'Harry' Antoniades (1974–2018).*

# Foreword

There has been stunning progress in treating viral hepatitis over the last decade. Despite that, the number of patients across the world with liver disease is increasing annually, and in the United Kingdom, this has had a disproportionate and adverse effect on younger patients, such that chronic liver disease in England is now the second and fourth most common cause of years lost in women and men, respectively. Almost all of the increase over the past two decades can be attributed directly to the epidemic of obesity in first-world countries, although in many parts of the world alcohol continues to play an important aetiological role. There is also a strong, disproportionate effect of socio-economic deprivation on the prevalence of liver disease.

So it was inevitable that the numbers of patients presenting with hepatocellular carcinoma (HCC) would rise in parallel with those developing chronic liver disease. The increased numbers presenting to liver specialists with primary liver cancer have been almost overwhelming, while the change in the demographics underlying these tumours has been striking. No more of the young male immigrant born in the African or Asian continents with Hepatitis B virus acquired perinatally driving cirrhosis as we were taught. Now it is the elderly, slightly overweight, male diabetic in the clinic who has never consumed alcohol to excess and who may not even have cirrhosis.

These remarkable lifestyle-driven increases in cases presenting with hepatocellular carcinoma have made clinicians and more recently basic scientists look more closely at every aspect of the disease from the molecular pathways that precede disease or modify the clinical course, through screening (still contentious) or early detection to curative or palliative treatment and end-of-life care.

The proportion of patients that can be offered curative therapy is small but increasing. Recent data suggest that this proportion is greater in those centres with greater experience and turnover. The options for curative therapy are limited and by no means novel but earlier diagnosis, better case selection, and more experience mean that these older approaches (surgery or liver transplantation or both) are being used more appropriately with improved outcomes. The many options for therapy intended to halt or slow the disease for patients with more advanced disease have also been used with increasing frequency and efficacy. But it is not clear which of these approaches is best for which patients nor is it clear if these approaches have additive benefit. Most centres report better survival now with non-curative therapy than a decade ago, reflecting greater availability of these approaches and again better selection based on growing experience. International meetings and the literature now report on potential pathways for novel approaches to primary liver cancer.

Those who deal with primary liver cancers will often be the same clinicians that are faced with benign tumours of the liver or with secondary malignancies.

HCC-UK was established 4 years ago to bring all of those interested in liver cancer. The faculty for this volume: *Liver Cancers: From Mechanisms to Management* are integral to HCC-UK and represent the best of UK specialist care in the field, so that every aspect of our current knowledge and clinical practice is covered.

Graeme Alexander
The Sheila Sherlock Liver Centre
The Royal Free Hospital
London, UK

# Preface

There has been a well-documented rise in the prevalence of advanced liver disease over the last few decades. The culmination of this has been an increase in patients with cirrhosis and its complications. One of the most feared of these was hepatocellular carcinoma (HCC). At one time, this diagnosis heralded a universally grim prognosis, and the treatment options, particularly cure, in the absence of surgical resection, was rarely achieved. But the development of new technologies and the availabilities of new treatments, in particular, liver transplantation, have revolutionized treatment for these patients. Yet, the majority of patients still remain undiagnosed until the disease is at an incurable stage. For these patients, provided that their liver function and performance status permits, there are treatments that can extend life, and novel treatments appear tantalizingly close, in particular immune therapies. In addition, forms of targeted radiotherapies are appearing on the horizon (e.g., stereotactic body radiotherapy – SBRT) and could provide further treatment options for clinicians. So as the horizons for HCC are broadening so are treatment options for cholangiocarcinoma and other forms of malignancy that involve the liver. The contribution to be made by different specialities in a multidisciplinary team involving surgery, transplantation surgery, hepatology, medical oncology, clinical oncology, and palliative care is vital to ensure the best possible outcome for these patients and cannot be overemphasized.

This book is aimed at the hospital specialist in training in the medical or surgical specialities, nurse specialists, and consultants and researchers who just want an approachable and usable management guide. The chapters have been written by experts in their fields and focuses primarily on hepatocellular carcinoma whilst having comprehensive sections on cholangiocarcinoma, neuroendocrine tumours, and colorectal cancer liver metastases. Many authors are members of HCC-UK which is a UK group of clinicians and researchers with an interest in HCC who wish to improve the care and outcome for these patients. Professor Graeme Alexander must be thanked for having the vision to set up this group, and the intention is to work together to deliver management changing high-impact publications in the future. There was some constraint on what could be included and so detailed chapters on endoscopic therapies and radiotherapy will have to wait for further editions.

I am grateful to all the contributors for the time and effort they put into producing their chapters and also to the production team at Springer in particular Maha and Evgenia. Finally, this book is dedicated to the memory of Dr. CG 'Harry' Antoniades who died suddenly this year. He was reader in medicine at Imperial College London, St Mary's Hospital. He was an exceptional clinician and researcher, as well as a great friend and colleague. He will be deeply missed by all those who knew him. He leaves behind his wife Rebecca (herself an oncologist) and two wonderful children Amelie and Theo. Our thoughts and prayers are with them, and this book is a small token to show the respect and esteem in which he was held.

Liverpool, UK
April, 2018

Tim Cross

# Contents

# Contributors

**Nicholas Bird, MBBS, MRCS** Hepatobiliary Surgery, Digestive Diseases unit, Aintree University Hospital, Liverpool, UK

**Alexa Childs** Department of Oncology, UCL Medical School, London, UK

**Jenny Cotton** Department of Medical Oncology, The Christie NHS Foundation Trust, Manchester, UK

Department of Medical Oncology, The Clatterbridge Cancer Centre, Wirral, UK

**Tim Cross, BMedSci (hons), MBBS, FRCP, MD** The Royal Liverpool Hospital, Liverpool, UK

Department of Molecular and Clinical Cancer Medicine, University of Liverpool, Liverpool, UK

**Rafael Diaz-Nieto, MD, PhD** Hepatobiliary Surgery, Digestive Diseases Unit, Aintree University Hospital, Liverpool, UK

**Mona Elshafie, MBChB, MSc, MD** Birmingham Neuroendocrine Tumour Centre, Queen Elizabeth Hospital, Birmingham, UK

**Jonathan C. Evans, MRCP, FRCR** The Royal Liverpool Hospital, Liverpool, UK

**Olusola O. Faluyi, MBChB (Hons), PhD, MRCP** Clatterbridge Cancer Centre, Wirral, UK

**Andrea Casadei Gardini** Department of Medical Oncology, Istituto Scientifico Romagnolo per Lo Studio e Cura Dei Tumori (IRST) IRCCS, Meldola, Italy

**Jessica C. Hale, MRCP** Clatterbridge Cancer Centre, Wirral, UK

**Matthew Hoare, MAMB, MRCP (UK), PhD** Cancer Research UK Cambridge Centre, University of Cambridge, Cambridge, UK

Department of Medicine, Addenbrooke's Hospital, University of Cambridge, Cambridge, UK

**Charles Imber, MD, FRCS, Mb, BCHir, BSc, Hons** Centre For HPB Surgery and Liver Transplantation, Royal Free Hospital, London, UK

**Nadya Fatima Jabbar, FRCR** Aintree University Hospital, Liverpool, UK

**Philip Johnson, MD, FRCP** Department of Molecular and Clinical Cancer Medicine, University of Liverpool, Liverpool, UK

**Robert Jones, BSc, MB, ChB, PhD** Department of Liver surgery, Aintree University Hospital NHS Foundation Trust, Liverpool, UK

**Shahid A. Khan, BSc (Hons), MBBS, PhD, FRCP** St Mary's Hospital (Imperial College), London, UK

**Nabil Kibriya, MBBS, FRCR** Kings College Hospital, London, UK

**Vinay Kumar Balachandrakumar, MBBS, MRCP (UK)** University of Liverpool, Liverpool, UK

**Angela Lamarca** Department of Medical Oncology, The Christie NHS Foundation Trust, Manchester, UK

**Yuk Ting Ma, PhD, FRCP** Department of Medical Oncology, Queen Elizabeth Hospital, Birmingham, UK

**Hassan Malik, MB, ChB, FRCS, MD** Department of Liver surgery, Aintree University Hospital NHS Foundation Trust, Liverpool, UK

**Aileen Marshall** The Sheila Sherlock Centre for hepatology and liver transplantation, The Royal Free Hospital, London, UK

**João Maurício** Northern Institute for Cancer Research, Newcastle University, Newcastle upon Tyne, UK

**Stephen McClements** St Mary's Hospital (Imperial College), London, UK

**Mairéad G. McNamara, MB, ChB, BMedSci, BSc, PhD** Department of Medical Oncology, The Christie NHS Foundation Trust, Manchester, UK

Division of Cancer Sciences, University of Manchester, Manchester, UK

**Tim Meyer, BSc, FRCP, PhD** UCL Cancer Institute, University College London, London, UK

**Andrew R. Moore, MB, ChB, PhD, MRCP** Liverpool Regional Neuroendocrine Tumour Service, Royal Liverpool University Hospital, Liverpool, UK

**James Pape, MB, ChB, MRCS** Centre For HPB Surgery and Liver Transplantation, Royal Free Hospital, London, UK

**Oliver Pickles** Department of Medical Oncology, Queen Elizabeth Hospital, Birmingham, UK

**Graeme J. Poston, DSc** Hepatobiliary Surgery, Digestive Diseases unit, Aintree University Hospital, Liverpool, UK

**Alberto Quaglia, MD, PhD, FRCPath** The Institute of Liver Studies, King's College Hospital, London, UK

**Leonard M. Quinn, MB, ChB (hons), MRCS** Hepatobiliary Surgery, Digestive Diseases unit, Aintree University Hospital, Liverpool, UK

**Helen Reeves, BMedSci, MBBS, PhD, FRCP** Northern Institute for Cancer Research, Newcastle University, Newcastle upon Tyne, UK

**Paul J. Ross, MBBS, PhD, FRCP** Department of Medical Oncology, Guy's Cancer, Guy's and St Thomas' NHS Foundation Trust, London, UK

Department of Oncology, King's College Hospital NHS Foundation Trust, London, UK

**Ian A. Rowe, MRCP, PhD** Liver Unit, St. James's University Hospital, Leeds, UK

Leeds Institute for Data Analytics, University of Leeds, Leeds, UK

**Vandana M. Sagar** Birmingham Neuroendocrine Tumour Centre, Queen Elizabeth Hospital, Birmingham, UK

**Bruno Sangro, MD, PhD** Liver Unit and HPB Oncology Area, Clinica Universidad de Navarra, IDISNA and CIBEREHD, Pamplona, Spain

**Tahir Shah, MBBS, FRCP, MD** Birmingham Neuroendocrine Tumour Centre, Queen Elizabeth Hospital, Birmingham, UK

**Dinesh Sharma, MBBS, MS, FRCS (Ed)** The Sheila Sherlock Centre for hepatology and liver transplantation, The Royal Free Hospital, London, UK

**Mikael H. Sodergren** Department of Surgery and Cancer, Imperial College London, London, UK

**Nicholas Stern, MB, ChB, MD, FRCP** Aintree University Hospital, Liverpool, UK

**Ray S. Tan, MBBS, MRCP** Department of Medical Oncology, Guy's Cancer, Guy's and St Thomas' NHS Foundation Trust, London, UK

**Eleanor J. Taylor** Liver Unit, St. James's University Hospital, Leeds, UK

**Juan W. Valle** Department of Medical Oncology, The Christie NHS Foundation Trust, Manchester, UK

Division of Cancer Sciences, University of Manchester, Manchester, UK

**David Vass** Hepatobiliary Surgery, Digestive Diseases unit, Aintree University Hospital, Liverpool, UK

**David White, FRCR** Aintree University Hospital, Liverpool, UK

**Caroline L. Wilson, BSc (hons), PhD** Faculty of Medical Sciences, Institute of Cellular Medicine, Newcastle University, Newcastle upon Tyne, UK

**Jen-Jou Wong** Department of Radiology, The Royal Lilverpool Hospital, Liverpool, UK

**Vincent S. Yip, MB, ChB, MD, FRCS** Department of Hepatobiliary and Pancreatic Surgery, Royal Liverpool & Broadgreen University Hospital, Liverpool, UK

# Part I
# Hepatocellular Carcinoma

# Chapter 1
# The Epidemiology of Hepatocellular Carcinoma

**Philip Johnson**

**Key Learning Points**

1. Hepatocellular carcinoma (HCC), the most common form of primary liver cancer, is predominantly a male disease, associated with increasing age and many types of chronic liver disease.
2. It is most prevalent in China and the Far East, Japan and sub-Saharan Africa.
3. This geographic variation is accounted for by the distribution of aetiological factors which include chronic hepatitis B virus infection (HBV), chronic hepatitis C virus (HCV) infection, alcoholic cirrhosis and obesity/metabolic syndrome—related to non-alcoholic fatty liver disease.
4. Vaccination against HBV and antiviral therapy for HCV will decrease the incidence of HCC in many populations and change the epidemiology.
5. In the West mortality from HCC is rising mainly due to fatty liver disease, consequent upon the increasing prevalence of obesity.

**Areas of Controversy and Uncertainty**

1. The long-term impact of obesity on the incidence of hepatocellular carcinoma in the West. The relationship between obesity-related HCC and cirrhosis is a major area of uncertainty.

P. Johnson (✉)
Department of Molecular and Clinical Cancer Medicine, University of Liverpool, Liverpool, UK
e-mail: Philip.Johnson@liverpool.ac.uk



T. Cross, D. H. Palmer (eds.), *Liver Cancers*,
https://doi.org/10.1007/978-3-319-92216-4_1

2. The long-term impact of antiviral treatment on the incidence of HCC both in the West (specifically hepatitis C) and the East (specifically hepatitis B).
3. The risk of HCC development after clearance of the hepatitis C virus by the action of direct-acting antiviral agents and the optimal strategy for surveillance amongst those who clear the virus.

## Introduction and Magnitude of the Problem

In an increasingly globalised world, understanding the epidemiology of HCC has important implications for the clinical management of HCC.

Worldwide, primary liver cancer or hepatocellular carcinoma (HCC) is the sixth most commonly occurring cancer and the second largest contributor to cancer-related mortality. Due to the aggressive nature of the tumour, the associated underlying liver disease, late presentation and the limited range of therapeutic options, incidence and mortality rates are very close. It is the commonest of the two main primary malignancies of the liver, the other major hepatic cancer being cholangiocarcinoma (CC) which accounts for between 5 and 10% of malignant primary liver tumours, although it is increasingly recognised that there can be overlap of the features of HCC and CC.

## Demography

The incidence of HCC can be broadly classified according to geographical region as high-, medium- and low-incidence areas (Fig. 1.1). The high-incidence areas include China, Southeast Asia, Japan and sub-Saharan Africa, with an incidence rate of over 20/100,000. Intermediate areas (incidence 5–20/100,000) include Southern Europe, and low-incidence areas include the USA, Scandinavia and Northern Europe [1].

In most areas of the world, the disease occurs predominantly in men over the age of 60 years, but the age at onset is significantly lower in sub-Saharan Africa. The reason for the male preponderance is unknown, but the regional variation in incidence is clearly accounted for by the geographic distribution of the major risk factors.

## Risk Factors

The most striking feature of the epidemiology of HCC is the wide geographical variation in incidence (Fig. 1.2) which largely reflects the global distribution of the major aetiological factors, as described below. However, the relative importance and thereby the geographical distribution are changing rapidly with the development of new therapies and public health initiatives.

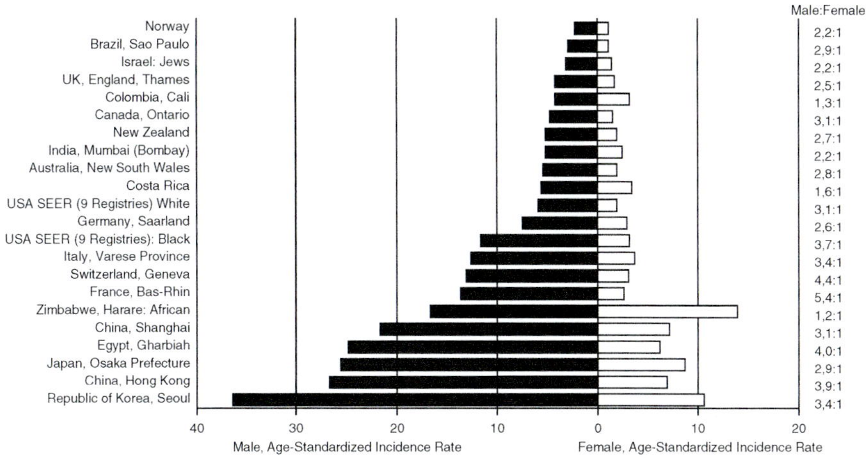


**Fig. 1.1** Age-adjusted incidences per 100,000 of liver cancer among men and women by region, 2003–2007. Age-adjusted to world standard (Available at http://ci5.iarc.fr)

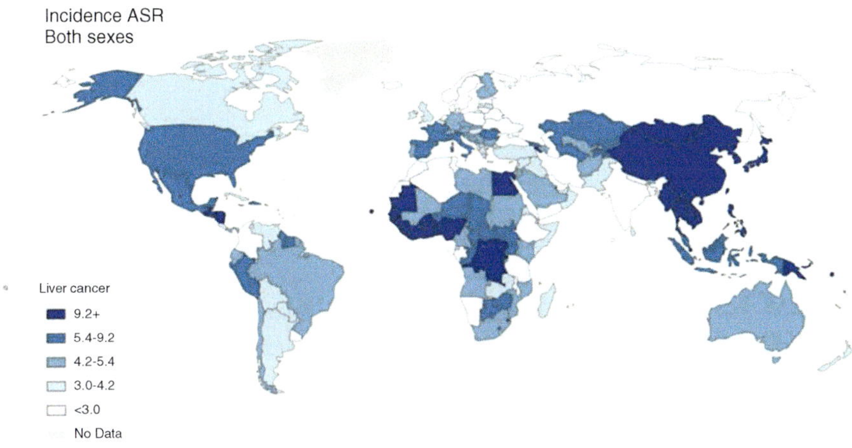


**Fig. 1.2** Geographic variation in liver cancer incidence (age-standardised) (Available from http://globocan.iarc.fr)

## The Hepatitis B Virus

The classic study of the natural history of hepatitis B virus infection and its relationship with HCC was reported from Taiwan [2]. This study followed up 22,707 HBV carriers for 5 years (Fig. 1.3). The annual incidence rate among those developing HCC was about 100-fold risk of the control group, thereby conclusively demonstrating the aetiological relevance of the HBV virus to HCC development and laying the basis for mass prevention strategies.

Fig. 1.3 The Taiwan prospective study of HCC development in patients with chronic hepatitis B virus infection. From Beasley et al. [2]

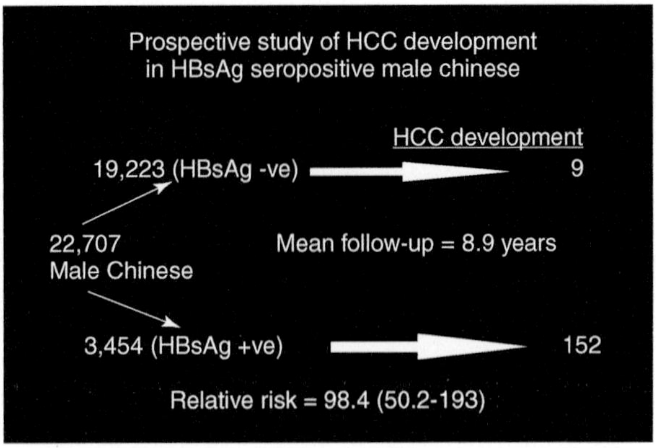


The natural history and global distribution of chronic HBV infection are now well documented [3, 4]. HBV is transmitted from mother to newborn at, or around, the time of birth, and this observation, combined with the Beasley study, led to a programme of mass vaccination against HBV, initiated in Taiwan in 1984 and supplemented by HBIG (hepatitis B immunoglobulin). The vaccine is extremely safe and effective, but, for a variety of reasons, vaccine-induced immunity coverage is much less than 100%, even in countries where universal vaccination is advocated.

The subsequent progress of this initiative in Taiwan and other countries and regions has been well documented. The latest analysis clearly shows that the prevalence of $HB_sAg$ seropositivity has fallen from around 10% to less than 2% among those born in the immunisation period, and there has been a dramatic decrease in the incidence of HCC although the full impact will not be realised for another 30 years, when the first vaccines reach their sixth decade [5]. In the West most HBV-related disease arises from intravenous drug abuse or is sexually transmitted. First-generation immigrant populations coming from high HBV incidence areas to the West also tend to be over-represented with respect to HCC.

Obviously immunisation will have no impact on those who are already HBV carriers, but current evidence suggests that antiviral therapy significantly reduces the incidence of HCC [6]. Nonetheless, and in marked contradistinction to the current situation in HCV, sustained virus control is difficult and expensive to achieve. Thus, the combination of immunisation and antiviral therapy is likely to alter the epidemiology of HCC dramatically over the coming decades, although the gap between what is medically possible and what is, in financial and political terms, deliverable remains wide.

All therapeutic interventions are small when compared to the impact of immunisation and other methods by which the hepatitis B virus can be eliminated or controlled.

## Hepatitis C Virus and the Changing Epidemiology of HCC in the West

Initially classified as 'non-A/non-B'virus infection, HCV was identified in 1989, and although such rigorous epidemiological studies as described above for HBV were never undertaken, case-control studies left little doubt that the virus was strongly associated with HCC. In the West HCV was acquired mainly though intravenous substance abuse or by blood transfusion. In Japan there was a major epidemic which led to around 35,000 cases developing per year for the 50 years following the end of the Second World War, after which there had been extensive use of infected blood [7].

In the last few years, effective therapy for HCV has been developed to the extent that complete "cure" can be obtained within a few months of treatment, and in several countries, the complete eradication of HCV is envisaged. After achievement of sustained virological remission, the risk of HCC decreases dramatically, further supporting the aetiological role of the virus [8].

## Alcohol

Alcoholic cirrhosis has long been considered a major risk factor for HCC accounting for a high proportion of cases in the West. However, it now seems likely that, whilst there is a significant increase in HCC among patients with a history of high alcohol intake, some of this is related to associated factors such as coexisting HBV and HCV infection, which were not recognised in earlier studies, and the increasing recognition that alcohol likely acts in a synergistic manner to encourage HCC in patients with other underlying causes [9, 10, 11–13].

## Aflatoxin

Aflatoxin B1 is a potent carcinogen derived from the mould *Aspergillus flavus* (hence aflatoxin) that grows in humid conditions on stored grain and ground nuts. It is a very likely contributor to the high incidence of HCC in sub-Saharan Africa and coastal regions of Southeast Asia and China [14]. Exposure to AFB1 is associated with a specific DNA mutation in the p53 gene (a 249ser mutation) [15]. It has a synergistic association with HBV in increasing the risk of HCC. The population attributable risk of AFB1 in sub-Saharan Africa is between 10 and 20%.

In general, in areas of the world where AFB1 exposure is high, chronic HBV infection is highly prevalent. As little can be done to alter the HBV chronic infection state, once established, eradicating AFB1 from the food supply is an important strategy to reduce HCC incidence. In parts of Africa and China where AFB1 eradication programmes have been implemented, significant reductions in HCC rates have been documented [16].

## Other Rarer Forms of Chronic Liver Disease

HCC is a recognised complication of all types of cirrhosis and chronic liver disease including primary biliary cirrhosis, Wilson's disease and alpha-1 antitrypsin deficiency. HCC is a major cause of mortality in haemochromatosis but can be prevented by venesection therapy if instituted before cirrhosis develops. This justifies careful screening of families with a history of haemochromatosis so as to achieve early diagnosis and to initiate appropriate therapy at a presymptomatic, pre-cirrhotic stage.

## Obesity/Metabolic Syndrome and NAFLD

There remain between 10 and 30% of cases in which no aetiological factors can be identified. Such cases were previously referred to as "cryptogenic". Over the past two decades, however, it has become apparent that in such cases there is a high incidence of obesity [17, 18] and diabetes. The associated liver disease is called non-alcoholic fatty liver disease (NAFLD) [19]. In a subgroup of this population, there is a fat-related inflammatory response that is likely to progress to serious liver disease—so-called non-alcoholic steatohepatitis (NASH). However, HCC may arise in NAFLD, without any associated chronic liver disease or cirrhosis [20]. Tobacco consumption probably imposes a risk, comparable to that of obesity.

## Implications of Epidemiology for Prevention

Epidemiological investigations have identified the relevant risk factors such that the major ones act as a target for preventative strategies. There is another and quite distinct epidemiological approach that may result in further preventative measures, and this relates to the analysis of large datasets that have been collected for purposes other than direct investigation of the prevention of HCC. This approach falls under the heading of "repurposing" of drugs. Thus, large-scale datasets reporting the incidence of HCCs in populations treated with various agents for purposes unrelated to their potential anticancer are an area of extensive research. Aspirin and non-steroidal anti-inflammatory drugs have well-documented activity in reducing the incidence of most gastrointestinal cancers, including HCC [21], and the evidence that statins have an equivalent effect is now substantial [22]. Antidiabetic drugs such as metformin have also been proposed, but the most recent meta-analyses are less convincing [23].

## The Changing Face of HCC Epidemiology

As suggested throughout this chapter, HCC is a preventable disease, and, over the last decade, evidence has emerged that preventative strategies are starting to have an impact on incidence. Chronic HBV infection rates, as a result of immunisation and antiviral treatment, are falling with resulting stabilisation or decrease in HCC rates across China and the Far East. In Japan and Southern Europe, the peak incidence of the post-war HCV epidemic is passing, and the later drug abuse-related epidemic in the West may be eradicated by direct-acting antiviral agents. Against these encouraging trends, it is sobering to note that HCC is now the most rapidly rising cause of cancer-related mortality at a time when the incidence of other cancers is falling by around 1–2% per annum (Fig. 1.4). The reason is clear. The major current aetiological factors are all related to the great addictions of Western societies, namely, alcohol, tobacco and, particularly, food. There is little prospect that this situation will change over the foreseeable future.

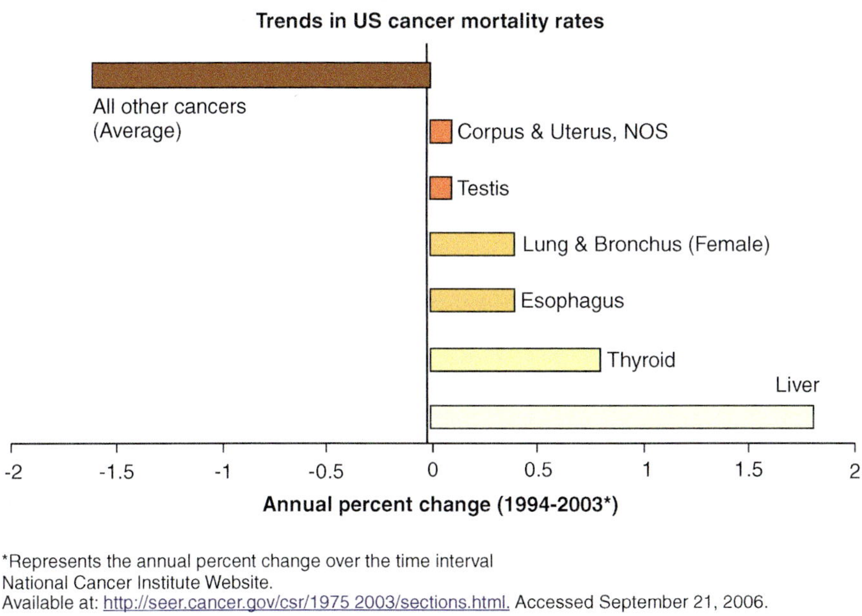


**Fig. 1.4** Change in cancer mortality rate in the USA. Note that "liver" is the most rapidly rising cause of cancer-related mortality at a time when the mortality from most cancers is decreasing

# References


1. Ferlay J, Parkin DM, Curado MP, et al. Cancer incidence in five continents, volumes I to X: IARC CANCERBase No. 10. 2014. [Internet]. Available at: http://ci5.iarc.fr. Accessed 25 Nov 2014.
2. Beasley RP, Hwang LY, Lin CC, Chien CS. Hepatocellular carcinoma and hepatitis B virus. A prospective study of 22 707 men in Taiwan. Lancet. 1981;2(8256):1129–33.
3. McMahon BJ. The natural history of chronic hepatitis B virus infection. Hepatology. 2009;49(5 Suppl):S45–55. [PubMed: 19399792]
4. Ott JJ, Stevens GA, Groeger J, Wiersma ST. Global epidemiology of hepatitis B virus infection: new estimates of age-specific HBsAg seroprevalence and endemicity. Vaccine. 2012;30(12):2212–9. PubMed: 22273662
5. Chiang CJ, Yang YW, You SL, Lai MS, Chen CJ. Thirty-year outcomes of the national hepatitis B immunization program in Taiwan. JAMA. 2013;310(9):974–6. PubMed: 24002285
6. Liaw YF, Sung JJ, Chow WC, Farrell G, Lee CZ, Yuen H, Tanwandee T, Tao QM, Shue K, Keene ON, Dixon JS, Gray DF, Sabbat J, Cirrhosis Asian Lamivudine Multicentre Study Group. Lamivudine for patients with chronic hepatitis B and advanced liver disease. N Engl J Med. 2004;351(15):1521–31.
7. Umemura T, Ichijo T, Yoshizawa K, Tanaka E, Kiyosawa K. Epidemiology of hepatocellular carcinoma in Japan. J Gastroenterol. 2009;44(Suppl 19):102–7.
8. El-Serag HB, Kanwal F, Richardson P, Kramer J. Risk of hepatocellular carcinoma after sustained virological response in Veterans with hepatitis C virus infection. Hepatology. 2016;64(1):130–7. https://doi.org/10.1002/hep.28535. Epub 2016 Apr 19
9. Hassan MM, Hwang LY, Hatten CJ, Swaim M, Li D, Abbruzzese JL, Beasley P, Patt YZ. Risk factors for hepatocellular carcinoma: synergism of alcohol with viral hepatitis and diabetes mellitus. Hepatology. 2002;36:1206–13.
10. Jepsen P, Ott P, Andersen PK, Sorensen HT, Vilstrup H. Risk for hepatocellular carcinoma in patients with alcoholic cirrhosis: a danish nationwide cohort study. Ann Intern Med. 2012;156:841–7.
11. Donato F, Tagger A, Gelatti U, Parrinello G, Boffetta P, Albertini A, Decarli A, Trevisi P, Ribero ML, Martelli C, Porru S, Nardi G. Alcohol and hepatocellular carcinoma: the effect of lifetime intake and hepatitis virus infections in men and women. Am J Epidemiol. 2002;155:323–31.
12. La Vecchia C. Alcohol and liver cancer. Eur J Cancer Prev. 2007;16:495–7. 52.
13. Morgan TR, Mandayam S, Jamal MM. Alcohol and hepatocellular carcinoma. Gastroenterology. 2004;127:S87–96.
14. Liu Y, Wu F. Global burden of aflatoxin-induced hepatocellular carcinoma: a risk assessment. Environ Health Perspect. 2010;118(6):818–24. PubMed: 20172840
15. Hsia CC, Kleiner DE Jr, Axiotis CA, Di Bisceglie A, Nomura AM, Stemmermann GN, Tabor E. Mutations of p53 gene in hepatocellular carcinoma: roles of hepatitis B virus and aflatoxin contamination in the diet. J Natl Cancer Inst. 1992;84:1638–41.
16. Chen JG, Egner PA, Ng D, et al. Reduced aflatoxin exposure presages decline in liver cancer mortality in an endemic region of China. Cancer Prev Res (Phila). 2013;6(10):1038–45.
17. Calle EE, Rodriguez C, Walker-Thurmond K, Thun MJ. Overweight, obesity, and mortality from cancer in a prospectively studied cohort of U.S. adults. N Engl J Med. 2003;348:1625–38.
18. Starley BQ, Calcagno CJ, Harrison SA. Nonalcoholic fatty liver disease and hepatocellular carcinoma: a weighty connection. Hepatology. 2010;51:1820–32. 47.
19. White DL, Kanwal F, El-Serag HB. Association between nonalcoholic fatty liver disease and risk for hepatocellular cancer, based on systematic review. Clin Gastroenterol Hepatol. 2012;10:1342–59.
20. Margini C, Dufour JF. The story of HCC in NAFLD: from epidemiology, across pathogenesis, to prevention and treatment. Liver Int. 2016;36:317–24.

21. Sahasrabuddhe VV, Gunja MZ, Graubard BI, et al. Nonsteroidal anti-inflammatory drug use, chronic liver disease, and hepatocellular carcinoma. J Natl Cancer Inst. 2012;104(23):1808–14.
22. Singh S, Singh PP, Singh AG, Murad MH, Sanchez W. Statins are associated with a reduced risk of hepatocellular cancer: a systematic review and meta-analysis. Gastroenterology. 2012;144(2):323–32.
23. Hagberg KW, McGlynn KA, Sahasrabuddhe VV, Jick S. Anti-diabetic medications and risk of primary liver cancer in persons with type II diabetes. Br J Cancer. 2014;111(9):1710–7.

# Chapter 2
# Surveillance for Hepatocellular Carcinoma

**Eleanor J. Taylor and Ian A. Rowe**

**Key Learning Points**

1. Surveillance for the development of HCC in patients at risk, particularly those with cirrhosis, is logical with the aim to reduce overall mortality.
2. Six-monthly ultrasound scans (with or without AFP testing) is the current standard of care defined by professional societies.
3. The overall benefits of surveillance are small in populations of patients with cirrhosis, accounting for a reduction in overall mortality over 5 years of surveillance of approximately 1–2%.
4. The effectiveness of surveillance is reduced by eligible patients not entering surveillance programmes and by patients ineligible for curative treatments entering such programmes.
5. There are harms associated with surveillance that need to be communicated to the patient, together with the benefits that might be achieved.

**Areas of Controversy and Uncertainty**

1. The magnitude of the benefit of surveillance in patients with cirrhosis is uncertain and is subject to confounding.

E. J. Taylor
Liver Unit, St. James's University Hospital, Leeds, UK

I. A. Rowe (✉)
Liver Unit, St. James's University Hospital, Leeds, UK

Leeds Institute for Data Analytics, University of Leeds, Leeds, UK
e-mail: I.A.C.Rowe@leeds.ac.uk



T. Cross, D. H. Palmer (eds.), *Liver Cancers*,
https://doi.org/10.1007/978-3-319-92216-4_2

2. Models that predict benefits of surveillance are based on confounded retrospective estimates.
3. The significance of the harms of surveillance is uncertain.
4. There is a rationale for developing a randomised controlled trial of surveillance to address this uncertainty, but this is not be supported by the expert consensus.

The majority of hepatocellular carcinoma (HCC) globally is associated with chronic viral hepatitis, and it occurs most frequently in individuals with cirrhosis [1]. In the developed world, HCC associated with cirrhosis is the predominant form of the disease, accounting for at least 80% of cases [2]. Outcomes after diagnosis of HCC remain poor, particularly when HCC is diagnosed at late stage. It is for these reasons that surveillance for HCC, using regular 6-monthly ultrasound scans, is proposed as a method to improve outcomes for patients with cirrhosis. The aim of that surveillance is to improve overall survival of patients with cirrhosis.

In this chapter we will discuss the rationale for surveillance and the evidence that supports it, rates and barriers to the uptake of surveillance at the population level, and the expected outcomes of surveillance given current diagnostic and treatment methods.

## The Rationale for Surveillance

Patients with chronic liver diseases, including viral hepatitis, alcohol-related liver disease and non-alcoholic fatty liver disease, as well as those with rarer metabolic diseases such as genetic haemochromatosis and autoimmune liver diseases, are at risk of developing cirrhosis. Treatment of the underlying cause of liver disease will usually prevent progression to cirrhosis and abrogate the risk of later developing complications of liver disease, including HCC. Those individuals who are not diagnosed with liver disease or those where treatment is for whatever reason unavailable or ineffective are at risk of disease progression through accumulation of liver fibrosis to cirrhosis. Once cirrhosis has developed, there is a risk of developing liver failure and also a risk of developing HCC. Since HCC is a major cause of mortality in this group, it is logical to consider surveillance to diagnose HCC early so that potentially curative treatments can be used to improve the overall survival of both the patient and the population with cirrhosis.

Typically surveillance is done using 6-monthly ultrasound scans and that is the method that is endorsed by the European Association for the Study of the Liver (EASL) as well as the United Kingdom National Institute for Health and Care Excellence (NICE) [3, 4]. There are however proponents for the addition of blood-based biomarkers of HCC development, most notably alpha-fetoprotein, to ultrasound to maximise early diagnosis. The additional benefits of AFP are frequently discussed and it is listed as optional in some guidelines [5]. Whilst there is a small increase in the sensitivity of surveillance in general for early HCC by incorporating AFP, this comes at the cost of increasing the numbers of false-positive surveillance assessments [6]. This will also inevitably increase the rates of surveillance-associated harms that are discussed later.

## The Target Population

Patients at risk of developing HCC are characterised as those with cirrhosis (from any cause) as well as those with advanced fibrosis from hepatitis C virus infection and those with hepatitis B virus (HBV) infection and associated risk factors including age, family history of HCC and active hepatitis. These groups are selected, largely on the basis of cost-effectiveness studies, as those with the most to gain from early diagnosis of HCC where the incidence is sufficient to warrant that intervention [3]. It is apparent that the annual incidence of HCC in each of the groups is different, ranging from 3% in those with hepatitis C cirrhosis to approximately 0.2% for those with HBV infection and associated risk factors. Given the low incidence in the non-cirrhotic HBV group, a number of investigators have tried to identify scores that will allow patients at high risk of HCC to be identified so that the whole group need not be entered into surveillance [7]. This is an attractive approach, but unless these scores can reliably identify groups with a *zero* risk of HCC development, it is challenging to implement given strong recommendations from the major professional associations [3, 5] for ongoing surveillance in this group.

## Evidence of the Benefits of Surveillance

There have been two randomised controlled trials of surveillance done in China. These studies are not applicable to current practice, either because they did not use current methods of surveillance (i.e., 6-monthly ultrasound examinations) or because they included patients without cirrhosis. There are also a number of methodological concerns regarding these studies [8]. Consequently, they cannot be used to justify surveillance in Western patients with cirrhosis today.

There are a large number of retrospective studies from Europe, the United States and the Far East that suggest benefits of surveillance. These have been systematically reviewed by two groups, one of whom pooled the data that were extracted in a meta-analysis. The conclusions of the two reviews were similar in that they each concluded that it was probable that surveillance allows earlier diagnosis of HCC but diverged on the impact on mortality. One review concluded that the quality of the published evidence was very low, and there was uncertainty as to whether surveillance improved survival in patients with cirrhosis [9]. The second review concluded that surveillance improved survival in patients with cirrhosis based on the outcomes of their meta-analysis [10], and this study has been used to support subsequent recommendations for surveillance in the American Association for the Study of Liver Diseases guideline for patients with HCC [5].

To understand the apparently contradictory findings of these reviews, it is critical to explore the evidence base further. The studies included in these reviews were all case control studies where the outcomes of patients with HCC were stratified by whether they had received surveillance or not. This design can therefore only assess whether surveillance improves outcomes in patients who have developed HCC and not those who have cirrhosis as a whole. Furthermore this design is subject to overestimation of the impact of surveillance since there will be confounding by a number of factors. These include confounding by the indication for surveillance where patients who are better suited to treatment for HCC are selected for surveillance, apparently improved survival as a consequence of lead time bias, as well as by length bias, each of which are well recognised in studies of other screening and surveillance programmes (Fig. 2.1). These factors are difficult to adjust for, and when adjustments for lead time bias in particular are made, there is a substantial reduction in the magnitude of the benefit that is apparent in those studies where this is done. Several studies have been published recently that aim to quantify the benefits of surveillance using a case control design with adjustments for lead time bias, and in those the absolute risk reduction in mortality at 3–5 years after the diagnosis of HCC is in the region of 10% [11, 12]. That is less than half of that reported in the meta-analysis and still subject to residual confounding from other sources.

It remains unclear from observational data therefore that surveillance using ultrasound will improve survival in patients with cirrhosis. Supportive evidence comes from both cost-effectiveness analyses and modelling studies of surveillance.

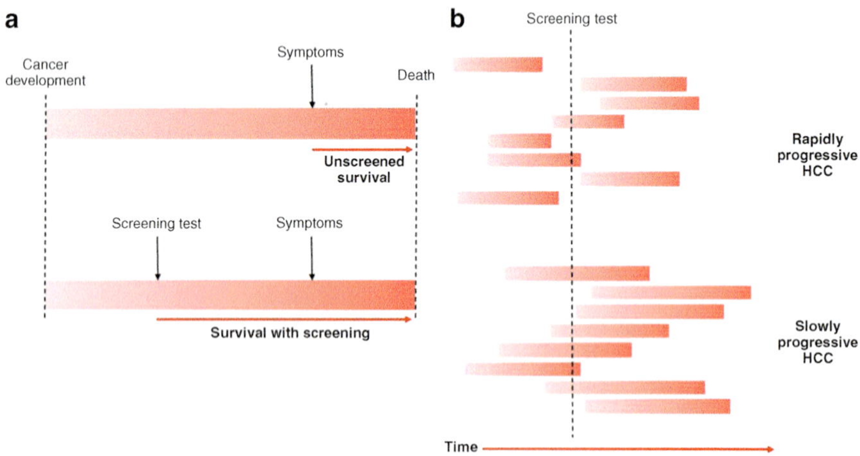


**Fig. 2.1** Lead time and length bias in cancer screening. Lead time bias (**a**) defines an apparent improvement in survival as a consequence of early diagnosis of cancer due to screening or surveillance in the case of HCC although there is no change in the natural history of that cancer through treatment. Length bias (**b**) identifies the likelihood that more indolent cancers are diagnosed by screening or surveillance before symptoms present. Each of these biases serves to overestimate the efficacy of screening or surveillance interventions

These use published data to provide estimates of the likelihood of events in populations with cirrhosis and draw from the published literature estimates of treatment efficacy and are therefore subject to the same biases as the original observational studies.

## Uptake of Surveillance at the Population Level

Despite low-quality evidence, surveillance is strongly recommended by all professional associations that represent physicians caring for patients with cirrhosis. Other expert bodies, including the US National Cancer Institute, do not recommend surveillance, but it is expected that most physicians would follow guidance issued by their professional societies. However, international studies, particularly from the United States and from the United Kingdom, suggest that only a minority of patients with cirrhosis receive surveillance. In the best characterised population, including individuals with cirrhosis due to HCV infection, rates of routine surveillance were calculated to be 42% in the first year after diagnosis and declined thereafter to 12% for individuals with at least 2 years of follow-up [13].

In the United Kingdom, a questionnaire study identified important deficits in surveillance for patients with cirrhosis. Whilst the majority of respondents reported that there was a surveillance programme in their hospital, there was often no mechanism to routinely recall the patient for follow-up imaging, and patients were not reliably informed of the reasons that surveillance was suggested [14].

## Barriers to Effective Surveillance

Clinical effectiveness of an intervention, such as surveillance for HCC, defines how well that intervention performs in the real world. Even for an intervention that is 100% efficacious, factors that limit its use mean that the clinical effectiveness is often much less than 100%. Where there are questions about the efficacy of surveillance when it is done, any factors that reduce its use or that impair its performance will inevitably further reduce its clinical effectiveness (Fig. 2.2). Barriers to patients entering surveillance, patients entering surveillance where there are contraindications to anticancer treatment such as advanced liver or non-liver co-morbidities, and

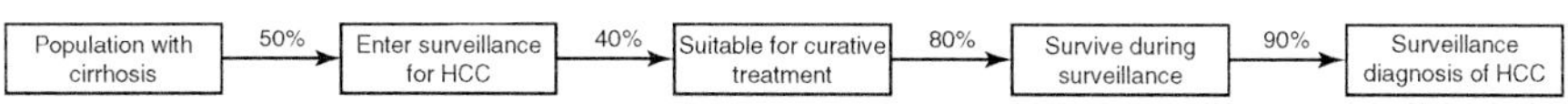


**Fig. 2.2** Factors affecting the clinical effectiveness of surveillance for HCC. Multiple steps before a diagnosis of HCC in surveillance diminish the overall benefit of surveillance in the population. In this illustration estimated over 5 years, only 14% (=100×0.5×0.4×0.8×0.9) of the population with cirrhosis are eligible to benefit from surveillance. If 10% of those eligible to benefit from surveillance develop HCC and there is a 10% absolute risk reduction in mortality from a diagnosis of HCC in surveillance, then the anticipated survival benefit at the population level is 0.14% (=14×0.1×0.1)

competing causes of mortality each reduce the clinical effectiveness of surveillance in this context.

Overall, the greatest barrier to a patient entering surveillance is not knowing that the patient has cirrhosis. Many patients with well-compensated cirrhosis are not diagnosed until complications (either liver failure or HCC) develop, and without that diagnosis, surveillance cannot be implemented. The principal factor that reduces the clinical effectiveness of surveillance for patients known to have cirrhosis, other than its efficacy, is patients not entering a surveillance programme. In the example shown in Fig. 2.2, the barriers to surveillance substantially reduce the number of individuals with cirrhosis who are eligible to benefit from that intervention. Since HCC only develops in a minority and surveillance has limited efficacy, the impact of surveillance at the level of the population with cirrhosis is minimal.

Several studies have evaluated physician's perspectives of surveillance and a number of themes have emerged [14, 15]. These largely relate to concerns about the lack of efficacy of surveillance and costs and availability of specialist ultrasonography. It is striking that these issues would be best addressed by the generation of high-quality prospective data that assess the effectiveness of surveillance. It is also striking that since fewer than half of patients with cirrhosis receive effective surveillance, making a cogent argument for a randomised controlled trial that compared surveillance with no surveillance. Such a trial would both increase the number of patients receiving high-quality surveillance and would provide a clear answer as to the (cost-) effectiveness of surveillance. In many ways it is therefore puzzling that this approach is not supported by many of the experts in the field (**Controversies box**).

## Expected Outcomes of Surveillance

### *Benefits*

For patients considering surveillance today, it is important that they receive balanced information about both the possible benefits and harms of that intervention so that they can make an informed decision to participate (or not). The possible benefits in patients who have developed HCC have been discussed above, but this tells only part of the story since the majority of patients with cirrhosis will never develop HCC and will undergo surveillance without any chance of benefit. For those patients there are only the risks of surveillance.

To derive a clearer perspective of the benefits of surveillance in the population with cirrhosis, one needs to consider the natural history of patients with compensated cirrhosis more closely. It is apparent that in viral hepatitis, where there are the best data, diagnosis of HCC is the most common early liver event in patients with compensated cirrhosis. It is also clear that these individuals remain at risk of death from other causes, including cardiovascular disease and extrahepatic malignancy. Critically, the balance of these competing risks is different, for instance, in patients with alcohol-related liver disease (ArLD) where the incidence of HCC is lower than in viral hepatitis with implications for the outcomes with surveillance.

Two groups, including ours, have developed models to identify the benefits of surveillance in the population with cirrhosis in the absence of a relevant and applicable randomised controlled trial [16, 17]. The approach to modelling is different, but the short-term outcomes are similar, showing a small, 1–2% decrease in overall mortality at 5 years after the onset of surveillance and assuming that surveillance is complete. This decrease is much smaller than is anticipated by the case control studies simply because the modelling studies take into account the majority of patients that do not develop HCC in the follow-up period. Critically, these estimates are made for patients with an incidence of HCC of 2.5% per annum and low rates of competing mortality from both liver and non-liver causes. If the models were refined to consider a population with a lower incidence of HCC and a higher rate of competing mortality (as would be expected in an ArLD population), the estimated mortality reduction would be smaller still.

## *Harms*

Considering the small benefit that surveillance offers at the population level, a patient considering entering surveillance will need information on the possible harms. Until recently there has been little attention focussed on this topic, and in a decision aid that aimed to assess feasibility of a randomised controlled trial, they were summarised as the possibility of a false alarm following a surveillance ultrasound [15]. It is now recognised that this is an oversimplification of the situation. In general, in the cancer screening literature, there are a number of potential harms recognised. These harms relate to physical and psychosocial harms from the test itself, harms resulting from false-positive screening tests and subsequent downstream testing as well as harms that result from false-negative testing.

Whilst a surveillance ultrasound scan is itself a safe intervention in the wider context, there are predictable harms that are likely to result. In prospective studies of surveillance [18], the false-positive rate for each ultrasound was in the region of 2%, meaning that approximately 1 in 50 individuals attending for ultrasound required additional testing with the attendant concerns that liver cancer had developed when it had not. In the United States, it has been reported that a quarter of patients in surveillance (over a short follow-up period of 2 years on average) required additional scans because of either a false-positive or indeterminate ultrasound scan [18]. This high rate of false-positive testing has further implications if the European Association for the Study of the Liver (EASL) recall policy [3] is applied. This policy mandates biopsy of 1–2 cm indeterminate lesions on cross-sectional imaging to determine the impact of this on patients in surveillance, and one of the modelling studies done to assess the benefits of surveillance also addressed this area. The study concluded that the harms of surveillance were more frequent than the benefits: 15% of individuals required additional testing, including 4% who (according to the EASL recall policy) underwent 'unnecessary' liver biopsy since that biopsy did not diagnose HCC [16].

False-negative testing, that is 'missing' cancer that is present, is also an issue in surveillance since only small HCC can be treated with curative intent. In the same prospective studies that required an ultrasound at baseline that did not identify HCC, 20% of those patients subsequently diagnosed with HCC had disease that had progressed beyond traditional curative criteria [19]. This is a substantial minority, and this partially explains why the efficacy of surveillance is not high.

Finally, there are clearly predictable harms that relate to concerns regarding the possible diagnosis of HCC in patients with cirrhosis. Patients with cirrhosis are (or should be) familiar with the possible complications of that disease. Six-monthly ultrasound scans will serve, in some patients at least, to emphasise the possibility that cancer might develop. Reports of quality of life in cirrhosis show significant impairments in many domains, and this might partially be explained by concerns regarding progression of liver disease and/or the development of HCC. For instance, in a report of patients undergoing surveillance in Texas, two thirds of patients were concerned they would develop HCC, and almost half were worried that they would die from HCC. This was despite half of patients already having advanced liver disease marked by the presence of ascites [20]. The majority of these patients will not develop HCC, and for those with ascites, there is no known survival benefit from surveillance, and the focus on HCC in this context is unwarranted and unhelpful.

## Improving Surveillance for the Future

Surveillance for HCC in patients with cirrhosis is logical but the evidence that supports it is of low quality. Surveillance is associated with frequent and sometimes significant physical harms and probably also psychosocial harms that are not well quantified. It is critical that we, as physicians caring for patients with liver disease, work together to improve surveillance and thereby improve outcomes of patients with cirrhosis. This might be achieved in a number of ways. First, there is a clear need to collect high-quality information regarding the current *effectiveness* of surveillance, including data on each of the parameters included in Fig. 2.2. That will allow specific targeted interventions with the greatest predicted benefit on outcomes. Second, there is a need to improve the *efficacy* of the surveillance intervention. Ideally, this would increase the sensitivity of the test and decrease the rate of false-positive testing. Currently, achieving this aim seems distant since although the addition of biomarkers to 6-monthly ultrasound might increase the sensitivity of the test, it is almost certain that this will also increase the false-positive rate and increase harm that accrues through surveillance. Finally, there is a need to better characterise the psychosocial harms of surveillance so that the process of information giving and consent can be optimised and the risk of HCC development put into context for patients with cirrhosis.

## References


1. Global Burden of Disease Mortality, Causes of Death Collaboration. Global, regional, and national age-sex specific all-cause and cause-specific mortality for 240 causes of death, 1990-2013: a systematic analysis for the Global Burden of Disease Study 2013. Lancet. 2015;385(9963):117–71.
2. El-Serag HB. Hepatocellular carcinoma. N Engl J Med. 2011;365(12):1118–27.
3. European Association for the Study of the Liver, European Organisation for Research and Treatment of Cancer. EASL-EORTC clinical practice guidelines: management of hepatocellular carcinoma. J Hepatol. 2012;56(4):908–43.
4. NICE. Clinical Guideline 50: Cirrhosis in over 16s: Assessment and management. 2016; https://www.nice.org.uk/guidance/ng50/evidence/full-guideline-2546537581. Accessed 12 Jul 2016.
5. Heimbach JK, Kulik LM, Finn R, et al. AASLD guidelines for the treatment of hepatocellular carcinoma. Hepatology. 2017;67(1):358–80.
6. Bruix J, Reig M, Sherman M. Evidence-based diagnosis, staging, and treatment of patients with hepatocellular carcinoma. Gastroenterology. 2016;150(4):835–53.
7. Wong VW, Janssen HL. Can we use HCC risk scores to individualize surveillance in chronic hepatitis B infection? J Hepatol. 2015;63(3):722–32.
8. Lederle FA, Pocha C. Screening for liver cancer: the rush to judgment. Ann Intern Med. 2012;156(5):387–9.
9. Kansagara D, Papak J, Pasha AS, et al. Screening for hepatocellular carcinoma in chronic liver disease: a systematic review. Ann Intern Med. 2014;161(4):261–9.
10. Singal AG, Pillai A, Tiro J. Early detection, curative treatment, and survival rates for hepatocellular carcinoma surveillance in patients with cirrhosis: a meta-analysis. PLoS Med. 2014;11(4):e1001624.
11. Mittal S, Kanwal F, Ying J, et al. Effectiveness of surveillance for hepatocellular carcinoma in clinical practice: A United States cohort. J Hepatol. 2016;65(6):1148–54.
12. Cucchetti A, Trevisani F, Pecorelli A, et al. Estimation of lead-time bias and its impact on the outcome of surveillance for the early diagnosis of hepatocellular carcinoma. J Hepatol. 2014;61(2):333–41.
13. Davila JA, Henderson L, Kramer JR, et al. Utilization of surveillance for hepatocellular carcinoma among hepatitis C virus-infected veterans in the United States. Ann Intern Med. 2011;154(2):85–93.
14. Cross TJ, Villanueva A, Shetty S, et al. A national survey of the provision of ultrasound surveillance for the detection of hepatocellular carcinoma. Frontline Gastroenterol. 2016;7:82–9.
15. Poustchi H, Farrell GC, Strasser SI, Lee AU, McCaughan GW, George J. Feasibility of conducting a randomized control trial for liver cancer screening: is a randomized controlled trial for liver cancer screening feasible or still needed? Hepatology. 2011;54(6):1998–2004.
16. Taylor EJ, Jones RL, Guthrie JA, Rowe IA. Modeling the benefits and harms of surveillance for hepatocellular carcinoma: Information to support informed choices. Hepatology. 2017;66(5):1546–55.
17. Yang JD, Mannalithara A, Piscitello AJ, et al. Impact of surveillance for hepatocellular carcinoma on survival in patients with compensated cirrhosis. Hepatology. 2017;68(1):78–88.
18. Atiq O, Tiro J, Yopp AC, et al. An assessment of benefits and harms of hepatocellular carcinoma surveillance in patients with cirrhosis. Hepatology. 2016;65(4):1196–205.
19. Trinchet JC, Chaffaut C, Bourcier V, et al. Ultrasonographic surveillance of hepatocellular carcinoma in cirrhosis: a randomized trial comparing 3- and 6-month periodicities. Hepatology. 2011;54(6):1987–97.
20. Farvardin S, Patel J, Khambaty M, et al. Patient-reported barriers are associated with lower hepatocellular carcinoma surveillance rates in patients with cirrhosis. Hepatology. 2016;65(3):875–84.

# Chapter 3
# Roles of the Immune System in the Development and Progression of Hepatocellular Carcinoma

**João Maurício, Helen Reeves, and Caroline L. Wilson**

**Key Learning Points**

1. The liver is constantly exposed to antigens and pathogen-derived molecules from the gut and has intrinsic tolerogenic mechanisms to ensure that chronic and systemic immune responses do not occur.
2. Hepatocellular carcinoma (HCC) is known to develop on a background of chronic liver disease and inflammation.
3. Despite evidence of immune responses against tumour-associated antigens (TAA), the HCC microenvironment fosters an immunosuppressive niche that escapes immune surveillance.
4. The inflammatory niche created in HCC is a critical target for immunotherapy, including vaccines, oncolytic immunotherapy, cell-based therapy, cytokines/cytokine inhibitors and immune checkpoint inhibitors.

**Areas of Controversy and Uncertainty**

1. There has been a steady increase in patients presenting with HCC arising in the absence of significant liver disease or underlying inflammation—the cause of which is uncertain.

J. Maurício · H. Reeves (✉)
Northern Institute for Cancer Research, Newcastle University, Newcastle upon Tyne, UK
e-mail: H.L.Reeves@ncl.ac.uk; helen.reeves@newcastle.ac.uk

C. L. Wilson
Faculty of Medical Sciences, Institute of Cellular Medicine, Newcastle University, Newcastle upon Tyne, UK



T. Cross, D. H. Palmer (eds.), *Liver Cancers*,
https://doi.org/10.1007/978-3-319-92216-4_3

2. Cancers arising in the absence of chronic liver disease tend to be associated with the metabolic syndrome. Obesity and type 2 diabetes may also affect immune responses, although these are less well studied.
3. Understanding how to activate a suppressed antitumour immune response safely and effectively is challenging.
4. The cancer immunotherapy era is an exciting one, but likely to be hindered by the present lack of biomarkers to guide selection of mono or combination therapies and monitor response.
5. The use of therapies activating aspects of the antitumour immune response in immunosuppressed patients will require careful consideration.

## Introduction

Hepatocellular carcinoma (HCC) accounts for 70–85% of the total primary liver cancer burden. It usually arises in a background of chronic liver disease consequent to hepatitis B virus (HBV)/hepatitis C virus (HCV) infection, alcoholic-related liver disease (ARLD) or non-alcoholic fatty liver disease (NAFLD), which is tightly linked to the metabolic syndrome and obesity [1]. While HCC is the fifth most common cancer in men and the ninth most common one in women, it is the second most common cause of cancer-related death worldwide [2], reflecting late-stage presentation and limited therapeutic options. Surgery, liver transplantation and local ablative therapies can be curative in early disease, but most patients are offered palliative treatments or supportive care. Currently, the only first-line FDA-approved treatment for advanced-stage HCC is sorafenib, a multikinase inhibitor, which offers a median overall survival (OS) benefit of just 10 weeks. Hence, there is a clear and urgent need for new therapies—with a recent focus in the oncology field on immune checkpoint inhibitors.

The liver is continually exposed to a multitude of antigens, gut-derived pathogens, toxins and environmental and bacterial products—entering the liver from the gastrointestinal tract via the portal vein. The liver has therefore developed constitutive tolerogenic mechanisms to prevent persistent gut-associated immune stimulation and systemic and chronic inflammation. A common feature underpinning HCC development, however, is chronic inflammation—consequent to the persistent hepatocyte injury associated with the aetiologies described above, which occurs in approximately 90% of the cases. The combination of chronic inflammation and the intrinsic tolerogenic properties of the liver creates an environment that facilitates cancer development, with progression promoted by additional immunosuppressive manipulation by the tumour itself.

In this chapter we will discuss some of the knowledge we have to date on how immune tolerance is evaded during liver disease and what we know about its contribution to HCC development and progression. We will also highlight some of the current therapeutic approaches designed to harness the immune system as a therapy for HCC.

## Pathobiology of HCC-Related Aetiologies

### *ARLD and NAFLD*

ARLD is the most common aetiology of HCC in industrialised countries, being responsible for 32–45% of cases [3]. However, in the last decades, the incidence of NAFLD-related HCC has been increasing worldwide, possibly because of the obesity and type 2 diabetes epidemic [4]. The mechanisms leading to HCC in either ARLD or NAFLD are similar, and several reviews have focused on these [1, 3–5]. A key aspect is the chronic damage and hence chronic stimulation of the immune system that overrides liver tolerance. Increased exposure to gut pathogens and persistent hepatotoxicity result in the production of regulatory miRNAs, pro-inflammatory mediators and damage-associated molecular patterns (DAMPs) that activate the immune response. Alcohol increases levels of miR-212 in gut epithelial cells, leading to decreased expression of ZO-1, a tight junction protein, disrupting gut integrity and allowing for translocation of bacterial endotoxins to the liver. There, the endotoxins impact Kupffer cells (liver-resident macrophages), hepatocytes and endothelial cells; Kupffer cells are activated, upregulate miR-155 and release pro-inflammatory mediators including tumour necrosis factor (TNF), contributing to hepatic inflammation. Additionally, alcohol induces oxidative stress: in hepatocytes, levels of miR-34a and miR-217 increase, resulting in hepatic steatosis via SIRT1 and, in endothelial cells, levels of miR-199a decrease, leading to endothelin-1 and hypoxia-inducible factor α (HIF-1 α) release, all contributing to the amplification of inflammation [3, 5].

In NAFLD, high-fat and carbohydrate (mainly fructose) intake can exacerbate cytokine production and increase hepatic de novo lipogenesis (via SREBP and ChREBP transcription factors), thus promoting lipid peroxidation and DNA damage. The underlying dysfunctional adipose tissue releases additional factors: TNFα and interleukin (IL)-6 enhance c-Jun N-terminal kinase (JNK)/nuclear factor kappa B (NF-κB) and Janus kinase (JAK)/signal transducer and activator of transcription (STAT)3 pathways, while leptin activates Akt/mTOR, leading to expression of genes involved in cell proliferation, migration and survival. Low levels of adiponectin hinder its anti-inflammatory activity and antagonising effect on leptin. In obesity, fatty liver may also be susceptible to carcinogens as a result of impaired ATP production, defective autophagy mechanisms, deregulation of energy and hormonal balance, hypoxia and systemic inflammation. Increased susceptibility of the steatotic liver to carcinogenic insults can be due to several local and systemic pathological changes that occur including metabolic imbalances and the "metabolic syndrome", hyperinsulinemia and the presence of insulin-like growth factor receptors in HCC, the systemic effects of dysregulated cytokines and adipokines, immune dysregulation and alteration in gut microbiota [1, 4].

## *HBV and HCV*

Viral hepatitis plays a significant role in up to 80% of all HCC globally, with HBV being responsible for two-thirds of all cases; HCV is responsible for 25% of HCC-related deaths. HCV is the primary cause of end-stage liver disease worldwide, and, unlike HBV-related acute hepatitis, it only resolves in about 10–40% of cases [6].

Histological changes are similar between both HBV and HCV infections, namely, hepatocyte death, inflammation, steatosis and progressive fibrosis, leading to cirrhosis and HCC. Specific mechanisms causing disease progression include expression of viral hepatitis B surface antigen (HBsAg) on the surface of hepatocytes, resulting in stimulation of the host's immune system, chronic inflammation, increased production of reactive oxygen species (ROS) and oxidative DNA damage. Integration of the viral DNA into the host genome can also result in genomic instability, chromosomal loss and abnormal gene activation. These effects are compounded by the ability of viral proteins to interfere with the regulation of cell cycle proteins and promote apoptotic escape. Moreover, persistent chemokines, cytokines, proteases and ROS produced by the inflammatory cell infiltrate promote the carcinogenic process further by inducing cell survival and proliferation [6].

## *Chronic Inflammation, Immune Suppression and HCC Progression*

In tumour-bearing hosts, cancer progression is driven by mechanisms promoting immune tolerance to tumour-associated antigens (TAA), including a failure to recognise malignant cells and suppression of the immune cells responsible for the death and clearance of the tumour. Despite a lack of knowledge concerning these pathways, available data thus far highlights the multiple immune responses implicated in HCC progression and allows for identification of promising new targets for future therapy [7, 8]. These cancer-related changes in the immune response comprise of changes in the number and/or function of immune cells, changes in cytokine levels and immune receptor/ligand expression, some of which will be reviewed here (Fig. 3.1).

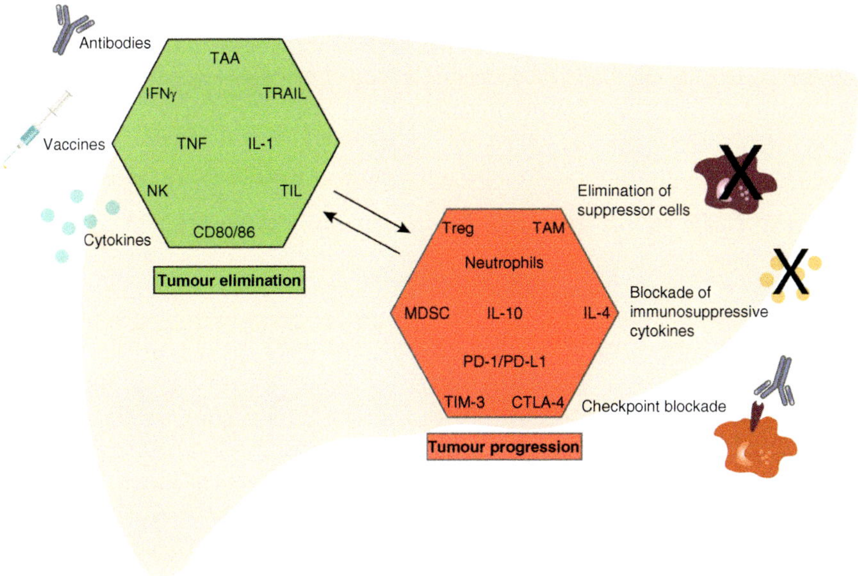


**Fig. 3.1** Crosstalk between multiple immune mechanisms determines the outcome of tumour cell death or growth. The different immunotherapy approaches are summarised and aim to promote tumour elimination or suppress tumour progression. Key: *TAA* tumour-associated antigen, *TIL* tumour-infiltrating lymphocytes, *NK* natural killer cell, *CD80/86* B7 costimulatory molecules expressed on the surface of antigen-presenting cells, *TRAIL* TNF-related apoptosis-inducing ligand, *IL-1* interleukin-1, *TNF* tumour necrosis factor, *IFNγ* interferon γ, *Treg* T regulatory cells, *MDSC* myeloid-derived suppressor cells, *TAM* tumour-associated macrophage, *CTLA-4* cytotoxic T-lymphocyte-associated protein 4, *PD-1* programmed death 1, *PD-L1* programmed death ligand 1, *TIM3* T-cell immunoglobulin and mucin domain-containing protein 3, *IL-4* interleukin-4, *IL-10* interleukin-10

## *Senescence and the Senescence-Associated Secretory Phenotype (SASP)*

Cellular senescence is a stress-response mechanism aimed at inducing proliferative arrest in a cell at risk of malignant transformation. In the liver, such process can be triggered by chronic inflammation, leading to recurring events of hepatocyte death, compensatory regeneration of hepatocytes and either replicative senescence or oncogene-driven senescence. A recent study by Eggert et al. [9] was designed to further address the implications of hepatocyte senescence in HCC development and progression. The SASP, which comprises of cytokines and chemokines secreted by senescent cells, is designed to recruit and activate myeloid cells and clear senescent hepatocytes, thus preventing tumorigenesis. However, this is dependent upon the context—SASP of senescent hepatocytes may also promote the growth of established HCC via recruitment of immunosuppressive immature myeloid cells which in turn inhibit NK-cell antitumour function, can dampen antitumour T cell responses and even promote tumour growth by production of growth factors, proteases and cytokines [9]. Hence, peritumoral tissue senescence contributes to accelerated tumour growth in mice and to decreased overall and recurrence-free survival in humans.

## *Immune Cells Involved in the Immunosuppressive HCC Niche*

### T Cells

The role of T cells in HCC is complex in that the outcome and prognosis differ depending on the type of T cell present and its ability to contribute to antitumour immunity. CD8+ T cells recognise antigens presented on major histocompatibility (MHC) complex I and kill tumour cells by secretion of cytolytic granules. CD4+ Th1 cells are able to kill tumour cells via the TNF-related apoptosis-inducing ligand (TRAIL) pathway. They secrete the cytokine interferon gamma (IFN-$\gamma$) which activates antigen-presenting cells (APC) and promotes CD8+ and NK-cell activation. CD4+ Th2 cells on the other hand are thought to be more immunosuppressive, producing the cytokines IL-4, IL-5, IL-10 and IL-13 involved in eosinophil recruitment and B-cell proliferation. CD4+ regulatory T cells (Treg) promote self-tolerance and prevention of autoimmunity, and these cells are often increased in patients' tumours and blood. Induced by transforming growth factor (TGF)-$\beta$, Treg cells can supress CD8+ and NK cytotoxic killing.

Significant changes in gene expression occur in the liver microenvironment, which influence HCC progression. A unique gene signature comprising 17 immune-related genes was shown to strongly predict the development of venous metastases and relapse in HCC patients [10]. Here, a global shift from a Th1 to a Th2 cytokine setting was observed, most likely compounded by the elevated expression of macrophage colony-stimulating factor (CSF1). In this immunosuppressive environment of the metastatic HCC, pro-inflammatory cytokines such as IL-1, TNF and IFN-$\gamma$ were significantly downregulated, whereas the anti-inflammatory cytokines such as IL-4, IL-5, IL-8, and IL-10 were strongly upregulated. These results centred on HBV-positive metastatic HCC. However, changes in the proportions of T-cell subtypes and function associated with HCC are well established in many mouse models of HCC and in human samples.

A recent study by Ma et al. [11] elucidated a role for CD4+ T cells in NAFLD-associated HCC. Here authors showed, in both mouse models and human samples, that dysregulation of lipid metabolism typical of NAFLD originates a selective loss of intrahepatic CD4+ but not CD8+ T cells, leading to accelerated hepatocarcinogenesis. CD4+ T cells had a greater mitochondrial mass than CD8+ T cells and produced higher levels of mitochondrial-derived ROS, which ultimately caused their death. Linoleic acid, a fatty acid accumulated in NAFLD, was found to be largely responsible for this mitochondrial dysfunction. The in vivo use of antioxidants reversed NAFLD-induced HCC. This novel link between obesity-associated lipid accumulation and selective CD4+ T-cell loss suggests a crucial role for CD4+ T cells in the disease progression from NAFLD to HCC.

In the chronically inflamed liver (particularly due to chronic viral infection) and HCC, it is common to find lymphocytic immune cell aggregates consisting predominantly of T and B cells, which form distinct structures known as ectopic lymphoid structures (ELS). The pro-tumorigenic role of ELS in HCC was recently reported, demonstrating that these lymphocyte structures—driven by NF-κB activation—provide a cellular and cytokine microniche that supports the growth and egress of malignant hepatocyte progenitor cells [12]. The authors identified HCC with similar chromosomal alterations, pointing towards a common source of malignant progenitor cells originating in ELS [12].

In HBV or HCV hepatitis-associated HCC, T- and B-cell production of the pro-inflammatory cytokines lymphotoxin (LT) α and β is markedly upregulated (alongside their receptor, LTβR) [13]. LTαβ acts mainly on hepatocytes expressing the LTβR, leading to elevated LT signalling, increased NF-κB activation and the release of chemokine C-C motif ligand (CCL)2, CCL7, chemokine C-X-C motif ligand (CXCL)1 and CXCL10 chemokines. The resulting increase in inflammatory cell recruitment leads to hepatocyte secretion of cytotoxic cytokines (IL-6, IL-1β, LTαβ), tissue damage, hepatocyte proliferation and death. In this scenario, hepatocytes are increasingly more predisposed to genomic instability leading to HCC. Furthermore, the authors also showed that LTβR inhibition in LTαβ-transgenic mice with hepatitis suppresses HCC formation [13].

## Neutrophils

Neutrophils are often thought to be innocent bystanders in cancer development and progression. However, controversial roles have emerged in recent years [14–16]. Friedlander and colleagues (2009) identified N1 antitumour neutrophils as being those that "fight infection and cancer", while N2 pro-tumour neutrophils—which display increased arginase and a loss of oxidative burst and phagocytic capacity—are present in the cancer microenvironment and promote tumour progression [17]. Subsequently, a study led by Wilson et al. [18] further highlighted the pro-tumour role of neutrophils using a diethylnitrosamine (DEN)-induced model of HCC. A tumour suppressor function for hepatocellular *nfkb1* that controls hepatocyte production of neutrophil chemokines was also described. The chemokine network comprising of S100A9, CXCL1 and CXCL2 was responsible for neutrophil recruitment to the liver, where neutrophils induced ROS-mediated telomere damage in hepatocytes and increased the development of HCC. In *nfkb1* knockout mice, several features were exacerbated—namely, steatosis, neutrophil recruitment, fibrosis, hepatocyte telomere damage and ultimately HCC. By antibody-mediated depletion of neutrophils or disruption of the chemokine network, these effects were abrogated and HCC development attenuated.

In another recent neutrophil study, researchers aimed at evaluating the role of tumour-associated neutrophils (TAN) in the progression of HCC and sorafenib resistance [19]. Here, they showed that CCL2 and CCL17 were highly expressed by TAN and peripheral blood neutrophils (PBN) when exposed to conditioned media from HCC cell lines. The number of CCL2+ or CCL17+ TANs correlated with tumour size, microvascular invasion, tumour encapsulation, tumour differentiation and stage. Also, patients whose tumours presented lower levels of CCL2+ or CCL17+ TAN had longer survival times than those with higher numbers of these cells. CCL2 enhanced the recruitment of macrophages, whereas CCL17 induced the recruitment of Treg cells (but not CD4+ CD25– or CD8+ lymphocytes). Mechanistically, the authors identified the PI3K/Akt and p38/MAPK signalling pathways as crucial mediators of the transformation of PBN into TAN in HCC. Regarding the neutrophil impact in sorafenib treatment, it was demonstrated that sorafenib-induced hypoxia activated NF-κB signalling, thus enhancing CXCL5 secretion by HCC cells, which initiated TAN recruitment. Depletion of TAN resulted in a reduction in tumour volume and enhancement of the effects of sorafenib [19].

### Myeloid-Derived Suppressor Cells (MDSC)

MDSC are a heterogeneous group of immature myeloid cells known for their immunosuppressive and pro-tumoural functions—they can induce tumour angiogenesis by vascular endothelial growth factor (VEGF) secretion, and they are able to disrupt both innate and adaptive antitumour activity [8, 20]. For example, Li et al. have shown that MDSC abrogate natural killer (NK)-cell cytotoxicity, NKG2D expression and IFN-γ production via membrane-bound TGF-β. Moreover, the authors demonstrated that depletion of MDSC restored NK function [21].

### Macrophages

Macrophages are known to exist in a continuous spectrum of phenotypes, although they are usually referred to by the simplified nomenclature of M1 (classically activated, antitumour) and M2 (alternatively activated, pro-tumour) macrophages [22]. The transition between pro- and antitumour phenotypes is fluid and dependent upon signals from the local microenvironment but can have a profound effect on tumoural immunity via production of pro/anti-inflammatory mediators and expression of inhibitory molecules against T cells and NK cells such as PD-L1. In a mouse model of HCC, TGF-β has been shown to skew macrophages towards an M2 pro-tumour phenotype, inducing the expression of IL-6, and T-cell immunoglobulin and mucin domain-containing protein 3 (TIM-3), which is an inhibitory receptor for T cells. TIM-3 expression by tumour-associated macrophages (TAM) also correlated with tumour grade and poor survival in HCC patients [23]. It appears that HCC cells can halt the maturation of infiltrating monocytes into macrophages by secreting cytokines that promote immunosuppressive TAM function, promoting evasion of antitumour immunity.

## Immunotherapy Approaches: Harness the Immune System to Modulate HCC Progression

Natural occurring adaptive immune responses towards HCC have been previously described and recently reviewed by Makarova-Rusher et al. [7]. Most patients develop adaptive immune responses against TAA, such as α-fetoprotein (AFP), telomerase reverse transcriptase (TERT), melanoma antigen gene-A (MAGE-A) and foetal oncoprotein glypican-3 (GPC3). However, the interactions between the HCC cells and the immune system mainly foster an immunosuppressive microenvironment that prevents antigen-mediated clearance of tumour cells via some of the mechanisms discussed above. A number of clinical trials have evaluated approaches aimed at enhancing the immune response against TAA or dampening the suppressive signals, as summarised in Table 3.1.

**Table 3.1** Immunotherapy clinical trials in HCC (https://clinicaltrials.gov/)

| Target/approach | Study features | Outcome |
|---|---|---|
| *Vaccines* | | |
| 4 AFP peptides | Single arm [24] | (2003) AFP-specific T-cell responses detected |
| DC + auto-tumour lysate | Single arm, 2 schedules [25] | (2005) PR (4) 12.9%, SD (17) 54.8%, 1-year OS 40.1 months |
| *Oncolytic viruses* | | |
| JX-594 oncolytic virus-carrying human GM-CSF genes | Dose-finding study (low vs high dose) [26] | (2013) ORR 15%, intrahepatic disease control rate 46% |
| *Adoptive cell transfer (ACT)* | | |
| Activated T cells + DC vaccine | Non-randomised [27] | (2014) RFS 24.5 vs 12.6 months ($p = 0.01$), OS 97.7 vs 41.0 months, p = 0.029 |
| CAR-T cell to GPC3 | NCT02723942. Randomised, phase I/II, 60 patients | Completed (2017)—NDA |
| PIK-PD-1 cells | NCT02632006. Randomised, phase I/II, 40 patients, advanced HCC | Completed (2017)—NDA |
| GPC3 redirected autologous T cells | NCT02715362. Single arm, phase I/II, 30 patients, advanced HCC | Ongoing |
| CIK | NCT02568748. Non-randomised, phase III, 20 patients, advanced HCC | Ongoing |

(continued)

**Table 3.1** (continued)

| Target/approach | Study features | Outcome |
|---|---|---|
| *Cytokines* | | |
| LY2157299 (small molecule inhibitor if TGF-β receptor I) | Randomised to 2 doses [29] | (2014) OS 36 weeks |
| *Immune checkpoint inhibitors* | | |
| Tremelimumab (anti-CTLA-4) | Single arm (HCV patients), 21 patients [30] | PR 17.6%, SD 58.8%, OS 8.2 months, TTP 6.48 months |
| Nivolumab (anti-PD-1) | Single arm [32] | NDA |
| Nivolumab (anti-PD-1) vs sorafenib | NCT02576509. Randomised, phase III, 726 patients, advanced HCC | Ongoing |
| *Combination therapies* | | |
| JX-594 oncolytic virus + anti-PD-1 antibody nivolumab as first-line treatment | NCT03071094. Single arm, phase I/II, 30 patients | Ongoing |
| Microwave ablation + T lymphocyte | NCT02851784. Non-randomised, phase II/III, 50 patients | Ongoing |
| JX-594 oncolytic virus + sorafenib vs Sorafenib alone | NCT02562755. Randomised, phase III, 600 patients | Ongoing |
| Precision T cells specific to multiple common TAA + TACE | NCT02638857. Randomised, phase I/II, 60 patients, advanced HCC | Completed (2017)—NDA |
| Irreversible electroporation + NK cells | NCT03008343. Randomised, phase I/II, 20 patients, recurrent HCC | Ongoing |
| RFA + CTL vs RFA alone | NCT02678013. Randomised, phase III, 210 patients, recurrent HCC | Ongoing |
| Radical surgery followed by DC-PMAT | NCT02632188. Randomised, phase I/II, 60 patients | Completed (2017)—NDA |
| Nivolumab or nivolumab in combination with other agents | NCT01658878. Non-randomised, phase I/II, 620 patients, advanced HCC | Ongoing |
| Resection + CTL vs resection alone | NCT02709070. Randomised, phase III, 210 patients | Ongoing |
| Carbon-ion radiotherapy + GM-CSF | NCT02946138. Single arm, phase II, 44 patients | Ongoing |
| Durvalumab (anti-PD-L1) + tremelimumab (anti-CTLA-4) vs durvalumab or tremelimumab alone | NCT02519348. Randomised, phase II, 440 patients, unresectable HCC | Ongoing |
| Neoadjuvant cabozantinib + nivolumab (anti-PD-1) | NCT03299946. Single arm, phase I, 15 patients | Ongoing |

**Table 3.1** (continued)

| Target/approach | Study features | Outcome |
|---|---|---|
| LY2157299 (TGF-β receptor I inhibitor) as monotherapy and in combination with sorafenib or ramucirumab (anti-VEGFR2) | NCT01246986. Non-randomised, phase II, 235 patients | Ongoing |
| Ramucirumab (anti-VEGFR2) + durvalumab (anti-PD-L1) | NCT02572687. Non-randomised, phase I, 114 patients, locally advanced and unresectable or metastatic disease | Ongoing |

*AFP* alpha fetoprotein; *CIK* cytokine-induced killer cells; *CTL* cytotoxic T lymphocytes; *CTLA-4* cytotoxic T lymphocyte antigen 4; *DC* dendritic cells; *DC-PMAT* dendritic cell-precision multiple antigen T cells; *GM-CSF* granulocyte-macrophage colony-stimulating factor; *GPC3* glypican-3; *NDA* no data available; *NK* natural killer cells; *ORR* objective response rate; *OS* overall survival; *PD-1* programmed cell death receptor 1; *PD-L1* programmed death ligand 1; *PIK-PD-1* pluripotent killer T cells expressing antibodies for programmed death 1; *PR* partial response; *RFA* radiofrequency ablation; *RFS* recurrence-free survival; *SD* stable disease; *TAA* tumour-associated antigens; *TACE* transarterial chemoembolisation; *TTP* time to progression; *VEGFR2* vascular endothelial growth factor receptor 2

## *Vaccines*

AFP was the first TAA to be targeted in the clinic for HCC treatment, in 2003. The clinical trial reported measurable (albeit transient) CD8+ T-cell responses following patient immunisation with a vaccine to four HLA-restricted AFP peptides [24]. Improvement in clinical outcomes in vaccine trials can be achieved by co-administering dendritic cells (DC)—which are professional antigen-presenting cells—pulsed with autologous tumour lysates [25].

## *Adoptive Cell Transfer*

Adoptive cell transfer (ACT) is an autologous infusion of ex vivo-selected, ex vivo-activated and ex vivo-expanded tumour-infiltrating lymphocytes (TIL), which are obtained from a patient's tumour or peripheral blood. Cytokine-induced killer cells (CIK) and genetically modified T cells can also be used, including TAA-specific T cells, e.g., GPC3 (Table 3.1). In a clinical trial developed by Shimizu K et al. [27], patients were treated with an autologous tumour lysate-pulsed DC vaccine and activated T-cell transfer, after curative resection. Preliminary data support remarkable differences in OS between patients submitted to surgery alone (41.0 months) and to combination treatment (97.7 months).

## *Oncolytic Viruses*

The use of oncolytic viruses as vectors for the delivery of transgenes is a relatively recent approach in the treatment of different types of cancer, including HCC. The JX-594 (Pexa-Vec) is an oncolytic poxvirus engineered to carry the human gene for granulocyte-macrophage colony-stimulating factor (GM-CSF) and has been used to stimulate antitumour responses. This particular virus selectively replicates in cancer cells due to a disruption of the viral thymidine kinase gene. Infected cells lyse and release TAA, which can be taken up by antigen-presenting cells, with the additional expression of GM-CSF heightening the antitumour immune responses. In liver cancer, a study in which patients were randomised to one of two doses of vaccinia demonstrated encouraging results, particularly for the higher dose. Notably, both doses produced equivalent response rates between injected and distant non-injected tumours, supporting the establishment of a systemic immune response [26]. An ongoing trial (NCT03071094) is set to evaluate the safety and efficacy of combining this oncolytic vaccinia with an immune checkpoint inhibitor (anti-PD-1) as a first-line treatment for advanced HCC.

## *Cytokines*

Inflammatory changes associated with liver disease and HCC often display a clear dysregulation in the balance between immunosuppressive (e.g., IL-10, IL-4, IL-5) and immune-activating (e.g., TNF, IFN-$\gamma$, IL-1) cytokines, promoting Treg expansion and a reduction in DC function. Trials with the immune modulator IFN$\alpha$ showed early promise which was not realised in a larger trial [28]. Treatments with cytokine inhibitors for the treatment of HCC are ongoing, with mixed results reported thus far. TGF-$\beta$ is known for regulating cell differentiation, proliferation and death, as well as for its immunosuppressive functions towards T cells, NK cells and neutrophils [8, 17]. In an ongoing phase II non-randomised clinical trial with a novel small molecule inhibitor of TGF-$\beta$ receptor I, LY2157299, preliminary results suggest AFP expression may influence response [29]. This molecule is currently being studied in a phase II, non-randomised trial as a single agent and in combination with sorafenib or ramucirumab, an anti-vascular endothelial growth factor receptor (VEGFR) 2 monoclonal antibody (NCT01246986).

## *Immune Checkpoint Inhibitors*

T cells and NK cells require organised activation and recognition signals before they are able to mediate tumour cell killing. However, essential inhibitory signalling also exists to prevent unwanted T- and NK-cell responses and “self-harm”.

Unfortunately, tumour cells can hijack this inhibitory pathway in order to evade immune cell destruction.

Cytotoxic T-lymphocyte-associated protein 4 (CTLA-4) is an inhibitory checkpoint receptor expressed on T cells, upregulated in patients with viral hepatitis. Upon contact with the activation molecules B7-1 and B7-2 expressed on antigen-presenting cells, CTLA-4 transmits co-inhibitory signals to the T cell, impairing its activity and preventing T-cell immunity [7, 8]. A CTLA-4-targeted antibody therapy has been clinically evaluated in a phase II, noncontrolled, multicentre clinical trial for patients with advanced HCC and chronic HCV infection. As a single agent, the trial reported a partial response rate of 17.6%, stable disease rate of 76.4% and median OS of 8.2 months, with evidence also of antiviral activity [30].

Another immune checkpoint pathway is that regulated by programmed cell death 1 receptor (PD-1). PD-1 is upregulated in T cells in HCC and its ligands—programmed death ligand 1 or 2 (PD-L1/PD-L2)—are involved in immune suppression of T cells by inducing their apoptosis or dysfunction [7, 8]. Monoclonal antibodies that target this pathway have been approved by the FDA as treatments for other cancer types, with encouraging results in patients with HCC [31, 32]. In September 2017, the Food and Drug Administration (FDA) granted accelerated second-line approval for nivolumab, for the treatment of HCC in patients who have progressed on sorafenib. Approval was based on a 154-patient subgroup of the CHECKMATE-040 (NCT01658878) trial. As a condition of accelerated approval, further trials will be required to verify the clinical benefit of the antibody for this indication. Ongoing clinical trials with immune checkpoint inhibitors in combination with other therapies are summarised in Table 3.1, e.g., phase I trial for ramucirumab and durvalumab (anti-PD-L1) in the setting of locally advanced and unresectable or metastatic gastrointestinal or thoracic malignancies, including HCC (NCT02572687) [8].

In addition to CTLA-4 and PD-1, there are other immune checkpoint inhibitors expressed on activated T cells and NK cells including KIR, TIM-3 and LAG-3 [8] and further highlight the promise of dual or triple therapy in patients with high expression of these receptors.

## Conclusions and Future Perspectives

As we begin to understand how the chronic inflammatory responses associated with chronic liver disease, associated with HCC-induced immune tolerance, we are entering an exciting era of immunotherapy—with perhaps tangible hope for the first time that effective anti-HCC therapies delivering long-term survival are on the horizon. How we will select and monitor these therapies and use them safely in different groups of patients is not yet clear, as the field is hampered by the lack of either tissue are circulating biomarkers to guide clinical decision making. Progress in these fields is also set to have a substantial impact on the future for patients with HCC.

## References


1. Marengo A, Rosso C, Bugianesi E. Liver cancer: connections with obesity, fatty liver, and cirrhosis. Annu Rev Med. 2016;67:103–17.
2. Knudsen ES, Gopal P, Singal AG. The changing landscape of hepatocellular carcinoma: etiology, genetics, and therapy. Am J Pathol. 2014;184(3):574–83.
3. Stickel F. Alcoholic cirrhosis and hepatocellular carcinoma. Adv Exp Med Biol. 2015;815:113–30.
4. Reeves HL, Zaki MY, Day CP. Hepatocellular carcinoma in obesity, type 2 diabetes, and NAFLD. Dig Dis Sci. 2016;61(5):1234–45.
5. Szabo G, Bala S. MicroRNAs in liver disease. Nat Rev Gastroenterol Hepatol. 2013;10(9):542–52.
6. Alison MR, Nicholson LJ, Lin WR. Chronic inflammation and hepatocellular carcinoma. Recent Results Cancer Res. 2011;185:135–48.
7. Makarova-Rusher OV, Medina-Echeverz J, Duffy AG, Greten TF. The yin and yang of evasion and immune activation in HCC. J Hepatol. 2015;62(6):1420–9.
8. Obeid JM, Kunk PR, Zaydfudim VM, Bullock TN, Slingluff CL Jr, Rahma OE. Immunotherapy for hepatocellular carcinoma patients: is it ready for prime time? Cancer Immunol Immunother. 2017;67(2):161–74.
9. Eggert T, Wolter K, Ji J, Ma C, Yevsa T, Klotz S, et al. Distinct functions of senescence-associated immune responses in liver tumor surveillance and tumor progression. Cancer Cell. 2016;30(4):533–47.
10. Budhu A, Forgues M, Ye QH, Jia HL, He P, Zanetti KA, et al. Prediction of venous metastases, recurrence, and prognosis in hepatocellular carcinoma based on a unique immune response signature of the liver microenvironment. Cancer Cell. 2006;10(2):99–111.
11. Ma C, Kesarwala AH, Eggert T, Medina-Echeverz J, Kleiner DE, Jin P, et al. NAFLD causes selective CD4(+) T lymphocyte loss and promotes hepatocarcinogenesis. Nature. 2016;531(7593):253–7.
12. Finkin S, Yuan D, Stein I, Taniguchi K, Weber A, Unger K, et al. Ectopic lymphoid structures function as microniches for tumor progenitor cells in hepatocellular carcinoma. Nat Immunol. 2015;16(12):1235–44.
13. Haybaeck J, Zeller N, Wolf MJ, Weber A, Wagner U, Kurrer MO, et al. A lymphotoxin-driven pathway to hepatocellular carcinoma. Cancer Cell. 2009;16(4):295–308.
14. Sagiv JY, Michaeli J, Assi S, Mishalian I, Kisos H, Levy L, et al. Phenotypic diversity and plasticity in circulating neutrophil subpopulations in cancer. Cell Rep. 2015;10(4):562–73.
15. Coffelt SB, Wellenstein MD, de Visser KE. Neutrophils in cancer: neutral no more. Nat Rev Cancer. 2016;16(7):431–46.
16. Powell DR, Huttenlocher A. Neutrophils in the tumor microenvironment. Trends Immunol. 2016;37(1):41–52.
17. Fridlender ZG, Sun J, Kim S, Kapoor V, Cheng G, Ling L, et al. Polarization of tumor-associated neutrophil phenotype by TGF-beta: "N1" versus "N2" TAN. Cancer Cell. 2009;16(3):183–94.
18. Wilson CL, Jurk D, Fullard N, Banks P, Page A, Luli S, et al. NFkappaB1 is a suppressor of neutrophil-driven hepatocellular carcinoma. Nat Commun. 2015;6:6818.
19. Zhou SL, Zhou ZJ, Hu ZQ, Huang XW, Wang Z, Chen EB, et al. Tumor-associated neutrophils recruit macrophages and T-regulatory cells to promote progression of hepatocellular carcinoma and resistance to sorafenib. Gastroenterology. 2016;150(7):1646–58 e17.
20. Medina-Echeverz J, Eggert T, Han M, Greten TF. Hepatic myeloid-derived suppressor cells in cancer. Cancer Immunol Immunother. 2015;64(8):931–40.
21. Li HQ, Han YM, Guo QL, Zhang MG, Cao XT. Cancer-expanded myeloid-derived suppressor cells induce anergy of NK cells through membrane-bound TGF-beta 1. J Immunol. 2009;182(1):240–9.
22. Noy R, Pollard JW. Tumor-associated macrophages: from mechanisms to therapy. Immunity. 2014;41(1):49–61.

23. Yan W, Liu X, Ma H, Zhang H, Song X, Gao L, et al. Tim-3 fosters HCC development by enhancing TGF-beta-mediated alternative activation of macrophages. Gut. 2015;64(10):1593–604.
24. Butterfield LH, Ribas A, Meng WS, Dissette VB, Amarnani S, Vu HT, et al. T-cell responses to HLA-A*0201 immunodominant peptides derived from alpha-fetoprotein in patients with hepatocellular cancer. Clin Cancer Res. 2003;9(16 Pt 1):5902–8.
25. Lee WC, Wang HC, Hung CF, Huang PF, Lia CR, Chen MF. Vaccination of advanced hepatocellular carcinoma patients with tumor lysate-pulsed dendritic cells: a clinical trial. J Immunother. 2005;28(5):496–504.
26. Heo J, Reid T, Ruo L, Breitbach CJ, Rose S, Bloomston M, et al. Randomized dose-finding clinical trial of oncolytic immunotherapeutic vaccinia JX-594 in liver cancer. Nat Med. 2013;19(3):329–36.
27. Shimizu K, Kotera Y, Aruga A, Takeshita N, Katagiri S, Ariizumi SI, et al. Postoperative dendritic cell vaccine plus activated T-cell transfer improves the survival of patients with invasive hepatocellular carcinoma. Hum Vaccin Immunother. 2014;10(4):970–6.
28. Chen LT, Chen MF, Li LA, Lee PH, Jeng LB, Lin DY, et al. Long-term results of a randomized, observation-controlled, phase III trial of adjuvant interferon Alfa-2b in hepatocellular carcinoma after curative resection. Ann Surg. 2012;255(1):8–17.
29. Faivre SJ, Santoro A, Kelley RK, Merle P, Gane E, Douillard J-Y, et al. A phase 2 study of a novel transforming growth factor-beta (TGF-β1) receptor I kinase inhibitor, LY2157299 monohydrate (LY), in patients with advanced hepatocellular carcinoma (HCC). J Clin Oncol. 2014;32(suppl 3):abstract LBA173.
30. Sangro B, Gomez-Martin C, de la Mata M, Inarrairaegui M, Garralda E, Barrera P, et al. A clinical trial of CTLA-4 blockade with tremelimumab in patients with hepatocellular carcinoma and chronic hepatitis C. J Hepatol. 2013;59(1):81–8.
31. El-Khoueiry AB, Sangro B, Yau T, Crocenzi TS, Kudo M, Hsu C, et al. Nivolumab in patients with advanced hepatocellular carcinoma (CheckMate 040): an open-label, non-comparative, phase 1/2 dose escalation and expansion trial. Lancet. 2017;389(10088):2492–502.
32. Sangro B, Crocenzi TS, Welling TH, Iñarrairaegui M, Prieto J, Fuertes C, et al. Phase I dose escalation study of nivolumab (Anti-PD-1; BMS-936558; ONO- 4538) in patients (pts) with advanced hepatocellular carcinoma (HCC) with or without chronic viral hepatitis. J Clin Oncol. 2013;31(suppl):abstr TPS3111.

# Chapter 4
# Mechanisms of Disease: The Damaged Genome in HCC

**Matthew Hoare**

## Abbreviations

| | |
|---|---|
| AFP | Alpha-fetoprotein |
| CNV | Copy number variation |
| DEN | Diethylnitrosamine |
| EGF | Epidermal growth factor |
| HCC | Hepatocellular carcinoma |
| HH | Hereditary haemochromatosis |
| HSC | Hepatic stellate cell |
| LINEs and SINEs | Long and short interspersed nuclear elements |
| NAFLD | Non-alcoholic fatty liver disease |
| NGS | Next-generation sequencing |
| SNP | Single nucleotide polymorphism |
| SNVs | Single nucleotide variants |

## Introduction

Hepatocellular carcinoma (HCC) remains one of the leading causes of cancer-related death worldwide, with a rising incidence across Europe and the United States [1, 2]. This relates, in part, to the epidemic of non-alcoholic fatty liver disease (NAFLD) as a consequence of increasing obesity and prevalence of the metabolic syndrome. The global annual death toll from HCC remains at similar levels to its

M. Hoare (✉)
Cancer Research UK Cambridge Institute, University of Cambridge, Cambridge, UK

Department of Medicine, University of Cambridge, Cambridge, UK
e-mail: Matthew.Hoare@cruk.cam.ac.uk



T. Cross, D. H. Palmer (eds.), *Liver Cancers*,
https://doi.org/10.1007/978-3-319-92216-4_4

incidence [3], which speaks of our lack of ability to cure most patients who present with this cancer.

Worldwide, the dominant risk factor for the development of HCC is chronic hepatitis B virus (HBV) infection, and more than 80% of new cases of HCC occur in Africa and East Asia where seropositivity rates for HBV are considerably higher than in Europe and the United States [4]. In Europe and the United States, the predominant risk factors include NAFLD, alcohol-related liver disease and hepatitis C virus (HCV) infection.

In recent years there has been an explosion of knowledge about the molecular mechanisms underpinning the development and progression of HCC [5]. Amongst these, our knowledge about the structure and function of the hepatocyte genome and how it changes from chronic liver disease (CLD) to cancer has revealed multiple potential avenues for future therapeutic exploration in a cancer that currently has few effective therapies. In this review we discuss the current state of knowledge about HCC-associated genomic changes, as well as changes in DNA methylation and their potential role in prognostication or therapy.

## Genetic Predisposition to HCC

As the majority of HCCs develop in patients with CLD, hereditary genetic syndromes driving the development of CLD are also associated with the subsequent development of HCC. Hereditary haemochromatosis (HH), an autosomal recessive disorder caused mostly by mutations of the *HFE* gene, results in the excessive tissue accumulation of iron, particularly in the liver [6]. CLD due to HH is associated with one of the highest attributable risks for HCC development with around 4% per annum developing a tumour [7]. A meta-analysis of studies of European patients found that the C282Y variant of *HFE* increased risk of HCC development in HH, but heterozygosity also increased the risk of development of HCC in patients with alcohol-related liver disease [7]. Other inherited genetic liver diseases such as Wilson's disease, porphyria or the glycogen storage disorders are less frequently associated with the development of HCC [8].

Non-disease-associated genetic variation can also predispose to, or predict, the subsequent development of HCC. Epidermal growth factor (EGF) signalling has been implicated in the pathogenesis of HCC [9]. Analysis of the EGF61*G genetic polymorphism, associated with an increased half-life, secretion and serum concentration of EGF, has shown that a G/G genotype is associated with a fourfold increased risk of HCC in cirrhotics, compared to the non-risk A/A genotype [10, 11]. This suggests that modulation of EGF signalling could represent a plausible therapeutic target to prevent HCC development in CLD. Candidate gene or pathway studies have highlighted numerous single nucleotide polymorphisms (SNPs) in oxidative stress, DNA repair and inflammatory pathways that are associated with the development of HCC [12]. Subsequent unbiased genome-wide association studies of an HBV-infected Chinese population identified a susceptibility locus on 1p36

[13], and a Japanese HCV-infected cohort identified a polymorphism at the MHC class 1-associated MICA locus [14] as predictive of HCC development. However, certain SNPs seem to lead to disease-specific risk effects: the *PNPLA3* SNP found in alcoholic and NAFLD-related liver disease can predict the development of HCC in these conditions [15, 16], but not in patients with HCV [17].

Clearly the use of non-disease-associated genetic features in clinical practice as either predictors or potential therapeutic targets for the prevention of HCC development in cirrhotic patients remains some way away, but could represent a cheap method of stratifying patients based on levels of risk of developing HCC.

## Mechanisms of Genomic Damage in Chronic Liver Disease

Whilst germline genetic variation contributes to the risk of developing HCC, the bulk of variation is derived from new somatic mutations arising during CLD. Approximately 70–90% of patients with HCC have a background of long-term, usually inflammatory, CLD leading to cirrhosis.

Understanding of the major drivers of acquired genetic changes can be obtained through exome or whole-genome sequencing analysis of cancer genomes. Population analyses of sequencing data allow us to understand particular mutagenic signatures that point to different mechanisms of genome injury [18]. A study of 27 HCCs from patients with viral hepatitis found T>C/A>G transitions, commonly seen in other cancers, but also identified C>A/G>T transversions and C>T/G>A transitions, specific for liver cancer and associated with chronic alcohol abuse [19]. A pan-cancer analysis of mutational signatures found six individual signatures in HCC, more than were seen with other cancers. This suggests that multiple and sometimes concurrent processes contribute to genomic damage in HCC [20]. However, population effects may predominate: Totoki el al. demonstrated that even in the context of common CLD aetiology, the most important associate of mutational signature was the genetic background of the patient [21], suggesting that genomes may become damaged in different ways even in the face of a common injurious agent.

### *Chronic Inflammation and Genome Instability*

Until recently it remained unclear how chronic liver inflammation drives carcinogenesis. However, recent discoveries suggest that inflammatory cytokines, and IL-6 in particular, may drive genomic instability leading to cancer-associated mutations.

In CLD the primary source of hepatic fibrosis is the activated hepatic stellate cell (HSC). Normally quiescent, in response to liver injury, they activate to become secretory myofibroblasts in an adaptive response to restore tissue homeostasis [22]. After activation, they undergo a secretome switch to an inflammatory state, secreting interleukins and chemokines [23] driving an immune-mediated response clearing the HSCs from the microenvironment. In CLD their chronic persistence becomes maladaptive and drives HCC development; in a mouse model of NAFLD, inflammatory, senescent HSCs led to the development of HCC. Abrogation of cytokine secretion, through genetic or antibody-mediated inhibition from persistent HSC, prevents HCC development [24].

Amongst the inflammatory cytokines, IL-6 has been implicated in the development of genomic damage. *Mdr2*$^{-/-}$ mice develop chronic cholestatic liver injury and subsequently HCC; transplantation of *IL-6*$^{-/-}$ bone marrow into these mice, leading to immune-specific loss of IL-6, delays HCC development compared to control animals [25]. The regenerative response to hemi-hepatectomy in *Mdr2*$^{-/-}$ mice is associated with the subsequent development of HCC. Depletion of IL-6 after hemi-hepatectomy reduces hepatocyte proliferation and prevents the development of HCC [26]. Importantly, blockade of IL-6 is also associated with reduced micronuclei formation and therefore may prevent genomic instability in hepatocytes. Consistently, blockade of IL-6 also reduces murine tumour formation after injection of the carcinogen diethylnitrosamine (DEN). Mechanistically, IL-6 reduces p53-dependent apoptosis and promotes β-catenin signalling through canonical IL-6 signalling, but also promotes angiogenesis through non-canonical IL-6 signalling to adjacent endothelial cells [27].

In a mouse model of impaired TGF-β signalling, treatment with IL-6 led CD133+ hepatic stem cells to undergo the epithelial-mesenchymal transition and become highly aggressive cancer stem cells, suggesting that not only can IL-6 drive genome instability, but also plasticity in the preneoplastic context [28]. These findings are consistent with studies in other tissues of the additive effect of IL-6 and tissue damage upon cellular reprogramming. Chronic tissue damage drives IL-6 secretion, crucial for cellular reprogramming in response to expression of the Yamanaka factors [29]. Inhibition of IL-6 signalling or prevention of damage-induced senescence, the source of endogenous IL-6, prevented cellular reprogramming. Therefore, chronic inflammation, and IL-6 in particular, within CLD is associated with extensive non-autonomous effects driving genetic instability and promoting cellular plasticity, potentially underpinning the development of HCC.

Interestingly, IL-6 signalling may underpin the tumorigenesis from other genomic mutations. As we shall see later, amplification of fibroblast growth factor 19 (*FGF19*) is a frequent occurrence in human HCC. HCCs with this lesion develop increased signalling through IL-6/STAT3 and become addicted to this pathway [30]. Pharmacological or genetic inhibition of IL-6 or downstream mediator Jak1 can prevent HCC development in the context of *Fgf19* amplification.

As a potential biomarker, IL-6 is significantly elevated in the serum of subjects with HCC, compared to matched cirrhotic controls [31, 32]. In a case-control study, Ohishi et al. found that retrospective analysis of serum IL-6 levels predicted the subsequent development of HCC in atomic bomb survivors [33].

Therefore, IL-6 represents a potentially interesting target as both a biomarker of HCC development and drug target to prevent development or progression of HCC in the context of chronic liver diseases.

## *Integration of Hepatitis B and Genomic Damage*

Whilst originally thought to reside as and episomal covalently closed circular DNA (cccDNA) within hepatocyte nuclei, there is now abundant evidence that HBV integrates into the human genome [34–36]. This preferentially occurs at dsDNA breaks [37] or at microsatellites, prone to genomic instability [38]. Integration can disrupt coding sequences, lead to viral-promoter-driven endogenous gene expression and chimeric viral-human transcripts and can induce copy number variation (CNV) [34]. Hepatocytes with integrated HBV genomes undergo clonal expansion [35], implying a positive selection pressure. Sung et al. studied 81 HBV-infected tumour-background liver pairs and identified clustering of integration sites at the *TERT* promoter as well as *MLL4* (encoding the lysine-methyltransferase KMT2B) and *CCNE1* genes (encoding the cell cycle mediator cyclin E1, regulated by the p53–p21 pathway) [34]. HBV integration into the *TERT* promoter has been confirmed in whole-genome sequencing studies [19, 21] and bait-capture studies [39], where integration was associated with upregulation of TERT expression.

Therefore, HBV infection leads to genomic damage through integration at sites that, as we shall see, can drive the development of HCC.

## *Chronic Inflammation and Endogenous Retrotransposons*

More than half of the human genome is comprised of mobile genetic sequences called transposable elements [40]. Although the majority are epigenetically silenced and no longer transpose, a small number retain the ability to transpose and induce genetic damage within somatic cells. One major class of these elements is the retrotransposons that include the long and short interspersed nuclear elements (LINEs and SINEs). LINE-1-mediated retrotransposition has been demonstrated to lead to insertional mutagenesis in human cancer: one of the first descriptions was of a LINE-1 insertion within the *MYC* gene in breast cancer [41].

More recently it has become clear that retrotransposons can drive mutagenesis in HCC. 20% of HCCs were found to have a LINE-1 insertion in the *MCC* gene, associated with downregulation and subsequent de-repression of β-catenin signalling [42]. Whilst LINE-1 insertions in established cancer have been demonstrated, whether retrotransposition can occur in pre-neoplasia, as a driver of genetic instability, is unknown. Interestingly, chronic inflammation, and IL-6 in particular, leads to a downregulation of DNA methylation of LINE-1 sequences that would normally repress transposition [43]. Whether chronic inflammation within the liver and subsequent LINE-1-mediated mutagenesis occurs, as an initiating event in HCC, is not known. Therapeutically, transposition can be inhibited with reverse transcriptase inhibitors such as lamivudine [44] suggesting a potential mechanism to reduce genome damage in CLD patients.

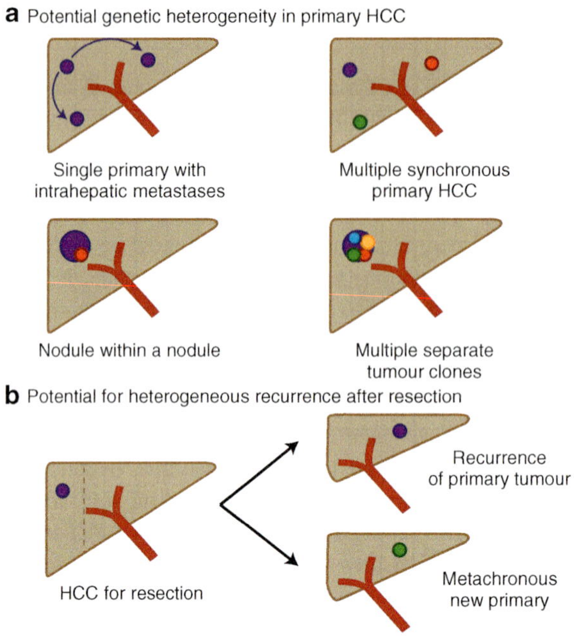


**Fig. 4.1** Genetic heterogeneity in HCC. (**a**) HCC develops on a background of chronic liver disease in the majority of cases, where the liver has undergone a cancerisation field effect. Therefore, in a multifocal tumour, it is currently radiologically impossible to distinguish between a single primary lesion with intrahepatic metastases and multiple synchronous, genetically-distinct primaries. Similarly, divergent clones with private genetic changes can arise within tumours, the so-called 'nodule within a nodule' or a large primary containing multiple separate, genetically-distinct clones resulting that genetic analysis of a single biopsy specimen will be insufficient to understand the complete genomic landscape of the tumour. (**b**) After hepatic resection for HCC, a new tumour deposit within the remnant liver cannot be assumed to be genetically identical to the original tumour, as it may represent a metachronous, genetically-distinct primary tumour. Adapted from Lu et al. [53]

progressive liver failure develop that can be rescued through re-expression of telomerase [64]. These findings suggest that the liver is susceptible to replicative senescence and subsequent declining function. This is potentially important if telomerase-modulating therapy is to be considered: telomerase inhibition to treat telomerase-expressing HCC may be complicated by declining function in the non-tumourous background liver.

Sequencing studies have found that acquired mutations in the core promoter sequences of *TERT*, leading to increased expression of telomerase [21, 65], are the most common somatic changes seen in HCC. Totoki et al. found that 68% of cases of HCC, from a variety of disease backgrounds, had SNVs or focal amplifications of the *TERT* promoter [21]. Similarly, Nault et al. found 59% of HCCs, but also a significant minority of preneoplastic hepatic adenomas [65] and dysplastic nodules

[66] had similar *TERT* promoter mutations, suggesting that these are amongst the earliest genetic lesions in the dysplasia to carcinoma sequence in the liver. Similarly to cancer-associated indels, HBV integration at the *TERT* promoter and subsequent activation have been demonstrated [21, 67], suggesting that telomerase activation is such an important event in HCC development that selection pressure drives multiple mechanisms of *TERT* re-expression in human HCC.

## *Mutation or Loss of p53*

p53 is one of the mostly commonly mutated or deleted genes in human cancer, suggesting that it is amongst the most important tumour suppressor proteins [68]. It controls the response to cellular stress or damage and underpins both apoptosis and senescence. Mutations of p53 have long been associated with HCC as aflatoxin B1, produced by food-contaminating *Aspergillus* sp., is associated with between 5 and 28% of the global burden of HCC cases [69]; aflatoxin exposure is associated with a highly specific R249S mutation of the *TP53* gene [70]. Subsequent sequencing studies of non-aflatoxin-associated cases have found a range of SNVs of *TP53* or larger indels on 17p [19, 21, 45, 46, 48–50], with the recent TCGA dataset suggesting that 33% of HCCs have mutated or lost p53 [48] (see Table 4.1). There is no clustering of mutations across the coding region to suggest specific domains are more important [71], but a spread of missense and truncating mutations that reduce expression and likely impair its function or chromatin-binding (Fig. 4.2a).

The canonical p53 pathway involves constitutive repression of p53 by MDM2 that is relieved by cellular stress driving proteasomal degradation of MDM2; release and subsequent chromatin-binding of p53 drive a highly conserved transcriptional programme, including the tumour suppressor and cell cycle regulator p21. Interestingly, whilst *MDM2* and *CDKN1A* (the gene encoding p21) are frequently mutated in other cancer types, they are rarely mutated in HCC. Similarly, the *TP53* family members, *TP63* and *TP73*, are also infrequently mutated stressing the importance of p53 loss in the pathogenesis of HCC (Fig. 4.2). Importantly, loss or mutation of *TP53* has a significant negative impact on prognosis after hepatic resection, with p53-null tumours significantly more likely to recur (TCGA data, Fig. 4.2c), have a higher alpha-fetoprotein (AFP) level and poorer differentiation grade [74, 75].

Mutations in *TP53* are not currently targetable, but there is significant interest in the potential of molecular chaperones designed to refold mutated p53 into a wild-type conformational structure and restore some level of p53 function [76]. Other potential therapeutic options include the use of hepatotropic adenoviral vectors to deliver and re-express wild-type p53 in liver tumours; one study has utilised trans-arterial embolisation to deliver these directly to tumour tissue with some success [77].

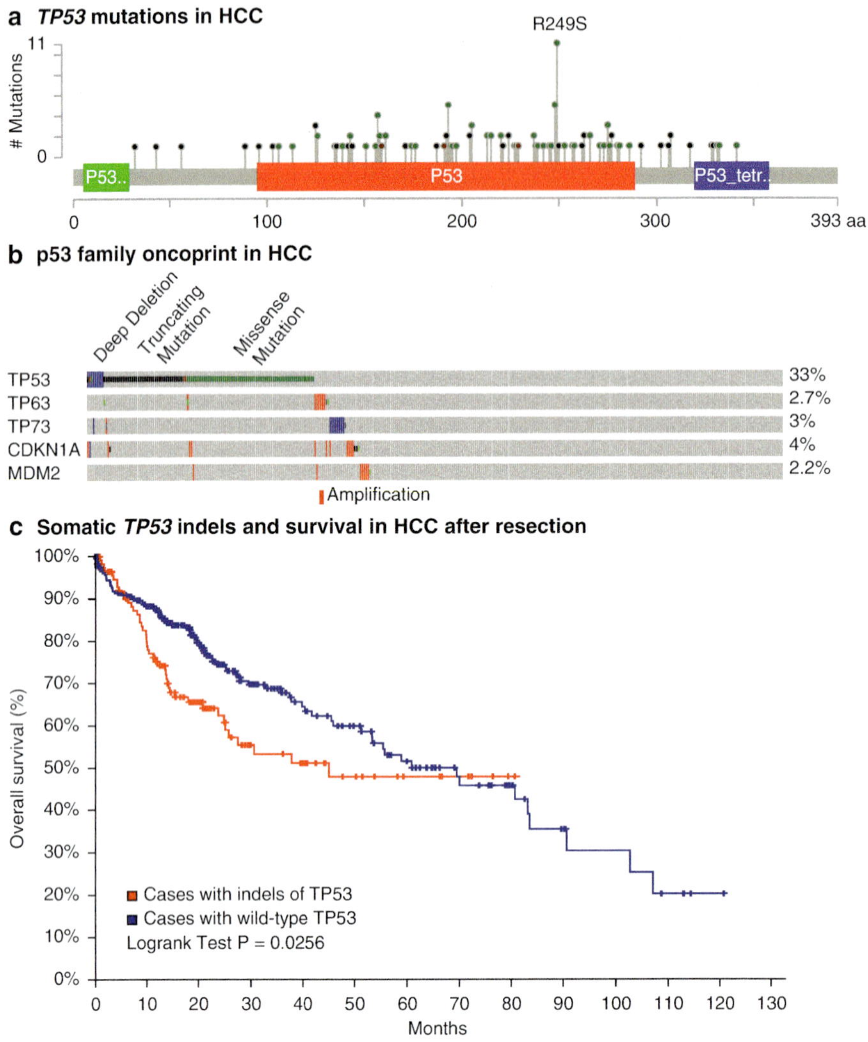


**Fig. 4.2** Mutations of *TP53* and their prognosis in HCC. (**a**) Distribution of somatic SNVs across the *TP53* gene, from samples in the TCGA dataset. p53 trans-activation domain in green, DNA-binding domain in red and tetramerisation domain shown in purple. There is a small cluster at amino acid 249 in the DNA-binding domain associated with exposure to aflatoxin B1. (**b**) Oncoprint of indels and larger-scale deletions of *TP53*, the *TP53* family members *TP63* and *TP73*, the p53-regulator *MDM2* and the canonical p53 transcriptional target p21 (*CDKN1A*) demonstrating alterations at significant frequency only occur in *TP53* itself. (**c**) Loss or indels of *TP53* in HCC are associated with a significantly worse prognosis after hepatic resection. Comparison by log rank test. Data and visualisation from the TCGA dataset [48] and cBioPortal (http://www.cbioportal.org) [72, 73]

## *Mutations in the Wnt/β-Catenin Pathway*

The association between mutations in *CTNNB1*, the gene encoding β-catenin and HCC was identified in the late 1990s when several groups found N-terminally clustered missense mutations in 30–40% of HCC cases from both Europe and Asia [78, 79]. These mutations were associated with increased nuclear localisation of β-catenin in tumour specimens [78, 80], reduced rates of large calibre vascular invasion and improved prognosis compared to HCC with wild-type *CTNNB1* [75, 81].

β-Catenin is normally held in the cytoplasm by a multimolecular complex containing APC, AXIN1 and GSK-3β. Upon binding of one of the Wnt family of extracellular proteins to the membrane-bound Frizzled receptor, GSK-3β is displaced from the complex releasing β-catenin to traverse to the nucleus, bind to LEF/TCF transcription factors and recruit transcriptional co-activators to Wnt target genes [82]. The stability of the β-catenin protein is controlled by phosphorylation at the N-terminus; mutations at this site are associated with greatly increased stability of the protein; thus mutations of CTNNB1 are clustered at this site [82].

Recent NGS studies have confirmed the earlier findings, with between 30 and 40% of HCCs found to have indels or deletions of *CTNNB1* (Table 4.1), but also a significant burden of genetic lesions in other members of the Wnt/β-catenin pathway, particularly *AXIN1* [21, 46, 48–50, 52]. Interestingly, nearly all studies have demonstrated a near mutual exclusivity between mutations of *TP53* and *CTNNB1*.

Therapeutic targeting of the Wnt/β-catenin pathway is not currently possible, with few agents progressing beyond phase 1 trials [83], but mouse models of β-catenin-driven colon cancer suggest that restoration of normal β-catenin function is associated with complete tumour regression in that context [84], raising hope that if therapeutic vulnerabilities could be established, effective treatments could be developed for this subtype of liver cancer.

## *Other High-Frequency Mutations in HCC*

All of the NGS studies have suggested that HCC contains frequent mutations of genes involved in regulation of chromatin structure and maintenance of the epigenome. Members of the SWI/SNF complex, responsible for nucleosome positioning, have been found to be recurrently mutated in a variety of human cancers and notably mutated at much higher frequency than components of other chromatin-modifying pathways [85]. Therefore, this pathway likely represents a conserved tumour suppressor mechanism. In HCC *ARID1A* and *ARID2* are mutated at frequencies of up to 26% and 11%, respectively [19, 21, 46, 48, 49, 52]. Subsequent functional genomic studies have found that *ARID1B* is crucial for oncogene-induced senescence and suppression of RAS-induced HCC development in a mouse model [86].

Members of the mixed-lineage leukaemia (MLL) family of histone methyltransferases are responsible for trimethylation of H3K4, associated with active transcription. MLL is also involved with signalling through the HGF-cMET pathway [87]. Sequencing studies have demonstrated that various members of the MLL family are mutated in HCC [19, 46, 48, 50].

## *Copy Number Variation in HCC*

In addition to small-scale genomic damage, multiple studies have demonstrated larger-scale chromosomal rearrangements, amplifications and deep deletions in HCC. Utilising array-based comparative genomic hybridisation in HCC, many groups have found amplifications and losses at key loci encoding putative oncogenes and tumour suppressor genes [18]. One of the first studies utilised a targeted oncogene panel array to demonstrate recurrent amplifications of *CCND1*, the gene encoding cyclin D1 required for G1 to S-phase transition, at 11q13 (the locus that also encodes *FGF19), TERC*, encoding the RNA component of telomerase and *MYC*, nearly ubiquitously dysregulated in human cancers [88]. Subsequent studies have confirmed these findings and demonstrated recurrent widespread CNV with gains at 1q, 8q and 20q and losses at 1p, 4q, 8p, 13q, 16q and 17p in HCC specimens from patients with different CLDs. In particular, loss of 8p and subsequent transcriptomic changes in HCC from a range of background diseases is associated with poor prognosis after resection [89].

The recently reported TCGA dataset has again confirmed many of the previously reported CNVs, but also given us much greater insight into the relative frequency of these changes in HCC (Table 4.2) [48]. Integrative analysis of indels and CNVs in HCC has shown how two key tumour suppressor pathways are inactivated by distinct mechanisms. As discussed earlier *TP53* is frequently mutated in HCC, predominantly through missense indels, whereas a second complementary pathway, the p16-Rb pathway, is inactivated through larger-scale deletions of either *CDKN2A* [90, 91] or *RB1* [92]. Therefore, it is likely that different mechanisms of genome injury are responsible for inactivation of these two tumour suppressor pathways.

P16, encoded by *CDKN2A* at the *INK4A/ARF* locus on 9p, is responsible for repression of CDK4 and CDK6, which in combination with cyclin D1 in turn repress Rb (see Fig. 4.3). Therapeutically novel agents such as palbociclib [93], a p16-mimetic that represses CDK4 and 6, show promise in HCC. However, it will be important to understand the pattern of loss of these different tumour suppressors in patients with HCC. CDK4/CDK6 inhibition will effectively repress cell cycle progression in the context of *TP53* mutations and loss of p16 through deep deletions of the *INK4A/ARF* locus or epigenetic repression of *CDKN2A*, but would be inactive in the context of deletions of *RB1*.

**Table 4.2** Recurrent copy number alterations in HCC from the TCGA dataset ($n = 442$). GISTIC-based copy number variation (CNV) analysis of HCCs in the TCGA dataset demonstrating common, recurrent chromosomal amplifications or deletions ranked by *q*-value. Data derived from cBioPortal (http://www.cbioportal.org/) showing the number of genes affected and selected proto-oncogenes or tumour suppressor genes at these cytobands

| Amp/ Del | Chr | Cytoband | Number of genes at this locus | Selected genes at this locus | *Q*-Value |
|---|---|---|---|---|---|
| Del | 13 | 13q14.2 | 2 | RB1 | 2.30E-37 |
| Del | 1 | 1p36.31 | 114 | TNFRSF4, TP73 | 1.20E-33 |
| Amp | 11 | 11q13.3 | 2 | CCND1, FGF19 | 3.40E-29 |
| Amp | 1 | 1q21.3 | 3 | | 2.10E-24 |
| Del | 4 | 4q35.1 | 5 | | 1.80E-23 |
| Del | 9 | 9p21.3 | 2 | CDKN2A CDKN2B | 3.10E-22 |
| Amp | 8 | 8q24.21 | 111 | MYC | 1.20E-21 |
| Del | 1 | 1p36.11 | 267 | HDAC1, LCK, ARID1A | 1.70E-20 |
| Del | 8 | 8p23.2 | 1 | | 2.10E-19 |
| Del | 6 | 6q27 | 4 | | 3.40E-15 |
| Amp | 17 | 17q25.3 | 7 | | 1.30E-14 |
| Amp | 3 | 3q26.31 | 1 | | 6.70E-11 |
| Amp | 5 | 5p15.33 | 6 | TERT | 1.10E-10 |
| Amp | 13 | 13q33.3 | 148 | ATP4B, FGF14 | 2.20E-10 |
| Del | 17 | 17p13.1 | 252 | | 4.00E-10 |
| Amp | 13 | 13q32.3 | 45 | | 6.80E-10 |
| Del | 10 | 10q23.31 | 3 | PTEN | 2.10E-09 |

## Damage to the Epigenome in HCC

In addition to extensive genomic damage in HCC, there is abundant evidence that epigenomic damage also occurs. As already discussed, DNA-sequencing studies have identified multiple changes to chromatin-regulator genes of the SWI/SNF complex and the MLL family, responsible for histone methylation.

The epigenome serves to regulate chromatin architecture and gene expression through (1) chemical modification of DNA, particularly methylation, (2) chemical modification of histones which define chromatin states and regulate transcription and (3) expression of non-coding RNAs such as long non-coding RNA and micro-RNAs that regulate gene expression post-transcriptionally. The epigenetics of HCC has been extensively reviewed elsewhere [94, 95]; therefore, only the role of DNA methylation in HCC will be discussed.

### *DNA-Methylation Changes in HCC*

Methylation of cytosine residues at CpG dinucleotides is stably transmitted to daughter cells at mitosis by methyltransferases of the DNMT family. Clusters of CpG sequences, termed CpG islands, are found adjacent to gene promoter sequences

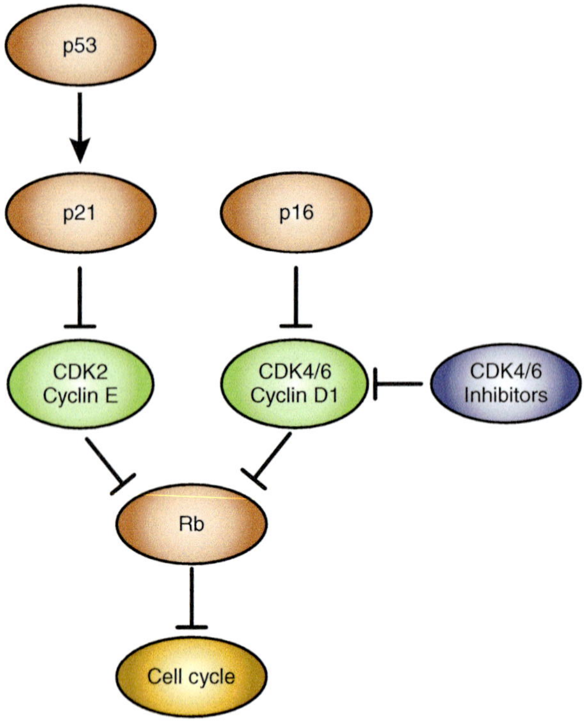


**Fig. 4.3** p53 and p16 signalling pathways. The p53-p21 and p16-Rb tumour suppressor pathways co-operatively regulate cell cycle progression. Both pathways are inactivated in HCC by distinct mechanisms. Novel therapies, such as the CDK4/CDK6 inhibitors will only work in the context of functional Rb

[96]. CpG island methylation is associated with transcriptional repression through sterically inhibiting the transcriptional machinery from accessing the chromatin, but also through recruitment of specific transcriptional inhibitors.

Global hypomethylation of CpG elements tends to occur as an early event in many human cancers [97], and this pattern may also be seen in HCC [98], where it seems to be associated with chromosomal instability. Several groups have defined locus-specific methylation patterns and found site-specific increases in DNA methylation with associated transcriptional repression in HCC [98–101]. Promoter methylation increases from normal liver to cirrhosis, dysplasia and then HCC [102]. Importantly, genome-wide studies have demonstrated a significant increase in DNA methylation at the *INK4A/ARF* locus [99, 100], consistent with previous candidate gene approaches demonstrating p16-promoter hypermethylation [90, 91]. Therefore, not only is p16 lost through deletion but also inactivated through epigenetic repression. Analysis of the prognostic implications of promoter DNA methylation shows that epigenetic repression of a small group of genes, including both *CDKN2A* and *APC* (a negative regulator of β-catenin), is associated with impaired prognosis compared to HCCs without promoter methylation at these loci [103]. Genome-wide analysis has identified a 36-gene methylation signature, including at *APC*, predictive of poor prognosis after hepatic resection [104]. Site-specific methylation also depends upon the β-catenin and p53 status of the HCC studied, implying distinct mechanisms of epigenetic change occur in tumours of different genotypes [105].

Whilst therapeutic targeting of the epigenome, and DNA methylation in particular, remains some distance away, in vitro reversal of HCC-associated DNA-methylation changes has identified novel tumour suppressor genes that had not previously been identified as their coding sequences were intact, eluding NGS studies [106].

Several groups have demonstrated the feasibility of analysing tumoral DNA-methylation changes from ctDNA [99, 107]. The ability to detect *CDKN2A*-specific or whole-genome DNA-methylation profiles suggests that in the future stratification by DNA and methyl-DNA sequencing will be possible to obtain information about mutations, as well as epigenetically regulated expression changes in HCC.

## Conclusions

CLD leads to extensive damage to the coding and non-coding DNA sequences of the hepatocyte genome, but also damage to the epigenome that regulates gene expression. Whilst tumour heterogeneity presents a significant problem for sequencing of single biopsies, the analysis of circulating tumour cells or ctDNA holds the promise of seeing the global mutational burden within tumours. We have only begun to understand the complex genomic architecture of HCCs and understand even less of the driver changes that underpin the initiation of this disease. However, with integration of this knowledge, we can start to target these genes and pathways to finally improve the prognosis of patients with HCC.

**Acknowledgements** MH is supported by a CRUK Clinician Scientist Fellowship (C52489/A19924).

## References

1. Konfortion J, Coupland VH, Kocher HM, Allum W, Grocock MJ, Jack RH. Time and deprivation trends in incidence of primary liver cancer subtypes in England. J Eval Clin Pract. 2014;20(4):498–504.
2. El-Serag HB, Kanwal F. Epidemiology of hepatocellular carcinoma in the United States: where are we? Where do we go? Hepatology. 2014;60(5):1767–75.
3. Jemal A, Bray F, Center MM, Ferlay J, Ward E, Forman D. Global cancer statistics. CA Cancer J Clin. 2011;61(2):69–90.
4. El-Serag HB. Epidemiology of viral hepatitis and hepatocellular carcinoma. Gastroenterology. 2012;142(6):1264–1273.e1.
5. Zucman-Rossi J, Villanueva A, Nault J-C, Llovet JM. Genetic landscape and biomarkers of hepatocellular carcinoma. Gastroenterology. 2015;149(5):1226–1239.e4.

6. Pietrangelo A. Hereditary hemochromatosis: pathogenesis, diagnosis, and treatment. Gastroenterology. 2010;139(2):393–408. –408.e1–2
7. Jin F, Qu LS, Shen XZ. Association between C282Y and H63D mutations of the HFE gene with hepatocellular carcinoma in European populations: a meta-analysis. J Exp Clin Cancer Res. 2010;29(1):18.
8. Villanueva A, Newell P, Hoshida Y. Inherited hepatocellular carcinoma. Best Pract Res Clin Gastroenterol. 2010;24(5):725–34.
9. Motoo Y, Sawabu N, Nakanuma Y. Expression of epidermal growth factor and fibroblast growth factor in human hepatocellular carcinoma: an immunohistochemical study. Liver. 1991;11(5):272–7.
10. Tanabe KK, Lemoine A, Finkelstein DM, Kawasaki H, Fujii T, Chung RT, et al. Epidermal growth factor gene functional polymorphism and the risk of hepatocellular carcinoma in patients with cirrhosis. JAMA. 2008;299(1):53–60.
11. Abu Dayyeh BK, Yang M, Fuchs BC, Karl DL, Yamada S, Sninsky JJ, et al. A functional polymorphism in the epidermal growth factor gene is associated with risk for hepatocellular carcinoma. Gastroenterology. 2011;141(1):141–9.
12. Nahon P, Zucman-Rossi J. Single nucleotide polymorphisms and risk of hepatocellular carcinoma in cirrhosis. J Hepatol. 2012;57(3):663–74.
13. Zhang H, Zhai Y, Hu Z, Wu C, Qian J, Jia W, et al. Genome-wide association study identifies 1p36.22 as a new susceptibility locus for hepatocellular carcinoma in chronic hepatitis B virus carriers. Nat Genet. 2010;42(9):755–8.
14. Kumar V, Kato N, Urabe Y, Takahashi A, Muroyama R, Hosono N, et al. Genome-wide association study identifies a susceptibility locus for HCV-induced hepatocellular carcinoma. Nat Genet. 2011;43(5):455–8.
15. Liu YL, Patman GL, Leathart JBS, Piguet AC, Burt AD, Dufour JF, et al. Carriage of the PNPLA3 rs738409 C >G polymorphism confers an increased risk of non-alcoholic fatty liver disease associated hepatocellular carcinoma. J Hepatol. 2014;61(1):75–81.
16. Trépo E, Nahon P, Bontempi G, Valenti L, Falleti E, Nischalke H-D, et al. Association between the PNPLA3 (rs738409 C>G) variant and hepatocellular carcinoma: Evidence from a meta-analysis of individual participant data. Hepatology. 2014;59(6):2170–7.
17. Guyot E, Sutton A, Rufat P, Laguillier C, Mansouri A, Moreau R, et al. PNPLA3 rs738409, hepatocellular carcinoma occurrence and risk model prediction in patients with cirrhosis. J Hepatol. 2013;58(2):312–8.
18. Shibata T, Aburatani H. Exploration of liver cancer genomes. Nat Rev Gastroenterol Hepatol. 2014;11(6):340–9.
19. Fujimoto A, Totoki Y, Abe T, Boroevich KA, Hosoda F, Nguyen HH, et al. Whole-genome sequencing of liver cancers identifies etiological influences on mutation patterns and recurrent mutations in chromatin regulators. Nat Genet. 2012;44(7):760–4.
20. Alexandrov LB, Nik-Zainal S, Wedge DC, Aparicio SAJR, Behjati S, Biankin AV, et al. Signatures of mutational processes in human cancer. Nature. 2013;500(7463):415–21.
21. Totoki Y, Tatsuno K, Covington KR, Ueda H, Creighton CJ, Kato M, et al. Trans-ancestry mutational landscape of hepatocellular carcinoma genomes. Nat Genet. 2014;46(12):1267–73.
22. Friedman SL. Hepatic stellate cells: protean, multifunctional, and enigmatic cells of the liver. Physiol Rev. 2008;88(1):125–72.
23. Krizhanovsky V, Yon M, Dickins RA, Hearn S, Simon J, Miething C, et al. Senescence of activated stellate cells limits liver fibrosis. Cell. 2008;134(4):657–67.
24. Yoshimoto S, Loo TM, Atarashi K, Kanda H, Sato S, Oyadomari S, et al. Obesity-induced gut microbial metabolite promotes liver cancer through senescence secretome. Nature. 2013;499(7456):97–101.
25. Kong L, Zhou Y, Bu H, Lv T, Shi Y, Yang J. Deletion of interleukin-6 in monocytes/macrophages suppresses the initiation of hepatocellular carcinoma in mice. J Exp Clin Cancer Res. 2016;35(1):131.
26. Lanton T, Shriki A, Nechemia-Arbely Y, Abramovitch R, Levkovitch O, Adar R, et al. Interleukin 6-dependent genomic instability heralds accelerated carcinogenesis following

liver regeneration on a background of chronic hepatitis. Hepatology. 2017;65(5):1600–11. Available from:. https://doi.org/10.1002/hep.29004.
27. Bergmann J, Müller M, Baumann N, Reichert M, Heneweer C, Bolik J, et al. IL-6 trans-signaling is essential for the development of hepatocellular carcinoma in mice. Hepatology. 2017;65(1):89–103.
28. Mitra A, Yan J, Xia X, Zhou S, Chen J, Mishra L, et al. IL6-mediated inflammatory loop reprograms normal to epithelial-mesenchymal transition(+) metastatic cancer stem cells in preneoplastic liver of transforming growth factor beta-deficient β2-spectrin(+/−) mice. Hepatology. 2017;65(4):1222–36.
29. Mosteiro L, Pantoja C, Alcazar N, Marión RM, Chondronasiou D, Rovira M, et al. Tissue damage and senescence provide critical signals for cellular reprogramming in vivo. Science. 2016;354:6315.
30. Zhou M, Yang H, Learned RM, Tian H, Ling L. Non-cell-autonomous activation of IL-6/STAT3 signaling mediates FGF19-driven hepatocarcinogenesis. Nat Commun. 2017;8:15433.
31. Porta C, De Amici M, Quaglini S, Paglino C, Tagliani F, Boncimino A, et al. Circulating interleukin-6 as a tumor marker for hepatocellular carcinoma. Ann Oncol. 2008;19(2):353–8.
32. Giannitrapani L, Cervello M, Soresi M, Notarbartolo M, La Rosa M, Virruso L, et al. Circulating IL-6 and sIL-6R in patients with hepatocellular carcinoma. Ann N Y Acad Sci. 2002;963:46–52.
33. Ohishi W, Cologne JB, Fujiwara S, Suzuki G, Hayashi T, Niwa Y, et al. Serum interleukin-6 associated with hepatocellular carcinoma risk: a nested case-control study. Int J Cancer. 2014;134(1):154–63.
34. Sung W-K, Zheng H, Li S, Chen R, Liu X, Li Y, et al. Genome-wide survey of recurrent HBV integration in hepatocellular carcinoma. Nat Genet. 2012;44(7):765–9.
35. Jiang Z, Jhunjhunwala S, Liu J, Haverty PM, Kennemer MI, Guan Y, et al. The effects of hepatitis B virus integration into the genomes of hepatocellular carcinoma patients. Genome Res. 2012;22(4):593–601.
36. Brechot C, Pourcel C, Louise A, Rain B, Tiollais P. Presence of integrated hepatitis B virus DNA sequences in cellular DNA of human hepatocellular carcinoma. Nature. 1980;286(5772):533–5.
37. Bill CA, Summers J. Genomic DNA double-strand breaks are targets for hepadnaviral DNA integration. Proc Natl Acad Sci U S A. 2004;101(30):11135–40.
38. Feitelson MA, Lee J. Hepatitis B virus integration, fragile sites, and hepatocarcinogenesis. Cancer Lett. 2007;252(2):157–70.
39. Toh ST, Jin Y, Liu L, Wang J, Babrzadeh F, Gharizadeh B, et al. Deep sequencing of the hepatitis B virus in hepatocellular carcinoma patients reveals enriched integration events, structural alterations and sequence variations. Carcinogenesis. 2013;34(4):787–98.
40. Kazazian HH, Moran JV. Mobile DNA in health and disease. N Engl J Med. 2017;377(4):361–70.
41. Morse B, Rotherg PG, South VJ, Spandorfer JM, Astrin SM. Insertional mutagenesis of the myc locus by a LINE-1 sequence in a human breast carcinoma. Nature. 1988;333(6168):87–90.
42. Shukla R, Upton KR, Muñoz-Lopez M, Gerhardt DJ, Fisher ME, Nguyen T, et al. Endogenous retrotransposition activates oncogenic pathways in hepatocellular carcinoma. Cell. 2013;153(1):101–11.
43. Gasche JA, Hoffmann J, Boland CR, Goel A. Interleukin-6 promotes tumorigenesis by altering DNA methylation in oral cancer cells. Int J Cancer. 2011;129(5):1053–63.
44. Jones RB, Garrison KE, Wong JC, Duan EH, Nixon DF, Ostrowski MA. Nucleoside analogue reverse transcriptase inhibitors differentially inhibit human LINE-1 retrotransposition. PLoS One. 2008;3(2):e1547.
45. Kan Z, Zheng H, Liu X, Li S, Barber TD, Gong Z, et al. Whole-genome sequencing identifies recurrent mutations in hepatocellular carcinoma. Genome Res. 2013;23(9):1422–33.
46. Schulze K, Imbeaud S, Letouzé E, Alexandrov LB, Calderaro J, Rebouissou S, et al. Exome sequencing of hepatocellular carcinomas identifies new mutational signatures and potential therapeutic targets. Nat Genet. 2015;47(5):505–11.

47. Huang J, Deng Q, Wang Q, Li K-Y, Dai J-H, Li N, et al. Exome sequencing of hepatitis B virus-associated hepatocellular carcinoma. Nat Genet. 2012;44(10):1117–21.
48. Cancer Genome Atlas Research Network. Electronic address: wheeler@bcm.edu, Cancer genome atlas research network. Comprehensive and integrative genomic characterization of hepatocellular carcinoma. Cell. 2017;169(7):1327–1341.e23.
49. Guichard C, Amaddeo G, Imbeaud S, Ladeiro Y, Pelletier L, Maad IB, et al. Integrated analysis of somatic mutations and focal copy-number changes identifies key genes and pathways in hepatocellular carcinoma. Nat Genet. 2012;44(6):694–8.
50. Cleary SP, Jeck WR, Zhao X, Chen K, Selitsky SR, Savich GL, et al. Identification of driver genes in hepatocellular carcinoma by exome sequencing. Hepatology. 2013;58(5):1693–702.
51. Jhunjhunwala S, Jiang Z, Stawiski EW, Gnad F, Liu J, Mayba O, et al. Diverse modes of genomic alteration in hepatocellular carcinoma. Genome Biol. 2014;15(8):436.
52. Li M, Zhao H, Zhang X, Wood LD, Anders RA, Choti MA, et al. Inactivating mutations of the chromatin remodeling gene ARID2 in hepatocellular carcinoma. Nat Genet. 2011;43(9):828–9.
53. Lu L-C, Hsu C-H, Hsu C, Cheng A-L. Tumor heterogeneity in hepatocellular carcinoma: facing the challenges. Liver Cancer. 2016;5(2):128–38.
54. Gerlinger M, Rowan AJ, Horswell S, Math M, Larkin J, Endesfelder D, et al. Intratumor heterogeneity and branched evolution revealed by multiregion sequencing. N Engl J Med. 2012;366(10):883–92.
55. Zhai W, Lim TK-H, Zhang T, Phang S-T, Tiang Z, Guan P, et al. The spatial organization of intra-tumour heterogeneity and evolutionary trajectories of metastases in hepatocellular carcinoma. Nat Commun. 2017;8:4565.
56. Jiang P, Chan CWM, Chan KCA, Cheng SH, Wong J, Wong VW-S, et al. Lengthening and shortening of plasma DNA in hepatocellular carcinoma patients. Proc Natl Acad Sci. 2015;112(11):E1317–25.
57. Ono A, Fujimoto A, Yamamoto Y, Akamatsu S, Hiraga N, Imamura M, et al. Circulating tumor DNA analysis for liver cancers and its usefulness as a liquid biopsy. Cell Mol Gastroenterol Hepatol. 2015;1(5):516–34.
58. Blackburn EH. Switching and signaling at the telomere. Cell. 2001;106(6):661–73.
59. d'Adda di Fagagna F, Reaper PM, Clay-Farrace L, Fiegler H, Carr P, von Zglinicki T, et al. A DNA damage checkpoint response in telomere-initiated senescence. Nature. 2003;426(6963):194–8.
60. Artandi SE, DePinho RA. Telomeres and telomerase in cancer. Carcinogenesis. 2010;31(1):9–18.
61. Calado RT, Brudno J, Mehta P, Kovacs JJ, Wu C, Zago MA, et al. Constitutional telomerase mutations are genetic risk factors for cirrhosis. Hepatology. 2011;53(5):1600–7.
62. Calado RT, Young NS. Telomere Diseases. N Engl J Med. 2009;361(24):2353–65.
63. Hartmann D, Srivastava U, Thaler M, Kleinhans KN, N'Kontchou G, Scheffold A, et al. Telomerase gene mutations are associated with cirrhosis formation. Hepatology. 2011;53(5):1608–17.
64. Rudolph KL, Chang S, Millard M, Schreiber-Agus N, DePinho RA. Inhibition of experimental liver cirrhosis in mice by telomerase gene delivery. Science. 2000;287(5456):1253–8.
65. Nault J-C, Mallet M, Pilati C, Calderaro J, Bioulac-Sage P, Laurent C, et al. High frequency of telomerase reverse-transcriptase promoter somatic mutations in hepatocellular carcinoma and preneoplastic lesions. Nat Commun. 2013;4:2218.
66. Nault J-C, Calderaro J, Di Tommaso L, Balabaud C, Zafrani ES, Bioulac-Sage P, et al. Telomerase reverse transcriptase promoter mutation is an early somatic genetic alteration in the transformation of premalignant nodules in hepatocellular carcinoma on cirrhosis. Hepatology. 2014;60(6):1983–92.
67. Paterlini-Bréchot P, Saigo K, Murakami Y, Chami M, Gozuacik D, Mugnier C, et al. Hepatitis B virus-related insertional mutagenesis occurs frequently in human liver cancers and recurrently targets human telomerase gene. Oncogene. 2003;22(25):3911–6.

68. Bieging KT, Mello SS, Attardi LD. Unravelling mechanisms of p53-mediated tumour suppression. Nat Rev Cancer. 2014;14(5):359–70.
69. Liu Y, Wu F. Global burden of aflatoxin-induced hepatocellular carcinoma: a risk assessment. Environ Health Perspect. 2010;118(6):818–24.
70. Bressac B, Kew M, Wands J, Ozturk M. Selective G to T mutations of p53 gene in hepatocellular carcinoma from southern Africa. Nature. 1991;350(6317):429–31.
71. Qi L-N, Bai T, Chen Z-S, Wu F-X, Chen Y-Y, De Xiang B, et al. The p53 mutation spectrum in hepatocellular carcinoma from Guangxi, China : role of chronic hepatitis B virus infection and aflatoxin B1 exposure. Liver Int. 2015;35(3):999–1009.
72. Cerami E, et al. The cBio cancer genomics portal: an open platform for exploring multidimensional cancer genomics data. Cancer Discov. 2012;2(5):401–4. PMID: 22588877
73. Gao J, et al. Integrative analysis of complex cancer genomics and clinical profiles using the cBioPortal. Sci Signal. 2013;6(269):23550210.
74. Hayashi H, Sugio K, Matsumata T, Adachi E, Takenaka K, Sugimachi K. The clinical significance of p53 gene mutation in hepatocellular carcinomas from Japan. Hepatology. 1995;22(6):1702–7.
75. Calderaro J, Couchy G, Imbeaud S, Amaddeo G, Letouzé E, Blanc JF, et al. Histological subtypes of hepatocellular carcinoma are related to gene mutations and molecular tumour classification. J Hepatol. 2017;67(4):727–38.
76. Bykov VJN, Wiman KG. Mutant p53 reactivation by small molecules makes its way to the clinic. FEBS Lett. 2014;588(16):2622–7.
77. Liu Y, Zhang Y, Bautista D, Tang S, Zhou J, Li C, et al. Trans-arterial p53-gene-embolization with gelatin sponge microparticles for hepatocellular carcinoma with BCLC stage B: single-center experience. Cell Biochem Biophys. 2015;71(1):99–104.
78. La Coste DA, Romagnolo B, Billuart P, Renard CA, Buendia MA, Soubrane O, et al. Somatic mutations of the β-catenin gene are frequent in mouse and human hepatocellular carcinomas. Proc Natl Acad Sci U S A. 1998;95(15):8847–51.
79. Miyoshi Y, Iwao K, Nagasawa Y, Aihara T, Sasaki Y, Imaoka S, et al. Activation of the beta-catenin gene in primary hepatocellular carcinomas by somatic alterations involving exon 3. Cancer Res. 1998;58(12):2524–7.
80. Van Nhieu JT, Renard CA, Wei Y, Cherqui D, Zafrani ES, Buendia MA. Nuclear accumulation of mutated β-catenin in hepatocellular carcinoma is associated with increased cell proliferation. Am J Pathol. 1999;155(3):703–10.
81. Mao TL, Chu JS, Jeng YM, Lai PL, Hsu HC. Expression of mutant nuclear beta-catenin correlates with non-invasive hepatocellular carcinoma, absence of portal vein spread, and good prognosis. J Pathol. 2001;193(1):95–101.
82. Polakis P. Wnt signaling and cancer. Genes Dev. 2000;14(15):1837–51.
83. Vilchez V, Turcios L, Marti F, Gedaly R. Targeting Wnt/β-catenin pathway in hepatocellular carcinoma treatment. World J Gastroenterol. 2016;22(2):823–32.
84. Dow LE, O'Rourke KP, Simon J, Tschaharganeh DF, van Es JH, Clevers H, et al. Apc restoration promotes cellular differentiation and reestablishes crypt homeostasis in colorectal cancer. Cell. 2015;161(7):1539–52.
85. Kadoch C, Hargreaves DC, Hodges C, Elias L, Ho L, Ranish J, et al. Proteomic and bioinformatic analysis of mammalian SWI/SNF complexes identifies extensive roles in human malignancy. Nat Genet. 2013;45(6):592–601.
86. Tordella L, Khan S, Hohmeyer A, Banito A, Klotz S, Raguz S, et al. SWI/SNF regulates a transcriptional program that induces senescence to prevent liver cancer. Genes Dev. 2016;30(19):2187–98.
87. Takeda S, Liu H, Sasagawa S, Dong Y, Trainor PA, Cheng EH, et al. HGF-MET signals via the MLL-ETS2 complex in hepatocellular carcinoma. J Clin Investig. 2013;123(7):3154–65.
88. Takeo S, Arai H, Kusano N, Harada T, Furuya T, Kawauchi S, et al. Examination of oncogene amplification by genomic DNA microarray in hepatocellular carcinomas: comparison with comparative genomic hybridization analysis. Cancer Genet Cytogenet. 2001;130(2):127–32.

89. Roessler S, Long EL, Budhu A, Chen Y, Zhao X, Ji J, et al. Integrative genomic identification of genes on 8p associated with hepatocellular carcinoma progression and patient survival. Gastroenterology. 2012;142(4):957–966.e12.
90. Liew CT, Li HM, Lo KW, Leow CK, Chan JYH, Hin LY, et al. High frequency of p16(INK4A) gene alterations in hepatocellular carcinoma. Oncogene. 1999;18(3):789–95.
91. Tannapfel A, Busse C, Weinans L, Benicke M, Katalinic A, Geissler F, et al. INK4a-ARF alterations and p53 mutations in hepatocellular carcinomas. Oncogene. 2001;20(48):7104–9.
92. Murakami Y, Hayashi K, Hirohashi S, Sekiya T. Aberrations of the tumor suppressor p53 and retinoblastoma genes in human hepatocellular carcinomas. Cancer Res. 1991;51(20):5520–5.
93. Bollard J, Miguela V, Ruiz de Galarreta M, Venkatesh A, Bian CB, Roberto MP, et al. Palbociclib (PD-0332991), a selective CDK4/6 inhibitor, restricts tumour growth in preclinical models of hepatocellular carcinoma. Gut. 2017;66(7):1286–96.
94. Ma L, Chua M-S, Andrisani O, So S. Epigenetics in hepatocellular carcinoma: an update and future therapy perspectives. World J Gastroenterol. 2014;20(2):333–45.
95. Wahid B, Ali A, Rafique S, Idrees M. New insights into the epigenetics of hepatocellular carcinoma. Biomed Res Int. 2017;2017:1609575.
96. Smith ZD, Meissner A. DNA methylation: roles in mammalian development. Nat Rev Genet. 2013;14(3):204–20.
97. Feinberg AP, Koldobskiy MA, Göndör A. Epigenetic modulators, modifiers and mediators in cancer aetiology and progression. Nat Rev Genet. 2016;17(5):284–99.
98. Nishida N, Kudo M, Nishimura T, Arizumi T, Takita M, Kitai S, et al. Unique association between global DNA hypomethylation and chromosomal alterations in human hepatocellular carcinoma. PLoS One. 2013;8(9):e72312.
99. Shen J, Wang S, Zhang Y-J, Kappil M, Wu H-C, Kibriyya MG, et al. Genome-wide DNA methylation profiles in hepatocellular carcinoma. Hepatology. 2012;55(6):1799–808.
100. Song M-A, Tiirikainen M, Kwee S, Okimoto G, Yu H, Wong LL. Elucidating the landscape of aberrant DNA methylation in hepatocellular carcinoma. PLoS One. 2013;8(2):e55761.
101. Hernandez-Vargas H, Lambert M-P, Le Calvez-Kelm F, Gouysse G, McKay-Chopin S, Tavtigian SV, et al. Hepatocellular Carcinoma Displays Distinct DNA Methylation Signatures with Potential as Clinical Predictors. PLoS One. 2010;5(3):e9749.
102. Lee S, Lee HJ, Kim J-H, Lee H-S, Jang JJ, Kang GH. Aberrant CpG island hypermethylation along multistep hepatocarcinogenesis. Am J Pathol. 2003;163(4):1371–8.
103. Nishida N, Kudo M, Nagasaka T, Ikai I, Goel A. Characteristic patterns of altered DNA methylation predict emergence of human hepatocellular carcinoma. Hepatology. 2012;56(3):994–1003.
104. Villanueva A, Portela A, Sayols S, Battiston C, Hoshida Y, Méndez-González J, et al. DNA methylation-based prognosis and epidrivers in hepatocellular carcinoma. Hepatology. 2015;61(6):1945–56.
105. Nishida N, Nishimura T, Nagasaka T, Ikai I, Goel A, Ajay G, et al. Extensive methylation is associated with beta-catenin mutations in hepatocellular carcinoma: evidence for two distinct pathways of human hepatocarcinogenesis. Cancer Res. 2007;67(10):4586–94.
106. Revill K, Wang T, Lachenmayer A, Kojima K, Harrington A, Li J, et al. Genome-wide methylation analysis and epigenetic unmasking identify tumor suppressor genes in hepatocellular carcinoma. Gastroenterology. 2013;145(6):1424–35.e1–25.
107. Wong IH, Lo YM, Zhang J, Liew CT, Ng MH, Wong N, et al. Detection of aberrant p16 methylation in the plasma and serum of liver cancer patients. Cancer Res. 1999;59(1):71–3.

# Chapter 5
# The Role of Histology in Hepatocellular and Cholangiocarcinoma

**Alberto Quaglia**

**Key Learning Points**

1. Liver biopsy has a critical role in the histological diagnosis of hepatocellular adenoma and hepatocellular carcinoma arising in patients with early stage chronic liver disease or normal/near-normal liver.
2. A biopsy sample of tumour should always be accompanied by a separate sample of background liver, taken well away from the lesion, and ideally submitted in a separate container.
3. Histological examination of surgically resected specimens is essential to confirm diagnosis and for prognosis in both hepatocellular and cholangiocellular tumours.
4. Intraoperative histological examination is critical to guide surgical intervention and attempt completeness of resection particularly for hilar cholangiocarcinoma.
5. Liver biopsy is the gold standard for the diagnosis of intrahepatic cholangiocarcinoma. Biliary brushing is increasingly used in the diagnosis of hilar and distal cholangiocarcinoma.

**Areas of Controversy and Uncertainty**

1. Liver biopsy may regain a role in the diagnosis and management of early hepatocellular carcinoma arising in patients with advanced stage chronic liver disease, by bringing together histological and molecular techniques.

A. Quaglia (✉)
The Institute of Liver Studies, King's College Hospital, London, UK
e-mail: alberto.quaglia@nhs.net



T. Cross, D. H. Palmer (eds.), *Liver Cancers*,
https://doi.org/10.1007/978-3-319-92216-4_5

2. The differential diagnosis between hepatocellular adenoma and well-differentiated hepatocellular carcinoma can be difficult, particularly when based on liver biopsy specimens. The use of the term "hepatocellular neoplasm of uncertain malignant potential" has been advocated in such instances.
3. The differential diagnosis between intrahepatic cholangiocarcinoma and metastatic adenocarcinoma should not rely exclusively on immunohistochemistry but needs to be based on clinico-pathological correlation.

Histopathologists retain a crucial role in the diagnosis of tumours, as eloquently expressed by Dr. Fletcher [1]: "... Molecular genetic techniques are meaningful if put into context and matched by morphology… proper professional interactions between histopathologists and molecular biologists are critical… claims that new modalities can replace histological interpretation need to be seen with suspicion...." Histology remains the gold standard for the classification and diagnosis of primary liver cancer. This chapter discusses the role of histology in hepatocellular carcinoma (HCC) and cholangiocarcinoma (ChC), with reference to biopsy and surgically resected specimens for each tumour type. The role of histology in the context of tumours with mixed hepatocellular and cholangiocellular differentiation is reviewed in Chap. 13. Paediatric liver tumours and in particular hepatoblastoma are outside the scope of this chapter.

## Hepatocellular Carcinoma

Advanced stage chronic liver disease [2] is the main risk factor for HCC, but HCC can occur in patients with chronic liver disease at an early stage and in patients with normal or near-normal livers. Liver biopsy for the diagnosis of early HCC in patients with advanced stage chronic liver disease is carried out rarely. This is the result essentially of five factors which came together in the early 2000s: (1) the generalised acceptance that cross-sectional imaging criteria based on arterial hypervascularity and venous or delayed phase washout were sufficient for the diagnosis of early HCC; (2) the limitations of histological interpretation based purely on morphological criteria in differentiating between large regenerative nodules and low-grade dysplastic nodules and between high-grade dysplastic nodules and well-differentiated HCC; (3) lack of high-throughput molecular data; (4) the perception that the morbidity, mortality and seeding risk related to the biopsy procedure outweighed the low diagnostic histological yield; and (5) the widespread application of local ablative therapies as a bridge to liver transplantation.

Times have changed, and although cross-sectional imaging retains its diagnostic role, its accuracy is now questioned and needs to be verified [3]; recommendation for bridging therapy is conditional due to the available limited evidence of its benefits [4]; histopathologists have additional immunohistochemical and molecular tools to place small hepatocellular lesions within a spectrum of malignant transformation and identify tumour subtypes including mixed variants; HCC molecular signatures are now available [5]; the value of molecular and histological data may offset the risk related to the biopsy procedure [3, 6]. A return to liver biopsy is therefore advocated based on the benefits of integrating histological and molecular data, as part of personalised medicine and clinical trial allocation [6].

Liver biopsy has a critical role in the diagnosis of HCC occurring in patients with chronic liver disease at an early stage or with normal or near-normal liver. HCC in this context has a bimodal distribution in terms of age of presentation, peaking at the second and seventh decades [7]. These tumours remain asymptomatic for a long time and tend to manifest when they reach a large size, because patients do not present earlier with symptoms of advanced stage chronic liver disease and do not often have high levels of serum alpha-fetoprotein. Common aetiological factors include hepatitis B virus infection, non-alcoholic steatohepatitis, genetic haemochromatosis and other metabolic disorders including glycogen storage disease, alpha-1-antitrypsin deficiency and porphyria, sex hormones and in particular anabolic steroids, vascular disorders such as Budd-Chiari and portosystemic shunts and toxins (e.g. aflatoxin B1). Fibrolamellar carcinoma is a subtype of HCC typically observed in young patients with no evidence of underlying liver disease. It has been shown to be associated with the DNAJB1-PRKACA fusion transcript.

The role of liver biopsy in these patients is diagnostic and usually to (1) establish whether the tumour is primary or secondary; (2) differentiate between HCC and ChC, except for tumours with a mixed hepatocellular and cholangiocellular phenotype; (3) confirm the clinical suspicion of fibrolamellar carcinoma; and (4) differentiate between hepatocellular adenoma and HCC. The histological differential diagnosis between HCC and hepatocellular adenoma may be difficult particularly with biopsy specimens, which may not be representative of the whole lesion. The use of the term "well-differentiated hepatocellular neoplasm of uncertain malignant potential" has been advocated, in selected circumstances [8, 9].

Knowledge of the state of the background liver and presence of an underlying disorder is critical to the histological interpretation of liver tumours. As a general rule, a biopsy sample of non-lesional liver should always be taken in adjunct to the lesional biopsy sample and should be submitted to the laboratory ideally in a separate container.

Histological examination of resection specimens remains a critical step in the management of patients with HCC. In the context of liver transplantation, a careful macroscopic analysis of the explanted liver is critical to identify histological features of prognostic value. Vascular invasion has been consistently shown to be associated with poor prognosis. Standardisation of the histological criteria for the identification of vascular invasion is necessary to ensure reproducibility. The term "cirrhotomimetic" refers to a rare variant of HCC characterised by minute tumour nodules of similar size of, and intermixed with, the parenchymal nodules of the background diseased liver. Except for those cases in which this pattern occurs in addition to one or more larger dominant tumours, cirrhotomimetic HCC cannot be identified on pre-transplantation imaging and is diagnosed exclusively by histology. A proportion of cirrhotomimetic HCC have a very poor prognosis [10]. Examination of the explanted liver reveals the effects of bridging local ablation therapy. Cholangiocellular differentiation is frequently identified in tumours treated with transarterial chemo-embolisation and may be associated with poor prognosis [11]. A careful examination of the explanted liver is necessary to confirm the tumour staging at the time of listing or detect interval tumour progression. It may also identify small lesions, undetected by pre-transplantation imaging, or large lesions resembling focal nodular hyperplasia or hepatocellular adenoma and mimicking HCC [12, 13]. More studies correlating the histological findings in explanted liver with antecedent imaging are needed to verify the accuracy of imaging techniques [3]. Correlation of histology with molecular data remains a powerful tool in the understanding of the pathogenesis and behaviour of HCC.

Histological examination of specimens removed at surgical resection of HCC is necessary for diagnostic and prognostic purposes. Extensive sampling may be necessary to confirm a diagnosis of HCC, particularly in the instance of well-differentiated hepatocellular lesions in which imaging and liver biopsy are not conclusive. Identification of vascular invasion, evaluation of the resection margin for completeness of rejection and the identification of additional small foci in the vicinity of a dominant lesion implying either intrahepatic tumour spread or multifocal disease may anticipate tumour recurrence in the liver remnant and/or extrahepatic spread. A recent study [14] on surgically resected HCC has shown the benefit of correlating histology with molecular profiling and clinical data. In that study, surgically resected HCC could be divided into two major groups based on their histological phenotype and molecular profile. One consisted of large well-differentiated cholestatic *CTNNB1*-mutated tumours arranged in a microtrabecular and pseudoglandular pattern. The other one consisted of *TP53*-mutated poorly differentiated tumours in a compact growth pattern and with frequent vascular invasion. In the same study, the scirrhous and steatohepatitic variants correlated with specific mutations and molecular pathways, and a novel subtype designated "macrotrabecular-massive" was characterised by vascular invasion, high alpha-fetoprotein levels, *TP53* mutation, *FGF19* amplification and poor survival.

## Cholangiocarcinoma

ChCs are adenocarcinomas composed of cells with a biliary phenotype and are generally classified according to their presumed site of origin in intrahepatic, hilar and distal ChC. The right and left hepatic duct confluence marks the point of separation between intrahepatic and hilar ChC. The biliary epithelial cells lining the bile ducts are considered to be the origin of hilar and distal ChC. Biliary intraepithelial neoplasia and intraductal papillary (biliary) neoplasms are the two well-characterised precursor lesions of ChC. Nakanuma et al. [15] have proposed that the similarities between biliary and pancreatic neoplasms, and in particular between ductal-type adenocarcinoma, mucinous cystic and intraductal papillary neoplasms, could be due to the common embryological origin shared by the extrahepatic biliary tree and the pancreas. Hilar ChC displays often an intestinal phenotype [16]. The pathogenesis of intrahepatic ChC is more complex. Cholangiocytes, progenitor/stem cells possibly residing in the canals of Hering and hepatocytes are now regarded as the possible cells of origin [17]. The term "cholangiolocellular carcinoma" refers to a type of intrahepatic ChC composed of tubulo-glandular structures with an appearance and immunohistochemical phenotype resembling cholangioles.

Intrahepatic ChC forms usually parenchymal nodular masses (mass-forming) in patients with normal or near-normal liver, and more rarely in the context of advanced stage chronic liver disease, not necessarily related to a chronic cholangiopathy. Histological identification of incidental small intrahepatic ChC in the livers removed at transplantation from patients with advanced stage chronic liver disease has shown that very early tumours of 2 cm or less on diameter are associated with a good prognosis and should not be a contraindication to liver transplantation [18]. Intrahepatic ChC can grow to a relatively large size before becoming symptomatic. In contrast, hilar and distal ChC become symptomatic earlier, due to biliary obstruction and jaundice. Intrahepatic ChC can be diagnosed exclusively by histology, on biopsy or surgical resection specimens. Intrahepatic ChC needs to be differentiated from HCC, particularly in patients with a normal or near normal liver, with metastatic adenocarcinoma and with benign biliary proliferations. The cells composing intrahepatic ChC can show an appearance very similar to that of hepatocytes and can mimic HCC quite closely. Immunohistochemical markers in support of hepatocellular differentiation include Hep Par 1, arginase 1, the identification of canaliculi expressing specific antigens such as the bile salt export pump (BSEP) and the identification of albumin by in situ hybridisation. Markers in support of cholangiocellular differentiation include CA19–9 and cytokeratin 19. None of these markers, however, is entirely specific. This is particularly true when trying to differentiate between ChC and metastatic adenocarcinoma, because there are no markers, to date, sufficiently specific of cholangiocellular differentiation. The role of liver biopsy in these instances is to confirm the presence of adenocarcinoma. Depending on the clinical context, immunohistochemistry may be used to investigate a possible site of origin but can be potentially misleading and needs to be interpreted in conjunction with a full clinical history, imaging and endoscopic findings when applicable. Subcapsular lesions identified during oncological abdominal surgery or staging laparoscopy are often sampled and submitted for intra-operatory diagnosis. Differentiation between metastatic adenocarcinoma and a primary benign biliary proliferation such as a microhamartoma or a biliary adenoma is straightforward in some cases. In patients with obstructive jaundice and ascending cholangitis, reactive biliary atypia and florid inflammation make it difficult to differentiate from ChC, and it may be preferable to defer the diagnosis to paraffin-embedded sections. Histological criteria in favour of intrahepatic ChC over benign biliary lesions such as bile duct adenoma include the presence of infiltrative features, an angulated profile of the tubule-glandular structures, the presence of mitoses, a high percentage of lesional nuclei staining for Ki67 and a nuclear atypia. Tubulin-beta 3 has been proposed as an immunohistochemical marker of biliary malignancy but needs further validation [19].

The diagnosis and grading of cystic mucinous neoplasms are purely histological. Liver biopsy is not advocated in this context, and the diagnosis is usually carried out on surgically resected specimens. Surgeons often request intraoperative histological diagnosis on frozen sections obtained from samples of cyst wall removed during cyst fenestration. False negatives are possible with this approach, because the histological changes necessary for the diagnosis of mucinous cystic neoplasm (e.g., the lining epithelium and the ovarian-like stroma) can be patchy, particularly in lesions with degenerative changes. Extensive sampling of the whole cystic lesion and examination of paraffin-embedded sections are necessary for a reliable diagnosis, proper grading of epithelial dysplasia and identification of foci of invasive ChC.

Liver biopsy has lesser of a role for the diagnosis of hilar and distal ChC. These lesions may be difficult to target, as they tend to be of relatively small size, may be difficult to delineate and targeted on imaging and have often a hard stromal component, which cannot be pierced easily by the biopsy needle. In contrast, biliary tract brushing carried out during endoscopic retrograde cholangiopancreatography (ERCP) is gaining role in the diagnosis of malignant biliary strictures. The procedure has high specificity but relatively low sensitivity. Its performance can be improved by the use of fluorescent in situ hybridisation (FISH) and digital image analysis (DIA) to identify chromosomal abnormalities and aneuploidy [20].

Histological examination of surgically resected specimen remains critical to confirm the diagnosis of intrahepatic, hilar and distal ChC and for prognosis. Involvements of surgical margins, lymphovascular and perineural invasion, satellite nodules, lymph node metastasis and poor differentiation are associated with poor prognosis. Intraoperative histological examination is particularly important during resection of hilar ChC in the attempt to achieve a complete resection.

## References


1. Fletcher CDM. Diagnostic histopathology of tumors. 4th ed. Edinburgh: Churchill Livingstone; 2013.
2. Hytiroglou P, Snover DC, Alves V, Balabaud C, Bhathal PS, Bioulac-Sage P, et al. Beyond "cirrhosis": a proposal from the International Liver Pathology Study Group. Am J Clin Pathol. 2012;137(1):5–9.
3. Mullhaupt B, Durand F, Roskams T, Dutkowski P, Heim M. Is tumor biopsy necessary? Liver Transpl. 2011;17(Suppl 2):S14–25.
4. Heimbach JK, Kulik LM, Finn R, Sirlin CB, Abecassis M, Roberts LR, et al. AASLD guidelines for the treatment of hepatocellular carcinoma. Hepatology. 2017;67(1):358–80.
5. Sia D, Villanueva A, Friedman SL, Llovet JM. Liver cancer cell of origin, molecular class, and effects on patient prognosis. Gastroenterology. 2017;152(4):745–61.
6. Torbenson M, Schirmacher P. Liver cancer biopsy–back to the future?! Hepatology. 2015;61(2):431–3.
7. Trevisani F, Frigerio M, Santi V, Grignaschi A, Bernardi M. Hepatocellular carcinoma in non-cirrhotic liver: a reappraisal. Dig Liver Dis. 2010;42(5):341–7.

8. Balabaud C, Bioulac-Sage P, Ferrell L, Kakar S, Paradis V, Quaglia A, et al. Well-differentiated hepatocellular neoplasm of uncertain malignant potential. Hum Pathol. 2015;46(4):634–5.
9. Bedossa P, Burt AD, Brunt EM, Callea F, Clouston AD, Dienes HP, et al. Well-differentiated hepatocellular neoplasm of uncertain malignant potential: proposal for a new diagnostic category. Hum Pathol. 2014;45(3):658–60.
10. Clayton EF, Malik S, Bonnel A, Mu Y, Olthoff K, Shaked A, et al. Liver transplantation and cirrhotomimetic hepatocellular carcinoma: classification and outcomes. Liver Transpl. 2014;20(7):765–74.
11. Zen C, Zen Y, Mitry RR, Corbeil D, Karbanova J, O'Grady J, et al. Mixed phenotype hepatocellular carcinoma after transarterial chemoembolization and liver transplantation. Liver Transpl. 2011;17(8):943–54.
12. Calderaro J, Nault JC, Balabaud C, Couchy G, Saint-Paul MC, Azoulay D, et al. Inflammatory hepatocellular adenomas developed in the setting of chronic liver disease and cirrhosis. Mod Pathol. 2016;29(1):43–50.
13. Quaglia A, Tibballs J, Grasso A, Prasad N, Nozza P, Davies SE, et al. Focal nodular hyperplasia-like areas in cirrhosis. Histopathology. 2003;42(1):14–21.
14. Calderaro J, Couchy G, Imbeaud S, Amaddeo G, Letouze E, Blanc JF, et al. Histological subtypes of hepatocellular carcinoma are related to gene mutations and molecular tumour classification. J Hepatol. 2017;67(4):727–38.
15. Nakanuma Y, Sudo Y. Biliary tumors with pancreatic counterparts. Semin Diagn Pathol. 2017;34(2):167–75.
16. Zen Y, Quaglia A, Heaton N, Rela M, Portmann B. Two distinct pathways of carcinogenesis in primary sclerosing cholangitis. Histopathology. 2011;59(6):1100–10.
17. Komuta M, Govaere O, Vandecaveye V, Akiba J, Van Steenbergen W, Verslype C, et al. Histological diversity in cholangiocellular carcinoma reflects the different cholangiocyte phenotypes. Hepatology. 2012;55(6):1876–88.
18. Sapisochin G, Facciuto M, Rubbia-Brandt L, Marti J, Mehta N, Yao FY, et al. Liver transplantation for "very early" intrahepatic cholangiocarcinoma: International retrospective study supporting a prospective assessment. Hepatology. 2016;64(4):1178–88.
19. Zen Y, Britton D, Mitra V, Pike I, Sarker D, Itoh T, et al. Tubulin beta-III: a novel immunohistochemical marker for intrahepatic peripheral cholangiocarcinoma. Histopathology. 2014;65(6):784–92.
20. Moreno Luna LE, Kipp B, Halling KC, Sebo TJ, Kremers WK, Roberts LR, et al. Advanced cytologic techniques for the detection of malignant pancreatobiliary strictures. Gastroenterology. 2006;131(4):1064–72.

# Chapter 6
# Diagnosis and Staging of Hepatocellular Carcinoma (HCC)

**Vinay Kumar Balachandrakumar, Nadya Fatima Jabbar, David White, and Nicholas Stern**

**Key Learning Points**

1. Patient outcomes in HCC is determined by stage of disease, tumour factors, patient factors and interventions available.
2. The patient's performance status should be calculated using the Eastern Cooperative Oncology Group (ECOG) system.
3. The possible poor impact of outcomes due to risk of liver failure needs to be highlighted as it may be greater than the risk of dying from cancer.
4. Treatment allocation should be made after initial assessment of the patient and multidisciplinary team (MDT) meeting decisions must be based on this assessment.

**Areas of Controversy and Uncertainty**

1. Limitations of staging system based on tumour location.
2. Incorporation of novel biomarkers within staging systems to better understand tumour biology, mechanisms of disease and treatment targets.
3. Role of routine use of liver biopsy in disease staging.

V. K. Balachandrakumar (✉)
University of Liverpool, Liverpool, UK

N. F. Jabbar · D. White · N. Stern
Aintree University Hospital, Liverpool, UK



T. Cross, D. H. Palmer (eds.), *Liver Cancers*,
https://doi.org/10.1007/978-3-319-92216-4_6

## Background

Liver cancer is the fifth most common cancer worldwide, second most common cause of cancer related deaths and accounts for 7% of all cancers. The incidence of HCC is growing worldwide and increases progressively with advancing age in all populations, with a peak age of 70 years. HCC has a strong male predominance with a male to female ratio of 2–2.5:1. The pattern of HCC has a strong geographical distribution, highest in East Asia and sub-Saharan Africa where around 85% of cases occur, and is very much linked to the prevalence of viral hepatitis (B and C). Obesity, diabetes and fatty liver disease have also been recognised to cause HCC throughout the world [1].

## Diagnosis

Improved imaging techniques have enabled earlier HCC diagnosis improving the chance to offer potentially curative treatment. This trend is expected to grow with the wider implementation of surveillance policies in developed countries. However, detection of nodules of <2 cm poses a challenge as they are difficult to characterise by radiological or pathological examination.

Defining nodules as pre-neoplastic lesions or early HCC has important implications. Dysplastic lesions should be followed up by regular imaging studies as one-third of them develop a malignant phenotype. Early tumours should be treated with curative intent: procedures such as resection, transplantation and percutaneous ablation.

HCC can be diagnosed radiologically in the presence of a cirrhotic liver with criteria as detailed below. In those cases which are equivocal or the background liver is non-cirrhotic, a histological diagnosis is needed.

## Radiological Criteria

Imaging holds a central role in the diagnosis of HCC, and to date, it is the only solid tumour for which non-invasive diagnosis is accepted [2]. Several imaging modalities including ultrasonography (US), computed tomography (CT) and magnetic resonance imaging (MRI) can be used in evaluating patients with chronic liver disease and suspected HCC. Dual phase contrast-enhanced CT or dynamic phase MRI are the current recommended modalities of choice for imaging diagnosis of HCC as per EASL and AASLD guidelines. These have the added benefit of providing information about the background liver, the hepatic vasculature as well as extrahepatic disease. MRI affords better characterisation of HCCs as the signal characteristics on several sequences aid the diagnosis, especially with equivocal cases. Additionally, MRI spares the patient repeated exposures to ionising radiation and iodinated contrast material. CT and MRI do have a significantly greater cost attached to them, whereas US is a cheap and relatively easily accessible modality for diagnosis.

The role of contrast-enhanced ultrasound (CEUS) in the diagnosis of HCC however is controversial and is not recommended in Western guidelines due to low specificity even though it has a high sensitivity but can be utilised when CT and MRI are inconclusive or contraindicated. Other limiting factors include interoperator variability, inability to image the entire liver during one contrast injection and limited views in obese patients [3–7].

## Diagnostic Hallmark of HCC

In order to understand the imaging characteristics of HCC and to be able to differentiate it from other nodules in the setting of the cirrhotic liver, it is important to understand the changes in the vascular supply and neovascularisation that occur through this dedifferentiation spectrum.

Regenerating nodules are supplied by the portal vein, and dysplastic nodules have primarily a portal venous supply but have an increasing amount of supply from the hepatic artery. HCCs are supplied by unpaired hepatic arteries, and thus they enhance in the arterial phase when the bulk of the contrast lies within the hepatic arteries. During the portal venous phase, as the contrast circulates through the portal venous system, the background liver parenchyma enhances, and as the HCC has no supply from the portal venous system, there is a "washout" of contrast. This arterial phase enhancement and washout during the portal venous phase are the hallmark of HCC.

Due to the difficulty in characterising small liver lesions (<1 cm), the radiological criteria for diagnosis apply to those nodules of at least 1 cm in diameter. Small HCCs, early HCCs and poorly differentiated HCCs may not show these typical features, and in such cases, the role of delayed phase imaging on MR with hepatobiliary contrast agents is central in aiding diagnosis. The differentiation between hepatobiliary and non-hepatobiliary agents is beyond the scope of this chapter but suffice to say that HCCs do not take up hepatobiliary contrast as they do not have functioning hepatocytes and are thus of low signal intensity on the delayed phase sequences. The caveat to this rule is that well-differentiated HCCs may take up the hepatobiliary contrast; in the latter cases, other ancillary features help in making the diagnosis (Figs. 6.1, 6.2, 6.3, 6.4 and Table 6.1).

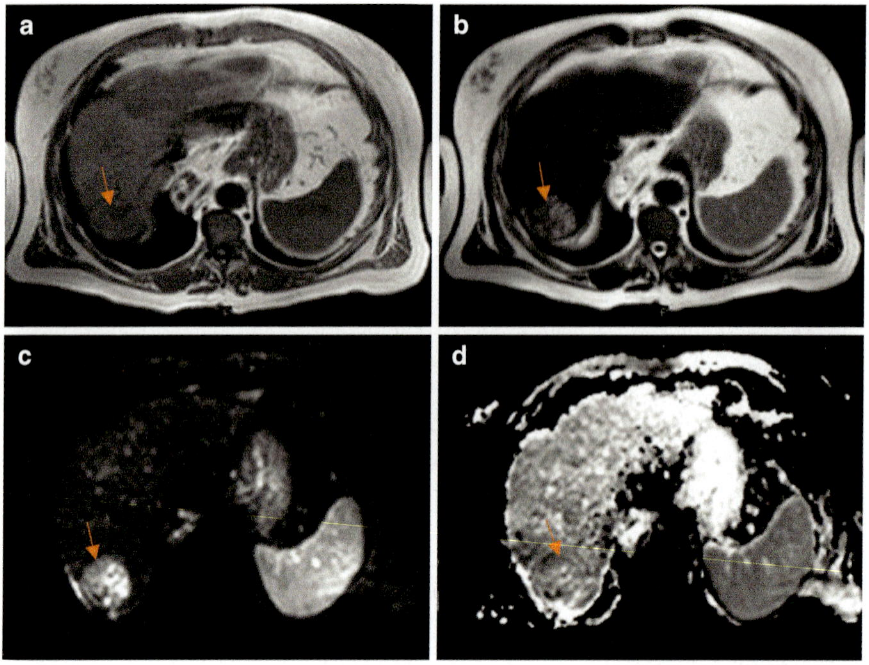


**Fig. 6.1** (**a**) Axial T1-weighted sequence showing an iso-hypointense well-defined lesion with a capsule and a central low signal area. (**b**) Axial T2-weighted sequence shows the internal heterogeneity of the lesion which has areas of low to intermediate signal intensity. (**c** and **d**) Diffusion-weighted and corresponding ADC map showing a high signal on the diffusion-weighted sequence with a corresponding low signal on the ADC map indicative of restricted diffusion within the lesion *and characteristics in keeping with a HCC*

## *Morphological and Other Features*

Presence of a capsule
Heterogeneity
Focus of calcification
Intralesional fat
Portal vein thrombus
Direct vascular invasion
Multifocality

## *CEUS*

Hypo-echoeic pre-contrast
Arterial enhancement and washout

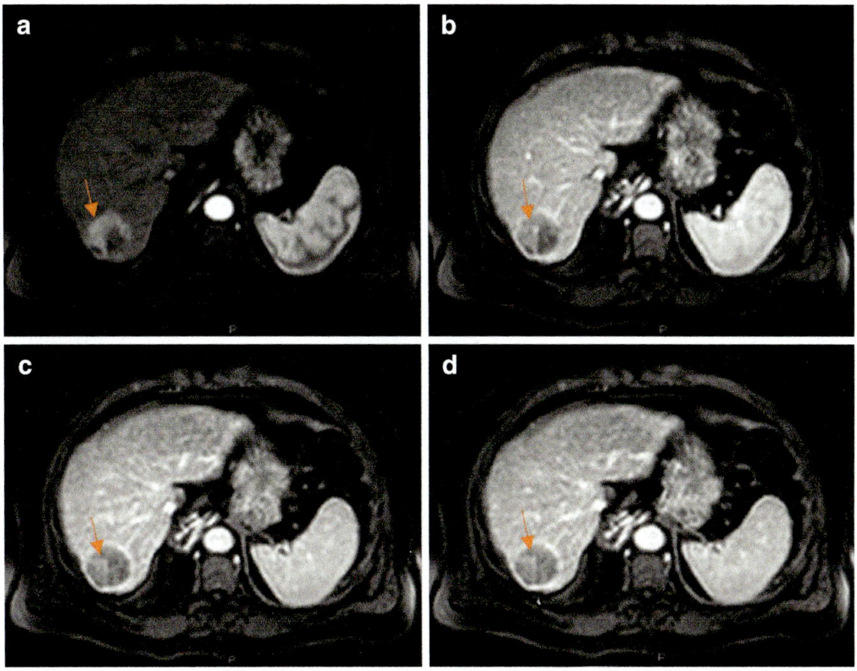


**Fig. 6.2** (**a**–**d**) Dynamic sequences through the liver showing arterial enhancement of the lesion with a gradual washout on the portal venous and delayed images *in keeping with features of HCC*. Note the capsular rim

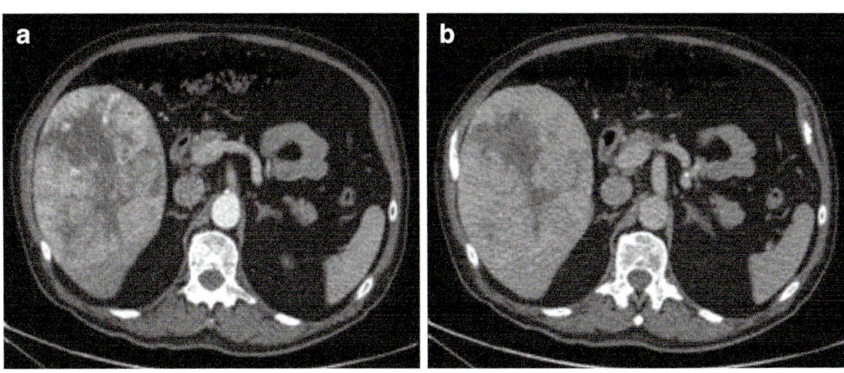


**Fig. 6.3** (**a**) Arterial phase CT showing a heterogeneous lesion with a necrotic centre. The periphery of the lesion enhances on the arterial phase. (**b**) Portal venous phase CT at the same level shows a washout of contrast *in keeping with features of HCC*

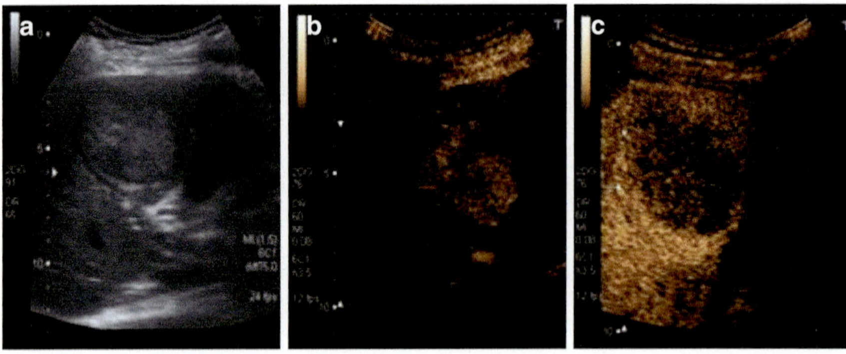

**Fig. 6.4** (**a**) Ultrasound image showing a 5 cm lesion within the right lobe of the liver. Contrast-enhanced ultrasound after administration of IV contrast showing (**b**) early and heterogeneous enhancement of the lesion at 13 s and (**c**) a rapid washout. The absence of uniform or continuous peripheral enhancement is highly suspicious of a malignant lesion. The early arterial enhancement and rapid wash out is characteristic of a HCC

## *CT*

Low attenuation on unenhanced CT

Arterial enhancement and portal venous phase washout

Foci of calcification

Capsule

Internal mosaic pattern

Vascular invasion

## *MR*

T1-Hypointense

Maybe hyperintense if they contain fat, copper, glycogen or iron

T2-hyperintense but less than benign lesions such as cysts and haemangiomas

May be isointense

In- and out-of-phase sequences: loss of signal depicting intralesional fat

Dynamic sequences: hyperintense on the arterial phase and hypointense during the portal venous phase

Hypointense during the hepatobiliary phase

Diffusion-weighted sequences: increased signal intensity as they restrict diffusion

**Table 6.1** Differential diagnosis and imaging characteristics [8–10]

| Lesions | T1 weighted | T2 weighted | Arterial phase sequences CT and MR | Portal venous sequences CT and MR | Delayed phase MR | 20 min post Gd-EOB-DTPA MR |
|---|---|---|---|---|---|---|
| Haemangioma | Iso- or hypointense | Hyperintense | Hyperintense | Hyperintense | Hyperintense | Hypointense |
| FNH | Hypointense | Iso- or hyperintense | Hyperintense | Isointense | Isointense | Hyperintense |
| Adenoma | Isointense | Iso- or hyperintense | Hyperintense | Isointense | Isointense | Hypointense |
| Hyper vascular metastasis | Hypointense | Hyperintense or variable | Hyperintense | Iso- or hypointense | Hypointense | Hypointense |
| Regenerating nodules | Iso- or hyperintense | Isointense | Isointense | Isointense | Isointense | Isointense |
| Dysplastic nodules | Isointense | Iso- or hyperintense | Hyperintense | Isointense | Isointense | Isointense |
| Cholangiocarcinoma | Hypointense | Iso- or hyperintense | Iso- or hyperintense | Iso- or hyperintense | Hyperintense | Hypointense |
| HCC | Variable | Hyperintense or variable | Hyperintense | Hypointense | Hypointense | Hypointense |

## Histological Diagnosis

A histopathological diagnosis of HCC is based on the World Health Organization (WHO) classification and International Consensus Group for Hepatocellular Neoplasia. Sensitivity of liver biopsy depends on the location, size of tumour and expertise. It can be difficult to determine the diagnosis of HCC on morphological criteria alone between HCC and high-grade dysplasia. Pathologists cannot always determine the pathological appearance of HCC or whether stromal invasion is present. A positive biopsy is useful to make a diagnosis of HCC, but a negative biopsy may not exclude the diagnosis. The risk of tumour seeding after liver biopsy is 2.7% with a median time interval between biopsy and seeding of 17 months [11]. This can clearly pose problems for patients potentially undergoing treatment with curative intent.

Immunohistochemistry can aid the histopathological diagnosis. Combinations of three different immunomarkers (glypican 3, HSP70 and glutamate synthetase) have demonstrated a sensitivity and specificity of 72% and 100%, respectively [1, 12]. Both the WHO and International Consensus Group of Hepatocellular Neoplasia have adopted this three-marker panel.

## Use of Alpha-Fetoprotein (AFP)

Alpha-fetoprotein has been used for the diagnosis of HCC and as part of surveillance algorithms. AFP is now felt to be insufficiently sensitive or specific to use as a surveillance assay. AFP can be elevated in intrahepatic cholangiocarcinoma (ICC) and in some metastases from colon cancer. Therefore, a mass in the liver with an elevated AFP does not indicate HCC. ICC is also more common in cirrhotics than in non-cirrhotics. Incidence of ICC is much lower than HCC, and given both are common in cirrhosis, they should be distinguished due to differences in treatment and outcomes [13].

## Surveillance Strategy for Indeterminate or Dysplastic Nodules

Most nodules smaller than 1 cm that can be detected in a cirrhotic liver are not HCCs. Therefore, a closer follow-up is recommended in these cases. An accepted rule is to consider any nodule >1 cm as an abnormal screening result warranting further investigation. These new nodules should prompt recall strategy for diagnosis with non-invasive or invasive (biopsy) criteria, as described above. If a diagnosis cannot be reached with non-invasive criteria due to atypical radiological appearance, then biopsy is recommended. If biopsy provides inconclusive results, then a closer follow-up every 3–4 months is recommended [1]. A second

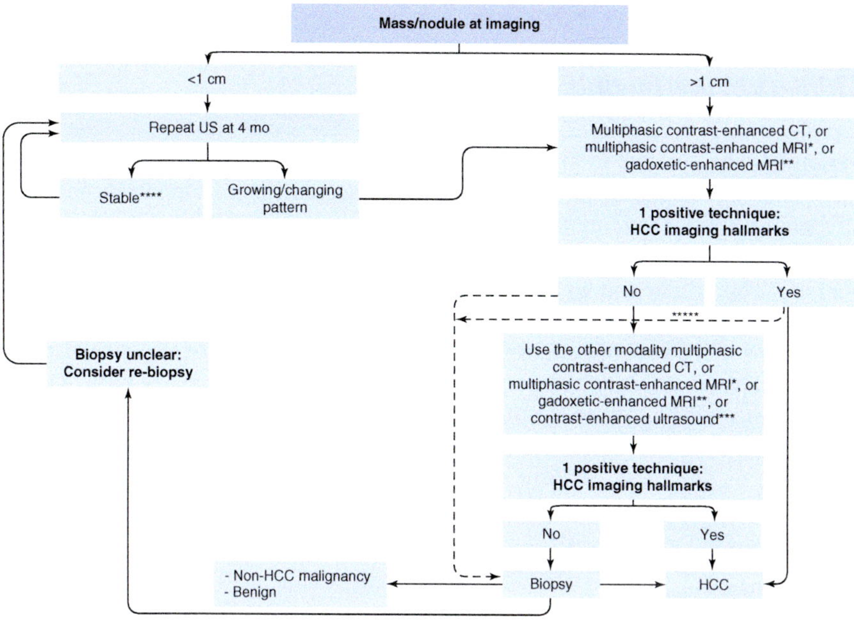


**Fig. 6.5** *Diagnostic algorithm and recall policy in cirrhotic liver.* *Using extracellular MR contrast agents or gadobenate dimeglumine. **Using the following diagnostic criteria: arterial phase hyperenhancement (APHE) and washout on the portal venous phase. ***Using the following diagnostic criteria: arterial phase hyperenhancement (APHE) and mild washout after 60 s. ****Lesion <1 cm stable for 12 months (three controls after 4 months) can be shifted back to regular six-month surveillance.****Optional for centre-based programmes

biopsy may be considered in case of growth or change in the enhancement pattern (Fig. 6.5).

## Staging

### *Staging of Liver Function, Performance Status and Tumour*

There are differing opinions on how best to stage and characterise HCC due to its characteristic clinical and biological variations. Despite recommendations produced by hepatologists, oncologists, surgeons and radiologists with multidisciplinary collaboration, there is still no single system used for classifying HCC.

As with any cancer, the aim of tumour staging in HCC is to estimate a patient's prognosis, which allows for appropriate therapy to be selected. The variations of HCC are not only because of various aetiological factors for cancer but also of the extent of impaired liver function. The contributions of cancer and hepatic dysfunction to overall prognosis were recognised with the first modern-era liver cancer staging system proposed at the Hepatocellular Carcinoma International Symposium in Kampala, Uganda, in 1971.

## Assessment of Liver Function

### *Child-Turcotte-Pugh (CTP)*

Initially, Child-Turcotte staging comprised clinical assessments of encephalopathy, ascites and nutritional status with laboratory measurements of serum bilirubin and albumin as a prognostic tool to predict mortality following variceal haemorrhage. This was reformed by Pugh with the replacement of nutritional status by prothrombin time. This simple and widely used system assesses liver function as a preoperative benchmark. However, the drawbacks are many, including laboratory variations, fluctuations in the key measurements and the subjective nature of the clinical grading of encephalopathy and ascites. It has been incorporated into many current scoring systems including the Barcelona Clinic Liver Cancer (BCLC) and Cancer of the Liver Italian Program (CLIP).

## Model for End-Stage Liver Disease (MELD)

The MELD score, initially developed to determine prognosis following a transjugular intrahepatic portosystemic shunt (TIPSS), is now widely used in the liver transplant arena to list donor liver allocation [14]. It is a logarithmic score that is comprised of international normalised ratio (INR), serum creatinine, total serum bilirubin and sodium. The advantage of the MELD score is its prediction of short-term mortality and is therefore able to identify the "sickest" patients for graft allocation. However, it fails to correctly classify a portion of patients with advanced cirrhosis. Patients with HCC need to have an adjusted MELD score.

## United Kingdom Model for End-Stage Liver Disease (UKELD)

The UKELD score is a scoring system used to predict the prognosis in patients with chronic liver disease. It is calculated using patients' international normalised ratio (INR), serum creatinine, serum bilirubin and serum sodium. This was developed in 2008 to aid clinicians in selecting patients for liver transplantation [15].

## Overview of Current Staging Systems

### *Barcelona Clinic for Liver Cancer (BCLC) Staging Algorithm*

The BCLC classification first published in 1999 was modified in 2018 and is considered the standard HCC system by the American Association for the Study of Liver Disease (AASLD) [13] and European Association for the Study of the Liver

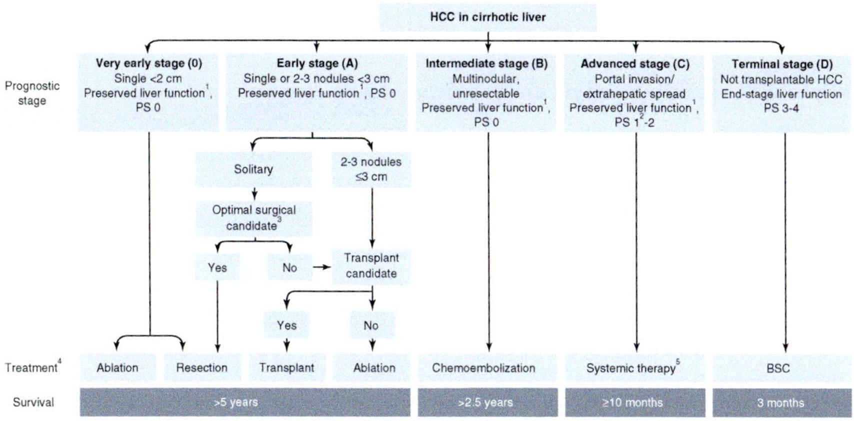


**Fig. 6.6** *Modified BCLC staging system and treatment strategy.* [1]"*Preserved liver function*" refers to Child-Pugh A without any ascites, considered conditions to obtain optimal outcomes. This prerequisite applies to all treatment options apart from transplantation, that is instead addressed primarily to patients with decompensated or end-stage liver function. [2]*PS 1* refers to tumour-induced (as per physician opinion) modification of performance capacity. [3]*Optimal surgical candidacy* is based on a multiparametric evaluation including compensated Child-Pugh class A liver function with MELD score <10, to be matched with grade of portal hypertension, acceptable amount of remaining parenchyma and possibility to adopt a laparoscopic/minimally invasive approach.[4] *The stage migration strategy* is a therapeutic choice by which a treatment theoretically recommended for a different stage is selected as best first-line treatment option. [5]As of 2017 Sorafenib has been shown to be effective in first line, while Regorafenib is effective in second line in case of radiological progression under Sorafenib

(EASL) [1]. BCLC takes into account the size and extent of the primary tumour, underlying liver function and physiological factors including performance status (PST). There is a treatment algorithm for each stage ranging from curative therapies such as resection or transplant for early-stage patients to best supportive care. BCLC had the best prognostic stratification when compared to six other used staging systems [16].

This system lacks discrimination within the intermediate-stage (BCLC-B) patients which forms a large proportion of the HCC population. The burden of liver disease which falls under BCLC stage B can differ greatly, from four small tumours to near-complete replacement of the liver by tumour, provided liver function is preserved and there is no vascular invasion, extrahepatic spread or compromised performance status, which would upstage to BCLC stage C or D. Therefore, in practice, some BCLB-B patients may no longer be eligible for liver-directed therapies and are generally treated following BCLC-C algorithms. The performance status (PST) is incorporated in the BCLC algorithm. The importance of patient fitness is underappreciated by clinicians and not accurately calculated using the ECOG system. A subdivision of BCLC stage B has been suggested which may help to stratify this heterogeneous group. In addition, scoring systems to predict the response to TACE or further TACE have been developed to help tailor treatment algorithms (HAP and ART scores) [17, 18] (Fig. 6.6).

## TNM Staging

The criteria are developed by the American Joint Committee on Cancer (AJCC) and the Union for International Cancer Control (UICC) and have been updated since the first edition in 1977; the seventh edition took effect in 2010. The TNM system evaluates primary tumour features (T), the presence or absence of nodal involvement (N) and distant metastasis (M). Additional information like the histologic grade (G) and fibrosis score (F) may be included based on Ishak classification but do not affect staging. The TNM system is based on histopathology and is appropriate in predicting survival for the minority of patients who have undergone curative surgery.

## Okuda Score

The Okuda system is a prognostic score which includes tumour features and degree of underlying cirrhosis which was introduced in 1985. The staging system is based on four factors which include tumour occupying greater or less than 50% of the liver, the presence or absence of ascites, serum albumin and bilirubin levels. The system's limitation is its rather crude classification of early-stage patients, and subsequent systems have refined Okuda stage I patients. It has a lower predictive capacity compared to the modern systems.

## Cancer of the Liver Italian Program (CLIP) Score

The CLIP score was proposed in 1998 and by combining Child-Pugh stage, tumour morphology, AFP level and the presence or absence of portal vein thrombosis, it includes both liver function and tumour characteristics. The CLIP score was first validated by the original investigators on a prospective cohort of HCC patients. The CLIP score is limited as it does not select the appropriate therapy for each patient.

## Japanese Integrated System (JIS)

In 2003, the Liver Cancer Study Group of Japan (LCSGJ) proposed the JIS score. The JIS score was developed from a cohort of Japanese patients and appeared superior at predicting survival compared to CLIP, particularly in patients with early-stage disease. The JIS system incorporates the Liver Cancer Study Group of Japan's modification of TNM system and the Child-Pugh score. Whilst it has been validated in Japan and in other Asian populations, the JIS has not been prospectively validated in a Western population. It is worth noting that the majority of patients with HCC in Japan have a background of hepatitis C cirrhosis.

## Chinese University Prognostic Index (CUPI)

The CUPI was developed at a single centre in Hong Kong based on a retrospective analysis of ethnic Chinese patients with high proportion of hepatitis B-related cirrhosis. The model included TNM staging, presentation with asymptomatic disease, AFP level, total bilirubin, serum alkaline phosphatase and clinical detection of ascites as significant prognostic factors. The CUPI is well-designed and easy to use. But it has not performed well in comparative studies in Western populations.

## Groupe d'Etude et de Traitement du Carcinome Hépatocellulaire (GRETCH)

The French scoring system, proposed by GRETCH in 1999, uses objective measures and an estimate of performance status to predict survival. This included performance status by Karnofsky score, serum bilirubin, serum alkaline phosphatase, AFP and presence or absence of portal obstruction by ultrasonography. The strength of the French classification is that its variables are available at the time of initial diagnosis and do not require imaging. Given the increasing use of imaging techniques for the diagnosis of HCC, this may impact the prognostic value of the staging system.

## Limitations of Current Staging Systems

The variation of HCC has made it hard to implement a generally accepted staging system. Although the staging systems consider the importance of underlying liver function and tumour characteristics, none of the systems consider the location and relation of the tumour to major vessels. Also, the worsening of the underlying liver disease is also difficult to calculate as patients can be clinically stable for a long time before having decompensated liver failure. The underlying liver disease and aetiology as well as the complex tumour biology of HCC are not accounted for by any of these systems. Many studies describe differences in cancer outcomes based on the aetiology of cirrhosis. This highlights challenges in distinguishing the prognostic impact of the extent and aetiology of underlying liver disease from that of tumour factors such as stage and tumour biology [19] (Table 6.2).

**Table 6.2** Comparison of current staging systems for HCC

| Comparison of HCC staging system | | | | |
|---|---|---|---|---|
| System | Hepatic function | AFP | PS | Tumour staging |
| *Europe-USA* | | | | |
| BCLC | CTP | No | Yes | Tumour size, number of nodules and PVT |
| TNM | No | No | No | Number of nodules, tumour size, presence of PVT and presence of metastasis |
| CLIP | CTP | <400 or ≥400 ng/mL | No | Number of nodules, tumour > or <50% area of liver and PVT |
| GRETCH | Bilirubin, ALP | <35 or ≥35 μg/L | Yes | PVT |
| *Asia* | | | | |
| Okuda | Ascites, albumin, bilirubin | No | No | Tumour > or < 50% area of liver |
| CUPI | Bilirubin, ascites, ALP | <500 or ≥500 ng/mL | Symptoms | TNM |
| JIS | CTP | No | No | TNM |

*AFP* alpha-fetoprotein; *PS* performance status; *CTP* Child-Turcotte-Pugh; *PVT* portal vein thrombosis; *ALP* alkaline phosphatase

## Novel Staging Systems

With evolving understanding of HCC genomics, it is now apparent that common molecular subclasses exist which are related with prognosis, which may be enriched in certain subsets according to aetiology of liver disease and could impact response to targeted therapies. Several recently proposed staging systems, which incorporate molecular biomarkers, of both tumour and cirrhosis, are discussed below.

## Genomic Signatures

Molecular signatures have been proposed to predict recurrence and cancer outcomes in surgically resected HCC:

- Molecular signatures
  - G3 signature
  - Poor survival signature
- Five-gene score

These are at a very early stage and require further research to determine their place in routine clinical practice [20].

Likewise, insulin-like growth factor-1 and vascular endothelial growth factor are being looked at as initial studies have suggested correlation with survival in patient with HCC [19].

## Conclusion

There is no consensus as to which staging system is the best in predicting the survival of patients with HCC. Attempts to better describe and classify this disease remain a challenge, particularly if we are able to identify patients who will have substantial benefit from interventions.

Because of its widespread presence in current HCC research, and recommendation in several international guidelines for the management of HCC, BCLC is used by many practitioners to guide clinical decision-making. This lays the framework for investigators and treating physicians alike to make best use of current data in treating a difficult cancer; however it should not be taken as evidence that BCLC is the most accurate system.

There is likely to be modifications in the staging systems of HCC given our growing understanding in tumour biology, advanced imaging techniques and better management of underlying liver diseases. As a complement to clinical staging, it is to be hoped that these evolving systems will allow us to advance our prognostic ability and deliver better care to patients diagnosed with HCC.

Whilst there are significant advantages to the patients of the diagnostic criteria which don't involve tissue acquisition (not needing a liver biopsy), we need to mention that this will lead to a small number of incorrect diagnoses. In addition this practice limits the HCC tissue available to further develop the area of development of biomarkers that may help us to predict the variability in the response of this tumour to treatment.

## References

1. EASL Clinical Practice Guidelines. Management of hepatocellular carcinoma. J Hepatol. 2018; https://doi.org/10.1016/j.jhep.2018.03.019.
2. Bota S, Piscaglia F, Marinelli S, Pecorelli A, Terzi E, Bolondi L. Comparison of international guidelines for noninvasive diagnosis of hepatocellular carcinoma. Liver Cancer. 2012;1(3–4):190–200.
3. Rimola J, Forner A, Reig M, Vilana R, de Lope CR, Ayuso C, et al. Cholangiocarcinoma in cirrhosis: absence of contrast washout in delayed phases by magnetic resonance imaging avoids misdiagnosis of hepatocellular carcinoma. Hepatology. 2009;50(3):791–8.
4. Jang HJ, Kim TK, Burns PN, Wilson SR. Enhancement patterns of hepatocellular carcinoma at contrast-enhanced US: comparison with histologic differentiation. Radiology. 2007;244(3):898–906.
5. Lencioni R, Mascalchi M, Caramella D, Bartolozzi C. Small hepatocellular carcinoma: differentiation from adenomatous hyperplasia with color Doppler US and dynamic Gd-DTPA-enhanced MR imaging. Abdom Imaging. 1996;21(1):41–8.

6. Lencioni R, Pinto F, Armillotta N, Bartolozzi C. Assessment of tumor vascularity in hepatocellular carcinoma: comparison of power Doppler US and color Doppler US. Radiology. 1996;201(2):353–8.
7. Lee JM, Trevisani F, Vilgrain V, Wald C. Imaging diagnosis and staging of hepatocellular carcinoma. Liver Transpl. 2011;17(Suppl 2):S34–43.
8. Choi JY, Lee JM, Sirlin CB. CT and MR imaging diagnosis and staging of hepatocellular carcinoma: part I. Development, growth, and spread: key pathologic and imaging aspects. Radiology. 2014;272(3):635–54.
9. Silva AC, Evans JM, McCullough AE, Jatoi MA, Vargas HE, Hara AK. MR imaging of hypervascular liver masses: a review of current techniques. Radiographics. 2009;29(2):385–402.
10. Khosa F, Khan AN, Eisenberg RL. Hypervascular liver lesions on MRI. AJR Am J Roentgenol. 2011;197(2):W204–20.
11. Silva MA, Hegab B, Hyde C, Guo B, Buckels JA, Mirza DF. Needle track seeding following biopsy of liver lesions in the diagnosis of hepatocellular cancer: a systematic review and meta-analysis. Gut. 2008;57(11):1592–6.
12. Di Tommaso L, Franchi G, Park YN, Fiamengo B, Destro A, Morenghi E, et al. Diagnostic value of HSP70, glypican 3, and glutamine synthetase in hepatocellular nodules in cirrhosis. Hepatology. 2007;45(3):725–34.
13. Bruix J, Sherman M. Management of hepatocellular carcinoma: An update. Hepatology. 2011;53(3):1020–2.
14. Botta F, Giannini E, Romagnoli P, Fasoli A, Malfatti F, Chiarbonello B, et al. MELD scoring system is useful for predicting prognosis in patients with liver cirrhosis and is correlated with residual liver function: a European study. Gut. 2003;52(1):134–9.
15. Neuberger J, Gimson A, Davies M, Akyol M, O'Grady J, Burroughs A, et al. Selection of patients for liver transplantation and allocation of donated livers in the UK. Gut. 2008;57(2):252–7.
16. Marrero JA, Fontana RJ, Barrat A, Askari F, Conjeevaram HS, Su GL, et al. Prognosis of hepatocellular carcinoma: comparison of 7 staging systems in an American cohort. Hepatology. 2005;41(4):707–16.
17. Kadalayil L, Benini R, Pallan L, O'Beirne J, Marelli L, Yu D, et al. A simple prognostic scoring system for patients receiving transarterial embolisation for hepatocellular cancer. Ann Oncol. 2013;24(10):2565–70.
18. Sieghart W, Hucke F, Pinter M, Graziadei I, Vogel W, Muller C, et al. The ART of decision making: retreatment with transarterial chemoembolization in patients with hepatocellular carcinoma. Hepatology. 2013;57(6):2261–73.
19. Subramaniam S, Kelley RK, Venook AP. A review of hepatocellular carcinoma (HCC) staging systems. Chin Clin Oncol. 2013;2(4):33.
20. Villanueva A, Hoshida Y, Battiston C, Tovar V, Sia D, Alsinet C, et al. Combining clinical, pathology, and gene expression data to predict recurrence of hepatocellular carcinoma. Gastroenterology. 2011;140(5):1501–12.e2.

# Chapter 7
# The Role of Liver Resection for the Treatment of Hepatocellular Carcinoma

Mikael H. Sodergren and Dinesh Sharma

**Key Learning Points**

1. Liver resection provides optimal outcomes for HCC in patients of good performance status with limited liver disease in the absence of portal hypertension.
2. Patient selection is crucial and should take place in a multidisciplinary care setting.
3. EASL/AASLD guidelines can guide clinicians regarding management decisions; however it is found too restrictive by clinicians, even in Western subgroups.
4. Where local expertise exists, the laparoscopic approach may lead to improved perioperative outcomes.
5. Recurrent disease should be treated aggressively, if possible, to optimise outcomes.

**Areas of Controversy and Uncertainty**

1. Liver resection for patients outside of the BCLC algorithm and criteria has been reported to improve oncological outcomes in select patient groups at specialist centres but should be approached with caution.

M. H. Sodergren
Department of Surgery and Cancer, Imperial College London, London, UK
e-mail: m.sodergren@imperial.ac.uk

D. Sharma (✉)
The Sheila Sherlock Centre for Hepatology and Liver Transplantation, The Royal Free Hospital, London, UK
e-mail: dinesh.sharma@nhs.net



T. Cross, D. H. Palmer (eds.), *Liver Cancers*,
https://doi.org/10.1007/978-3-319-92216-4_7

2. The objective evaluation of portal hypertension to stratify risk for surgery varies between groups, and novel dynamic imaging methods offer potentially promising solutions.
3. The role of robotics surgery is not clearly defined, and this approach requires further evaluation in the context of surgery for HCC.
4. ALPPS in patients with HCC is associated with high mortality, and further assessment is required prior to routine application outside clinical trials or registries.

## Introduction

The incidence of HCC is increasing in the UK and many other countries. Surgery in the form of liver resection or transplantation remains the mainstay of curative treatment for HCC, even though selected patients with small tumours may also be cured with ablation. Liver resection and transplantation are not necessarily two binary choices in most patients and, despite all the debates, are often complementary treatment modalities ideally suited to different patient groups. Thus characterisation of patient and tumour characteristics to guide decision making is vital to achieve the best outcome for patients, and these aspects will be discussed as pertaining to selection for liver resection in this chapter.

Even as recently as 20–30 years ago, long-term survival following liver resection for HCC was rare. Significant advances have been made in early diagnosis, patient selection and preoperative investigations to exclude those with underlying liver dysfunction and likely poor outcomes. Operative techniques and anaesthetic/critical care management have been refined resulting in a <10% need for perioperative blood transfusion and a treatment-related mortality of 1–3%, even in cirrhotic patients. The 5-year survival following surgical resection for HCC can today exceed 50%.

On these bases, all patients diagnosed with HCC should be referred to a multidisciplinary centre with access to hepatologists, pathologists, surgeons, interventional radiologists, palliative care specialists and oncologists. Although transplantation is discussed in other chapters, it is important to acknowledge the role of liver resection as a bridge to transplantation in selected patients, particularly in the context of long waiting lists for grafts.

## Preoperative Assessment

The selection of patients for surgical resection should be made on a patient-by-patient basis in a tertiary centre multidisciplinary team setting and involves consideration of the following three factors in the context of current guidelines and available evidence:

## *Tumour Staging*

Assessment of size, number and extent of tumour nodules with relationship to vascular structures, along with exclusion of extrahepatic disease, is the aim of a thorough tumour staging. Staging and surgical planning should be completed by evaluation of dynamic multiphase computed tomography (CT) or magnetic resonance imaging (MRI) scans. Intraoperative ultrasound may further aid in detecting smaller nodules and should be routinely be used for this purpose and to aid anatomical resection. Further tumour classification can be performed using the American Joint Committee on Cancer (AJCC) tumour/node/metastasis (TNM) system, fibrosis score and histological grade.

## *Liver Function and Portal Hypertension: Assessing Liver Remnant*

The Child-Pugh score is the conventional measure used in BCLC guidelines. The score divides patients into three groups (A, B and C) based on serum albumin, bilirubin and prothrombin time/INR, and presence and severity of ascites and encephalopathy, correlating with severity of chronic liver disease as illustrated in Table 7.1. Platelet count (<100,000/mm$^3$) is a further useful parameter, particularly in combination with splenomegaly, to indicate clinically significant portal hypertension. Further radiological indicators of portal hypertension and decompensated liver disease include morphological liver changes and the presence of varices/collaterals and/or ascites. In Western countries the hepatic vein pressure gradient is used to evaluate portal hypertension via hepatic vein catheterisation. A gradient of

**Table 7.1** Child-pugh score and interpretation

| *Classification* | *1* | *2* | *3* |
|---|---|---|---|
| Serum bilirubin (μmol/L) | <34 | 34–51 | >51 |
| Serum albumin (g/L) | >35 | 28–35 | <28 |
| Presence of ascites | Absent | Controllable | Refractory |
| Encephalopathy | Absent | Minimal | Severe |
| INR | <1.7 | 1.7–2.3 | >2.3 |
| *Interpretation* | | | |
| *Points* | *Class* | *Life expectancy* | *Perioperative mortality* |
| 5–6 | A | 15–50 years | 10% |
| 7–9 | B | Candidate for transplant | 30% |
| 10–15 | C | 1–3 months | 82% |

*Score* 5–6 (Child's A), 7–9 (Child's B), 10–15 (Child's C)

<10 mmHg in combination with a normal bilirubin is an excellent indicator for low risk of post-hepatectomy liver failure [1]. The indocyanine green retention rate at 15 min ($ICG_{R15}$) is more commonly used in Eastern practice. ICG is an inert, water-soluble, fluorescent tricarbocyanine, with a protein binding close to 95%, which in healthy individuals shows a high hepatic extraction rate (>70%). There are now commercially available transcutaneous non-invasive pulse dye densitometry systems that can be used at the bedside. Generally most liver resection in cirrhotic patients are deemed safe with $ICG_{R15} < 15\%$ in the context of an adequate FLR [2].

The use of the model for end-stage liver disease (MELD) score is controversial in the context of liver resection for HCC. However the prognostic value in surgery for HCC is not well established, and there are concerns regarding the narrow range (9–14) in which the score is applied. Emerging methods of preoperative assessment of liver function include transient elastography, 99mTc-labeled GSA scintigraphy and functional MRI using Gd-EOP-DTPA contrast enhancement. Although further data are required prior to routine clinical implementation, liver stiffness on transient elastography has been found to correlate with postoperative liver failure after hepatectomy for HCC. Novel imaging such as 99mTc-GSA allows not only for measurement of total liver function but also enables quantitative segmental assessment of liver function, which may be valuable in high-risk patient groups.

In addition to function, an assessment of liver remnant volume is essential prior to surgery. In the context of cirrhosis, it is recommended that the future liver remnant (FLR) should be at least 40%; however this should be considered on an individual basis taking account other patient factors. There is no benefit for the use of preoperative chemo-embolisation or portal vein embolisation in patients who meet criteria for surgical resection. However portal vein embolisation may render unresectable patients operable due to an increase in FLR and allows for evaluation of regenerative capacity. When the liver does not regenerate after PVE, most agree that major hepatectomy should be contraindicated to avoid severe postoperative liver failure. Should trans-arterial embolisation be appropriate, it is desirable that this is performed prior to portal vein embolisation [3].

## *Patient Fitness*

Prior to being offered liver resection for HCC patients should undergo a thorough clinical assessment with identification of any significant cardiac, pulmonary or renal co-morbidities. Any suggestion in the history of underlying co-morbidities should be extensively investigated. ASA score has been found to accurately predict mortality of patients with liver cirrhosis undergoing abdominal surgery and should be accurately documented. Even in patients of good performance status, pre-existing co-morbidities may contraindicate surgical resection. In the authors' institution, cardiopulmonary exercise testing is sometimes used as an adjunct to other conventional assessments of fitness such as the stairs test in determining suitability for surgery in borderline cases.

BCLC guidelines suggest that surgery should only be offered to patients with Eastern Cooperative Oncology Group (ECOG) performance status (PS) of 0; however many studies have shown PS to be least respected BCLC criteria. Age in itself should not be a contraindication to surgery. Limited evidence suggests that there may be a higher incidence of serious complications in this group; however disease-free survival and mortality appear similar to younger cohorts [4]; therefore careful patient selection is essential, and particular caution should be applied for patients outside BCLC guideline criteria.

## Patient Selection

### *Guidelines/Criteria for Resection*

The Barcelona Clinic Liver Cancer (BCLC) staging system utilises tumour stage, physical status, liver function and cancer-related symptoms to recommend treatment allocations. It has been externally validated and used in many clinical trials of HCC treatment and therefore has also been used in the current European Association for Study of the Liver (EASL) and American Association for the Study of Liver Diseases (AASLD) guidelines for the treatment of HCC [5, 6], which are illustrated in Fig. 7.1. Using these guidelines resection is recommended as the primary treatment in patients with a single tumour (previously in smaller tumours though the

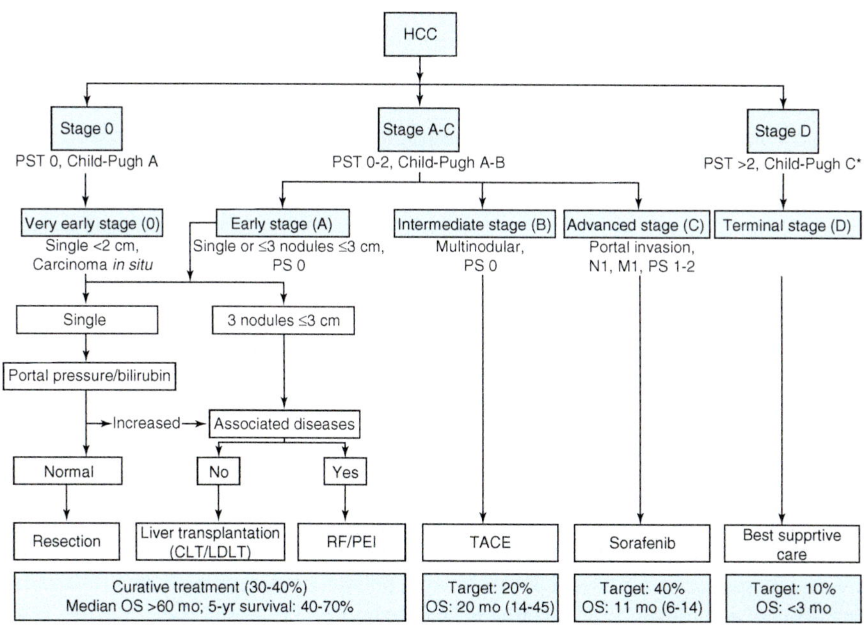


**Fig. 7.1** AASLD-EASL-EORTC treatment algorithm for HCC

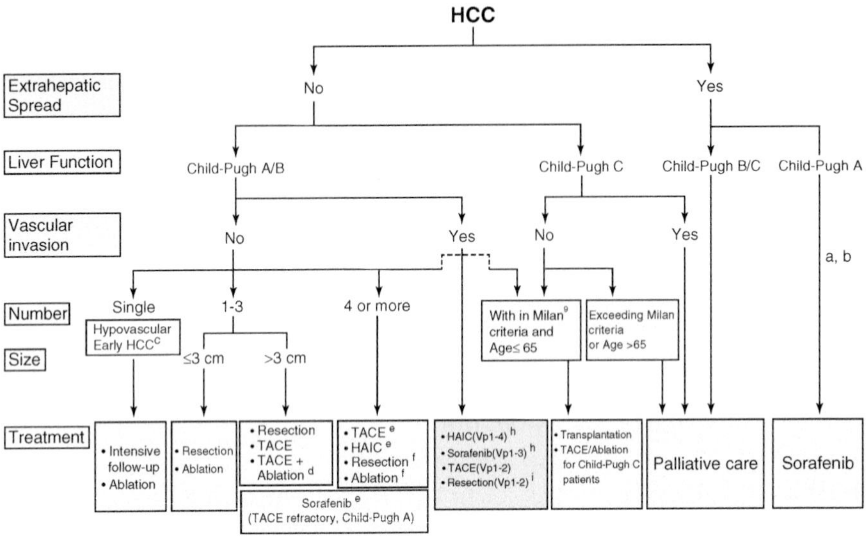


**Fig. 7.2** JSH Liver Cancer Study Group of Japan consensus-based treatment algorithm Kudo [7]

later versions have removed this restriction), Child-Pugh Class A liver function with normal bilirubin, no evidence of portal hypertension (hepatic vein pressure gradient <10 mmHg or platelet count >100,000) and good performance status. It is worth noting that Eastern guidelines differ from those used in Western countries and on the whole adopts a more aggressive treatment approach. Regarding the role of resection, the Liver Cancer Study Group of Japan published guidelines [7], illustrated in Fig. 7.2, and recommended potentially curable therapy with resection and ablation to be attempted even in the presence of four or more nodules. Furthermore they recommend TACE or resection in the case of minor vascular invasion (Vp1 or Vp2) for which sorafenib would be the recommended treatment under Western guidelines. However, it is worth noting that in the East, the incidence of HCC in non-cirrhotic patients (40%) and HBV is much greater than that in Western countries (5%).

## *Extended Criteria Resections*

It is well known that clinical practice sometimes deviates from the BCLC recommendations, often found to be too restrictive at the authors' institution especially for intermediate or advanced disease, and there is a growing body of evidence that suggests liver resection to be safe in selected patients with portal hypertension and well-compensated liver function, thereby including these patients on a curative treatment pathway. Criteria have been extended to patients with macrovascular invasion as well as multiple or large HCCs, in addition to portal hypertension, with superior reported outcomes to palliative therapies in selected patients [8]. There are however no randomised data to guide patient selection for these controversial indications, and a meta-analysis of patients with clinically significant portal hypertension undergoing resection for HCC has shown a significant increase in 3- (OR 2.09, 95% CI: 1.52–2.88) and 5-year (OR 2.07, 95% CI 1.51–2.84) mortality and of clinical decompensation (OR 3.04, 95% CI 2.02–4.59) after surgery [9]. An analysis from ten high-volume centres of 2046 patients showed that only 50% of patients were operated within BCLC recommendations with 36% and 14% of patients in BCLC stage B or C undergoing surgery. The reported 5-year overall survival after resection in BCLC groups A, B and C was 61%, 57% and 38%, respectively, with 5-year disease-free survival of 21%, 27% and 18% [10]. These survival curves are illustrated in Fig. 7.3.

## *A Pragmatic Approach to HCC Resections*

We would consider liver resection first in all standard risk resection patients, i.e., those with Child-Pugh A cirrhosis with a hepatic wedge pressure gradient of 10 mmHg or less and a good ICG clearance with a $PDR_{15}$ of >15 with an $R_{15}$ of <15, with adequate liver remnant ideally >40%—especially for major resections. Despite ongoing debate we feel a liver transplant for these patients does not necessarily guarantee the best outcome and potentially deprives others in the UK setting.

Patients who are not within the standard risk category for resection will be considered for liver transplantation if appropriate (if they are within existing criteria and fit).

Radiofrequency ablation will be considered as a possible curative treatment modality if neither resection nor transplantation is feasible or appropriate with standard risk.

In patients for whom a low or standard risk resection, liver transplantation or radiofrequency ablation (in that order of consideration) is *not* feasible or appropriate, then a higher risk resection (for instance with multiple nodules or with some portal hypertension or poor liver function or macrovascular invasion, as in Fig. 7.4) may be considered as long as the size of resection is thought to be compatible with the impairment of liver synthetic function or portal hypertension. This would be discussed on a case-by-case basis by the multidisciplinary team. The approach would of course vary in a different geocultural environment.

## Anaesthetic Considerations

There are several important measures that can be taken by the anaesthetist to improve outcomes of liver resection for HCC. Intraoperatively a low central venous pressure (CVP), preferably <5 cm $H_2O$, is important in limiting blood loss. This can be achieved by a combination of diuretics or nitroglycerine, reduction in tidal volume and positive end-expiratory pressure and placing the patient in the reverse Trendelenburg position as well as minimal intravenous fluid infusion.

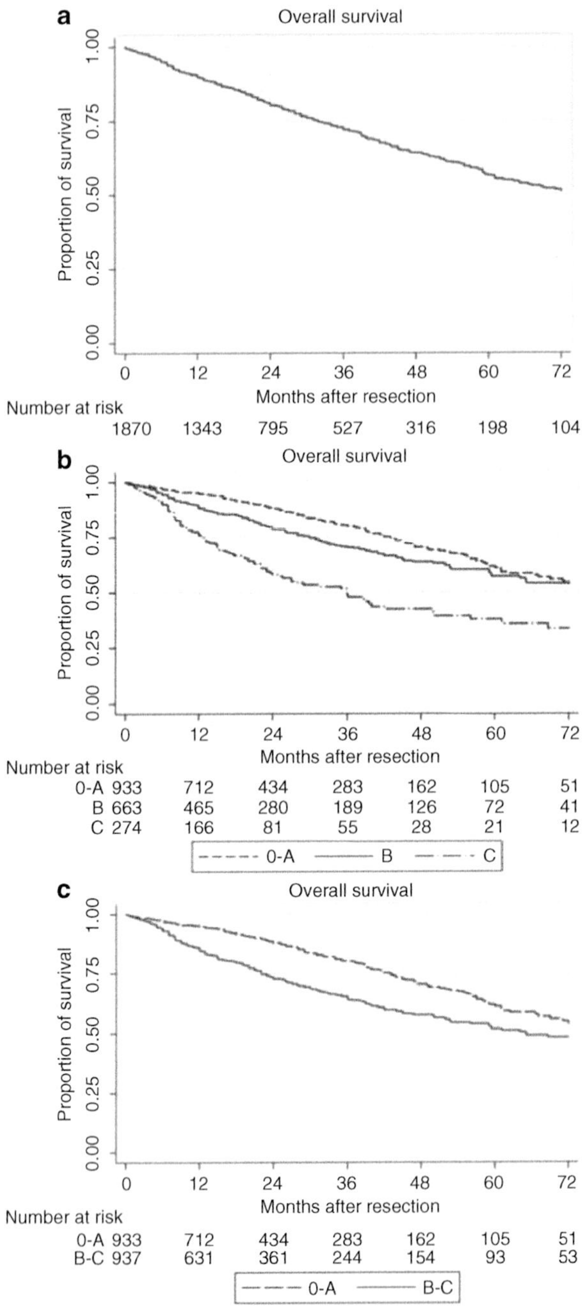


**Fig. 7.3** Survival after resection. (**a**) Overall survival of 2046 patients resected for HCC. (**b**) Overall survival stratified according to the BCLC classification ($P = 0.000$). (**c**) Overall survival of patients in the very early and early stages (BCLC 0-A) versus patients in the intermediate and advanced stages (BCLC B-C) ($P = 0.000$) Torzilli [10]

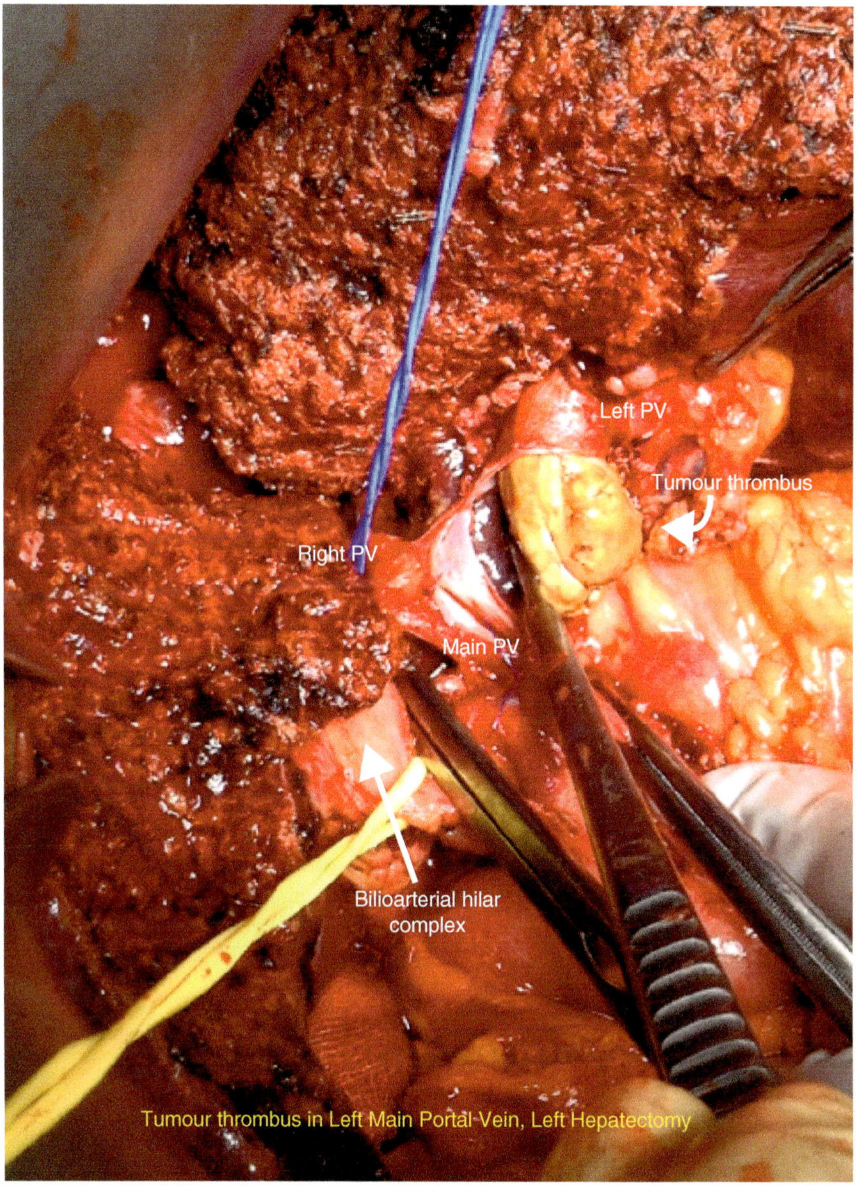


**Fig. 7.4** Liver resection with macroscopic portal vein extension

## Surgical Technique

### Anatomical Resection or Not?

The aim of liver resection in patients with HCC and CLD is that it should be curative with resection of tumour vascular territories and also preserve as much liver volume as possible to prevent postoperative liver failure. EASL guidelines recommend anatomical resection of HCC, whereby the lines of resection match the limits of one or more functional segments of the liver. This is based on evidence suggesting superior oncological outcomes in addition to a reduction in the risk of bleeding and biliary fistula. Although there are no randomised data, a meta-analysis including 1829 patients from 12 non-randomised comparative trials did not show any benefit of anatomical compared with non-anatomical resection in 1-, 3- and 5-year survival, recurrence rate, postoperative morbidity or blood loss [11]. It is the authors' practice to perform an anatomical resection for tumours >2 cm, and for smaller tumours in anatomically favourable positions, a wedge with adequate margin is often sufficient [12]. Modifying techniques to maximise parenchymal preservation preserving adequate margins are often the key in these patients.

### Anterior Approach

The anterior approach, as described by Professor Belghiti [13], has been advocated for large right-sided tumours. This technique involves transection of the liver parenchyma to the IVC without mobilisation of the liver with the theoretical advantage of less tumour seeding. A prospective randomised controlled trial compared the anterior and conventional approach on 120 patients with large (>5 cm) HCCs. The anterior approach group had less blood transfusion requirements and a significantly longer overall survival (68.1 v 22.6 months; $p = 0.006$) [14].

### Parenchymal Transection

As in liver resection for other indications, there is no good evidence to indicate that a single method of parenchymal transection, application of fibrin sealants or intermittent inflow occlusion is beneficial in surgery for HCC. There is also no evidence to suggest that using special equipment for liver resection is of any benefit in decreasing the mortality, morbidity, or blood transfusion requirements [15]. Surgeons should use techniques in which they have been trained and can demonstrate acceptable outcomes.

## *Laparoscopic Approach*

Laparoscopic HCC resections are gaining popularity as the approach is more widely adopted across centres. It is important that patients for laparoscopic resection are selected based on the technical capabilities of the surgeon and centre, and the proper mentoring takes place during the learning curve. A summary of published meta-analyses concluded that the laparoscopic approach was associated with improved short-term outcomes (blood loss, complication rates and hospital length of stay) without compromising long-term oncological outcomes. It is worth noting that there are no randomised data; however a number of trials are in progress. Furthermore, their analysis suggested that the incidence of postoperative ascites and liver failure is decreased in the selected group of laparoscopic liver resections [16]. A further meta-analysis of cirrhotic patients up to Child-Pugh B undergoing laparoscopic compared with open liver resection for HCC confirmed these perioperative benefits [17].

## *Robotic Approach*

Although still very much in its infancy, the application of robotic surgery to HCC resection can theoretically yield similar advantages in short-term outcomes to the laparoscopic technique. The only comparative study between robotic and open liver resection for HCC included 183 patients undergoing robotic hepatectomy who were compared using propensity scoring with a cohort of 275 open resections. The robotic group required longer operating time (343 vs 220 min), shorter hospital stays (7.5 vs 10.1 days) and lower dosages of postoperative patient-controlled analgesia (350 vs 554 ng/kg). The 3-year disease-free survival of the robotic group was comparable with that of the open group (72.2% vs 58.0%; $p = 0.062$), as was the 3-year overall survival (92.6 vs 93.7%; $p = 0.431$) [18]. The associated financial costs of robotic surgery still pose a limitation to its adoption, and it is unclear if this approach is associated with any significant advantages over laparoscopic rather than open resection.

## *Associating Liver Partition with Portal Vein Ligation for Staged Hepatectomy (ALPPS)/TAE/PVE*

ALPPS is still considered an experimental technique in which a first-stage procedure consisting of physical liver splitting and portal vein ligation is followed by a second stage of resection of the HCC and associated liver segments. The advantage seen in colorectal liver metastases is that of rapid hypertrophy for the FLR. There are only limited data describing outcomes of ALPPS for HCC; however an analysis of 35 patients in the international ALPPS registry showed an impressive FLR hypertrophy of 47% following the first stage of the procedure that was associated with a 31% peri-operative mortality rate. The majority of these patients were in the intermediate-stage category of the BCLC algorithm [19]. Further evaluation is required prior to routine use of ALPPS for HCC resection, and it is the view of the authors that ALPPS may be a procedure best reserved for carefully selected patients who have bilateral disease.

### *Combined Resection with RFA for Bilobar HCC*

For patients with multiple or bilobar HCC in whom resection is contraindicated due to inadequate FLR, combined resection and radiofrequency ablation (RFA) may yield better results than alternative treatments. A single-centre study compared patients with bilobar liver HCCs who underwent resection ($n = 89$), combination of resection and RFA ($n = 114$) and TACE ($n = 161$). The results showed that 1-, 3- and 5-year survival was better in both resection and combined resection, and RFA groups compared with TACE and survival and disease-free survival were comparable between both surgical groups. They concluded that resection combined with RFA provided a chance for cure in patients with bilobar HCC, and provided liver function is preserved, aggressive treatment can improve prognosis [20].

## Ruptured Hepatocellular Carcinoma

Ruptured HCC occurs in approximately 10% of patients and is a potentially life-threatening complication with a mortality rate of up to 50%. The initial concern is often haemostasis, and this can be achieved in a number of ways including TACE, bland embolisation and laparotomy with packing or liver resection. When possible hepatic resection has the best outcome and should be the treatment of choice however following haemostasis. The test of time is often useful to determine the biology of the tumour prior to embarking on definitive treatment. A case-controlled propensity matched study of 34 Western patients presenting with rupture was compared with a cohort of HCC patient who did not present with rupture. There was no difference in overall and disease-free survival between these groups; however underlying cirrhosis was associated with significantly worse prognosis. Rupture in itself was not found to be a risk factor for survival in selected patients who undergo hepatectomy [21].

## Liver Resection for Recurrent Hepatocellular Carcinoma

Intrahepatic recurrence of HCC following resection or ablation is common, up to 70% at 5 years following primary resection comprising of both local recurrence and de novo disease. Factors associated with an increased risk of recurrence include hepatitis C diagnosis, preoperative aspartate aminotransferase (AST) greater than twice normal, large intraoperative blood transfusion and preoperative serum alpha-fetoprotein (AFP) of more than 10,000 ng/mL. Unlike in primary HCC, there are no consensus guidelines to inform management decisions, and treatment options include repeat hepatectomy, RFA, TACE or transplantation. A meta-analysis comparing hepatectomy, RFA and TACE including 2764 patients suggested a trend towards improved survival following repeat hepatectomy compared with TACE (HR = 1.61; $p = 0.056$) with similar outcomes to RFA (HR = 1.03; $p = 0.897$). Short disease-free interval and multiple and larger hepatic metastases were all found to be negative prognostic factors [22].

## Conclusion

It is crucial that patients with HCC are treated in appropriate centres that have the infrastructure and expertise available to manage this complex disease and ideally who can offer all treatment modalities. The treatment approach followed at the authors' institution has been outlined. Surgical resection should be offered to patients who are of good performance status with limited liver disease (single lesion with Child-Pugh A cirrhosis with normal bilirubin and absence of portal hypertension). The EASL/AASLD guidelines provide a good framework on which to base treatment strategies. Resection contemplated for more advanced disease or cirrhosis may be carefully considered in a case-by-case basis by an expert multidisciplinary team. However, despite retrospective nature of studies, it is likely that careful patient selection may permit curative liver resection in groups outside the BCLC recommendations such as those with multiple tumours, portal hypertension or even macrovascular invasion. Available data regarding operative risks, alternative treatments and oncological prognosis must be frankly discussed with the patient. Low CVP during surgery may aid in reducing blood loss. The standard surgical approach is that of an anatomical open liver resection with a minimum of 40% FLR in cirrhotic patients. Portal vein ligation/embolisation may be useful in specific cases to increase the FLR and decrease risk of postoperative liver decompensation. The anterior approach may be useful for large lesions and may have some oncological benefits. The laparoscopic approach is gaining popularity, particularly for anterior/left-sided segmental liver resection, and appears to be associated with improved perioperative outcomes. Techniques such as robotic surgery and ALPPS are still considered experimental and should not be practised routinely outside clinical trials or registries. Ruptured HCC, once haemostasis has been established, should be treated under the same oncological pathway as non-ruptured tumours including consideration of surgical resection for appropriate patients. A large number of patients will experience recurrence of HCC after resection. They should be re-evaluated for radical treatment with both reoperation and RFA producing improved outcomes to TACE or supportive treatment.

## References


1. Boleslawski E, Petrovai G, Truant S, Dharancy S, Duhamel A, Salleron J, et al. Hepatic venous pressure gradient in the assessment of portal hypertension before liver resection in patients with cirrhosis. Br J Surg. 2012;99(6):855–63.
2. Lam CM, Fan ST, Lo CM, Wong J. Major hepatectomy for hepatocellular carcinoma in patients with an unsatisfactory indocyanine green clearance test. Br J Surg. 1999;86:1012–46.
3. Ogata S, Belghiti J, Farges O, Varma D, Sibert A, Vilgrain V. Sequential arterial and portal vein embolizations before right hepatectomy in patients with cirrhosis and hepatocellular carcinoma. Br J Surg. 2006;93:1091–8.
4. Huang J, Li BK, Chen GH, et al. Long-term outcomes and prognostic factors of elderly patients with hepatocellular carcinoma undergoing hepatectomy. J Gastrointest Surg. 2009;13(9):1627–35.
5. Bruix J, Sherman M, American Association for the Study of Liver D. Management of hepatocellular carcinoma: an update. Hepatology. 2011;53(3):1020–2.
6. European Association for the Study of the L, European Organisation for R, Treatment of C. EASL-EORTC clinical practice guidelines: management of hepatocellular carcinoma. J Hepatol. 2012;56(4):908–43.
7. Kudo M, Matsui O, Izumi N, et al. JSH consensus-based clinical practice guidelines for the management of hepatocellular carcinoma: 2014 update by the liver cancer study group of Japan. Liver Cancer. 2014;3(3-4):458–68.
8. Guglielmi A, Ruzzenente A, Conci S, et al. Hepatocellular carcinoma: surgical perspectives beyond the Barcelona clinic liver cancer recommendations. World J Gastroenterol. 2014;20(24):7525–33.
9. Berzigotti A, Reig M, Abraldes JG, Bosch J, Bruix J. Portal hypertension and the outcome of surgery for hepatocellular carcinoma in compensated cirrhosis: a systematic review and meta-analysis. Hepatology. 2015;61(2):526–36.
10. Torzilli G, Belghiti J, Kokudo N, et al. A snapshot of the effective indications and results of surgery for hepatocellular carcinoma in tertiary referral centers: is it adherent to the EASL/AASLD recommendations?: an observational study of the HCC east-west study group. Ann Surg. 2013;257(5):929–37.
11. Tang YH, Wen TF, Chen X. Anatomic versus non-anatomic liver resection for hepatocellular carcinoma: a systematic review. Hepato-Gastroenterology. 2013;60(128):2019–25.
12. Eguchi S, Kanematsu T, Arii S, Okazaki M, Okita K, Omata M, Ikai I, Kudo M, Kojiro M, Makuuchi M, et al. Comparison of the outcomes between an anatomical subsegmentectomy and a non-anatomical minor hepatectomy for single hepatocellular carcinomas based on a Japanese nationwide survey. Surgery. 2008;143:469–75.
13. Belghiti J, Guevara OA, Noun R, Saldinger PF, Kianmanesh R. Liver hanging maneuver: a safe approach to right hepatectomy without liver mobilization. J Am Coll Surg. 2001;193(1):109–11.
14. Liu CL, Fan ST, Cheung ST, Lo CM, Ng IO, Wong J. Anterior approach versus conventional approach right hepatic resection for large hepatocellular carcinoma: a prospective randomized controlled study. Ann Surg. 2006;244(2):194–203.
15. Moggia E, Rouse B, Simillis C, et al. Methods to decrease blood loss during liver resection: a network meta-analysis. Cochrane Database Syst Rev. 2016;10:CD010683.
16. Morise Z, Ciria R, Cherqui D, Chen KH, Belli G, Wakabayashi G. Can we expand the indications for laparoscopic liver resection? A systematic review and meta-analysis of laparoscopic liver resection for patients with hepatocellular carcinoma and chronic liver disease. J Hepatobiliary Pancreat Sci. 2015;22(5):342–52.
17. Twaij A, Pucher PH, Sodergren MH, Gall T, Darzi A, Jiao LR. Laparoscopic vs open approach to resection of hepatocellular carcinoma in patients with known cirrhosis: systematic review and meta-analysis. World J Gastroenterol. 2014;20(25):8274–81.

18. Chen PD, Wu CY, Hu RH, et al. Robotic versus open hepatectomy for hepatocellular carcinoma: a matched comparison. Ann Surg Oncol. 2016;24(4):1021–8.
19. D'Haese JG, Neumann J, Weniger M, et al. Should ALPPS be used for liver resection in intermediate-stage HCC? Ann Surg Oncol. 2016;23(4):1335–43.
20. Zhang T, Zeng Y, Huang J, Liao M, Wu H. Combined resection with radiofrequency ablation for bilobar hepatocellular carcinoma: a single-center experience. J Surg Res. 2014;191(2):370–8.
21. Pinsker N, Papoulas M, Sodergren M, Quaglia A, Suddle A, Jassem W, Melendez HV, Prachalias A, Srinivasan P, Menon K, Heaton N, et al. Outcomes following liver resection for ruptured and non-ruptured hepatocellular carcinoma–a propensity matched analysis. In: 19th Annual Scientific Meeting of the Association-of-Upper-Gastrointestinal-Surgeons-of-Great-Britain-and-Ireland. Wiley-Blackwell. 2016; p. 17, ISSN: 0007-1323.
22. Erridge S, Pucher PH, Markar SR, Malietzis G, Athanasiou T, Darzi A, et al. Meta-analysis of determinants of survival following treatment of recurrent hepatocellular carcinoma. Br J Surg. 2017;104:1433–42.

# Chapter 8
# Liver Transplantation for the Treatment of Hepatocellular Carcinoma

**Aileen Marshall**

## Introduction

Liver transplantation is established as an effective treatment for patients with chronic liver diseases. Patients with primary liver cancer have been part of the patient group since the first human liver transplants were performed in the 1960s. The first report from Thomas Starzl of three successful liver transplants included one paediatric patient with hepatic cell carcinoma [1]. This patient survived for 13 months and died of metastatic disease.

During the 1970s and 1980s as liver transplant programmes grew, HCC remained an indication for transplant but with no clear selection criteria intended to optimise the outcome for those recipients. It became evident that tumour recurrence post-transplant was a frequent occurrence, was difficult to treat, and had a high mortality. Rapid HCC reoccurrence and death at a time when survival following liver transplant for other indications was improving tempered enthusiasm to offer liver transplantation to patients with HCC.

The importance of HCC stage to influence risk of recurrence was recognised. A seminal paper published by Mazzaferro and colleagues in 1996 defined size and number criteria that demonstrated a low risk of recurrence and patient and graft survival comparable to other transplant indications [2]. The cohort of 48 patients, predominantly HCV or HBV positive, had either a single HCC $\leq$ 5 cm or up to 3 HCC all in one lobe and the largest $\leq$3 cm. Radiological evidence of extrahepatic disease or tumour invasion into a branch of the portal vein were exclusion criteria. In this cohort 4/48 patients had HCC recurrence and 4 year recurrence-free survival was 83%, representing a significant improvement compared to historical

A. Marshall (✉)
The Sheila Sherlock Centre for Hepatology and Liver Transplantation, The Royal Free Hospital, London, UK
e-mail: aileen.marshall@nhs.net

 
T. Cross, D. H. Palmer (eds.), *Liver Cancers*,
https://doi.org/10.1007/978-3-319-92216-4_8

series. Known as the Milan criteria, these size and number criteria were widely adopted worldwide and remain the basis for patient selection for liver transplantation until now.

Whilst implementation of the Milan criteria renewed HCC as an indication for liver transplantation, it is clear that one snapshot of tumour stage at one time point does not capture the variability of tumour biology and prognosis for HCC. At one end of the spectrum, there are patients with early-stage disease who still experience post-transplant recurrence, and at the opposite end, there are patients with HCC beyond the Milan criteria who had long-term recurrence-free survival. The challenge has been to optimise identification of patients who will benefit most from liver transplantation. Histologically, the presence of microvascular invasion is the most important predictor of recurrence. Microvascular invasion is defined as tumour present within a blood vessel with a muscular wall >1 cm from the tumour margin [3]. Additional factors impacting recurrence risk are grade of differentiation and the presence of satellite nodules. All these factors can only be assessed fully following transplantation so cannot be used in patient selection for transplantation.

The keys themes of research regarding patient selection for liver transplantation have been:

1. Expansion of size and number criteria beyond Milan.
2. Pre-transplant radiological and serological parameters that predict post-transplant prognosis.
3. Change in radiological or serological parameters over time.
4. Response to locoregional treatment.

## Pre-transplant Radiological Criteria

Table 8.1 summarises the proposed expansions to Milan criteria [4–8]. The first proposal to modestly expand criteria was based on retrospective analysis of 70 patients receiving liver transplants between 1988 and 2000 at the University of California, San Francisco (UCSF). They identified that overall survival was 90% at 1 year and 72.5% at 5 years for patients with 1 HCC < 6.5 cm, or up to 3 HCC, largest <4.5 cm and total tumour diameter <8 cm [4]. In contrast, patients exceeding these criteria had 50% 5 year survival. These data were obtained using histopathology and subsequently were validated prospectively using pre-transplant radiology in 168 patients and reporting 1- and 5-year recurrence-free survival of 92.1% and 80.7% [9].

In a study of 1556 patients exceeding Milan criteria, Mazzaferro and colleagues proposed the concept of the "Metroticket" using HCC size and number [7]. The up-to-seven criteria combine number of HCC with the size of the largest lesion so that as number increases, the permitted size of the largest HCC decreases. Predicted survival following transplantation decreases as the combined score increases, and it was suggested that this graded approach could be used to identify patients with

**Table 8.1** Selection criteria for liver transplantation for patients with hepatocellular carcinoma. *TTD* total tumour diameter, *OS* overall survival, *RFS* recurrence-free survival

| Reference | Name | Criteria | Outcome |
|---|---|---|---|
| Mazzaferro et al. [2] | Milan | $1 \leq 5$ cm OR $3 \leq 3$ cm | 83% 4-year RFS |
| Yao et al. [4] | UCSF | $1 \leq 6.5$ cm OR<br>$3 \leq 4.5$ cm AND TTD $\leq 8$ cm | 75.2% 5-year OS |
| Zheng et al. [5] | Hangzhou | TTD $\leq 8$ cm OR<br>TTD $\geq 8$ cm and Grade I/II differentiation and AFP $\leq 400$ ng/ml | 72.3% 5-year OS |
| Lee et al. [6] | Asan | Up to 6 HCC $\leq 5$ cm and no macrovascular invasion | 76.3% 5-year OS (LDLT only) |
| Mazzaferro et al. [7] | Up-to-seven | Sum of size of largest HCC and number of HCC $< 7$ | 71.2% 5-year OS |
| Takada et al. [8] | Kyoto | Up to 10 HCC $\leq 5$ cm AND PIVKA-II $< 400$ mAU/ml | 87% 5-year OS (LDLT only) |

HCC beyond Milan criteria yet acceptable 5-year post-transplant survival. A revised "Metroticket 2.0" model has just been published that also incorporated AFP.

Similarly, in populations where living donor transplant is more commonly performed, expansion of size and number criteria have been proposed that are reported to provide similar 5-year survival to the Milan criteria (Table 8.1) [6, 8].

Positron emission tomography (PET) is a combination of morphological and functional imaging that relies on uptake of compounds by metabolically active cells. FDG-PET has become part of the diagnostic algorithm for many solid cancers, but not HCC as a large proportion of HCC are non-avid. However, it may have usefulness as a prognostic marker. In a Japanese cohort of patients receiving liver donor transplant for HCC, pre-transplant PET-positive status was associated with microscopic vascular invasion and with higher post-transplant recurrence [10].

In the UK, the liver transplant selection criteria are based on the Milan criteria with minor modifications. A patient can be offered transplant if there is one HCC < 5 cm or up to 5 HCC, largest ≤3 cm. The presence of extrahepatic disease, radiological evidence of macrovascular invasion and AFP > 1000 IU/ml are exclusion criteria. In addition, patients with a single HCC 5–7 cm in size that is stable over 6 months can be offered transplantation.

## Pre-transplant Serum Biomarkers for HCC

Alpha-fetoprotein (AFP) is the most well-known and widely used biomarker, originally linked to HCC in 1970. As a diagnostic marker for HCC, AFP is limited by poor sensitivity and specificity. However, as a prognostic marker, numerous studies have shown that a high pre-transplant AFP has been associated with an increased risk of HCC recurrence. A systematic review and meta-analysis of published studies found the hazard ratio for recurrence was 2.69 (2.08–3.47) if the AFP was >400 IU/ml [11]. In the UK, the cut-off for AFP has been reduced from 10,000 IU/ml to 1000 IU/ml.

Serial measurement of AFP pre-transplant also gives prognostic value; three separate studies have identified that rising AFP whilst awaiting transplantation is associated with adverse outcome. In Canadian patients, AFP increasing by >50 μg/l per month was associated with 1-year recurrence-free survival of 40% [12]. A French single-centre study reported 5-year recurrence-free survival 47% in patients who had a pre-transplant AFP rising by 15 μg/l per month [13]. Similarly, a multi-centre European study found that 5-year recurrence-free survival using the same cut-off was 53.8% [14]. This study also showed that increasing AFP pre-transplant conferred an increased risk of dropout from the transplant waiting list.

Des-gamma-carboxy prothrombin (DCP), also known as protein induced by vitamin K absence (PIVKA), has been studied predominantly in Eastern populations. It is proposed as a diagnostic marker and to provide prognostic value for patients with HCC treated with liver resection. In transplant populations, a meta-analysis of five published studies of HCC recurrence following liver transplantation showed a strong correlation between pre-transplant DCP and post-transplant HCC recurrence (HR 5.99, 3.27–10.98) [11].

## Novel and Molecular Biomarkers in Liver Transplant Patients

Given the limitations of existing radiological criteria and serum biomarkers, there is a great deal of interest in novel and molecular biomarkers as both diagnostic and prognostic markers. As yet, none have been shown to perform well enough to be implemented into clinical decision-making. A combination of clinical and serum biomarkers (GALAD; Gender, Age, L3-AFP, AFP and DCP) has been shown to improve sensitivity in HCC diagnosis, but this combination has not been evaluated as a prognostic marker in liver transplant patients.

### *Non-coding RNA*

Non-coding RNA, including long non-coding RNA (lncRNA) and microRNA (miRNA), are molecules that have been discovered to play a critical role in the regulation of gene expression. In recent years, non-coding RNA have been extensively investigated for their role in carcinogenesis, as diagnostic markers and in cancer therapeutics. Thousands of human miRNA are described with specific tissue patterns and with specific alterations in many cancers. MiRNA are detectable in serum which make them attractive biomarkers. A small number of studies, reviewed in [15], found associations between pre-transplant miRNA profile and post-transplant recurrence. However, miRNA expression is also likely to be altered by the type and stage of background liver disease or by comorbidities.

The earliest studies used standard extraction techniques to detect miRNA in serum. It now appears that miRNA are found within circulating exosomes, small membrane bound vesicles that are released into the circulation via fusion with the cell membrane. Exosomes are thought to play a role in cell-cell communication of genetic material. Therefore, extraction of miRNA from exosomes may improve the sensitivity and specificity of detecting circulating cancer-derived miRNA. Using this technique, decreased exosomal mir718 was found to be associated with more HCC aggressiveness and recurrence post-transplant [16].

Tissue expression of two lncRNA (MALAT1 and HOTAIR) has been reported in two cohorts to be associated with post-transplant recurrence. Circulating lncRNA are now reported to be detectable in circulating exosomes, but as yet there is no date on circulating lncRNA in patients with HCC.

## Circulating Tumour Cells and Circulating Cell-Free Tumour DNA

Circulating cancer cells and cell-free DNA have been described in several different cancers, and in some cases, detection of circulating cells or DNA can lead to early detection of recurrence or relapse following treatment. The extraction of such cells relies on expression of cell surface markers, e.g., the stem cell marker EPCAM, or detection of a known cancer mutation. For HCC, detection of p53 mutation in cell-free DNA has been described. At present, it is not known whether these markers have a role in prognostication, early detection of recurrence or treatment decisions. In the future it may be possible to identify an individual's cancer mutation profile using a biopsy or surgical specimen and then use that patient's tumour-specific mutations to detect recurrence.

## Pre-transplant Locoregional HCC Treatment and Downstaging

In the UK approximately 22% of patients who receive a liver transplant have HCC [17]. In common with other Western countries, most patients receiving liver transplants for HCC will receive an organ from a deceased donor. The overall median waiting time is 135 days, but there is a large range. For all patients, 18% are still waiting 1 year after listing, and 5% are still waiting at 2 years. Given the uncertainty about how long the patient will wait, it is common practice to offer locoregional treatment (LRT) such as transarterial (chemo) embolisation (TA(C)E) or radiofrequency ablation (RFA) where possible. Some patients with decompensated liver disease will not be able to receive LRT. There are no randomised controlled clinical trials comparing outcomes in patients who do not receive LRT whilst on the transplant waiting list; however the United Network for Organ Sharing (UNOS) data from North American transplant centres does demonstrate better post-transplant outcomes in patients who are able to receive LRT.

Application of LRT to patients with HCC beyond Milan criteria has led to the concept of downstaging, that is, using LRT to reduce the tumour size or number to within accepted transplant criteria. In this context a response to LRT is thought to be a surrogate marker for favourable tumour biology and hence an acceptable risk of post-transplant recurrence. The published data is limited by heterogeneity in patient selection, downstaging protocols, outcome assessment and study quality. A systematic review of these studies concluded that the overall downstaging was achieved in 40% of patients, and post-transplant recurrence was 16% [18].

Protocols and clinical outcomes have been published by two well-established downstaging programmes conducted in UCSF [19] and French transplant centres [20]. The UCSF group recently reported long-term outcomes in 118 patients initially outwith UCSF criteria entered into a downstaging protocol. Sixty-four patients were successfully downstaged and received a transplant; of this group 7.5% had HCC recurrence. Duvoux and colleagues have used pre-transplant AFP, tumour size and tumour number to categorise patients as "low risk" or "high risk" (Table 8.2) for recurrence and then re-categorise patients according to the response to LRT. Patients who are initially high risk but following LRT meet low-risk criteria have the same HCC recurrence, 14.3% over 4 years, as patients with low-risk HCC throughout. Patients who are low risk and then progress to high risk had 58% 4-year recurrence, and patients who were high risk throughout had 65% 4-year recurrence.

In the UK, there is a pilot programme to offer liver transplant to patients who achieve downstaging to a Duvoux score of ≤2 and demonstrate stable tumour characteristics over 6 months. At present, 12 patients are registered and have received transplants in this ongoing pilot.

**Table 8.2** Duvoux criteria for liver transplantation for patients with hepatocellular carcinoma incorporating AFP. Patients with score ≤ 2 are categorised as "low risk" and score > 2 high risk for post-transplant recurrence [20]

| Variable | Points |
|---|---|
| Largest Diameter (cm) | |
| ≤3 | 0 |
| 3–6 | 1 |
| >6 | 4 |
| Number of nodules | |
| 1–3 | 0 |
| ≥4 | 2 |
| AFP (ng/ml) | |
| ≤100 | 0 |
| 100–1000 | 2 |
| >1000 | 3 |

## Types of Donor Liver

Most patients receiving a liver transplant receive a whole organ from a deceased donor after brain death is confirmed. As the demand for organ transplant exceeds supply, surgical innovations have been introduced to expand the donor pool.

These are:

1. Deceased donors after cardiac or circulatory death (DCD).
2. Split liver transplant, when the whole organ is separated and right and left lobes transplanted into two recipients. Usually the left lobe is transplanted into a paediatric recipient and the right lobe into an adult. Left lobe transplant into adult recipient has been reported with successful outcome.
3. Adult-to-adult living donor liver transplant (LDLT). Again it is usually the right lobe that is donated and transplanted into an adult recipient. In some countries, such as Japan, deceased donors are very limited, and the most frequent transplants are LDLT.

During DCD organ retrieval, there is an additional period when the liver is exposed to warm ischaemia. There is a higher incidence of primary non-function and ischaemic biliary injury, leading to an ischaemic cholangiopathy, in patients receiving DCD transplants. As many patients with HCC undergoing transplants have preserved synthetic liver function and performance status compared to patients with decompensated cirrhosis, this group is more likely to receive a transplant from one of these more marginal donors.

Inferior survival for patients with HCC receiving DCD organs has been demonstrated using UNOS data [21]. Analysis of over 76,000 patients receiving transplants between 1995 and 2011 compared outcomes in patients transplanted for HCC or non-HCC and also patients receiving DBD or DCD donor livers in each group. Patients with HCC had lower 5-year survival compared with non-HCC recipients whether receiving DBD or DCD donors with the lowest 5-year survival in the HCC/DCD group (Table 8.3). This may be influenced by differences in recipient characteristics as patients transplanted for HCC were older and more were hepatitis C positive. Furthermore, the time period studied includes the introduction of DCD transplantation. In general, outcome improves with time, so this study includes patients transplanted at the start of DCD programmes who would be expected overall to have an inferior outcome.

**Table 8.3** 1-, 3- and 5-year post-transplant survival in patients comparing patients receiving DBD or DCD donor liver transplants and comparing HCC with non-HCC indication, UNOS data [21]

| Group | 1 Year | 3 Years | 5 Years |
|---|---|---|---|
| HCC-DBD | 84.29% | 72.23% | 63.77% |
| Non-HCC–DBD | 86.50% | 78.97% | 73.24% |
| HCC-DCD | 75.98% | 63.87% | 55.86% |
| Non-HCC–DCD | 85.79% | 76.76% | 70.52% |

UK transplant centres presented data for patients receiving liver transplants over a 5-year period at the national British Liver Transplant Group meeting, Sept. 2017 (Data unpublished). The proportion of patients with HCC receiving DCD transplants numerically exceeded each centre's overall DCD rate. Overall, currently 28% of UK patients receive a DCD transplant. In the seven UK centres, the proportion of HCC patients receiving a DCD transplant ranged from 18 to 49%. The two centres with the highest proportion of DCD transplants also reported lowest 5-year survival. In UK recipients, the two commonest causes of graft loss are liver-related and recurrent HCC.

At present, the standard process for organ retrieval incorporates a period of cold storage prior to organ implantation. A novel innovation is to use normothermic machine perfusion (NMP) prior to implantation of the donor liver. This allows the function of the donor organ to be observed, through measuring such factors as lactate and ALT, which is not the case with standard retrieval. This has two main advantages: to avoid transplanting an organ that does not function well and also may allow transplantation of donor livers that appear too high risk but during observation function adequately. Theoretically, NMP has potential to expand the donor pool and improve transplant outcomes, and studies are underway to evaluate the technology.

## Effect of Immunosuppression on Outcome Following Liver Transplant for HCC

Immune surveillance is now known to be critically important as a physiological mechanism to prevent the development and progression of solid organ cancers. Therefore, in patients receiving liver transplants for HCC, immunosuppression could influence the risk of recurrence and death from recurrence. The goal of immunosuppression is to prevent rejection but also to minimise the side effect. The most frequent initial immunosuppression regime consists of a combination of corticosteroids, azathioprine or mycophenolate, and a calcineurin inhibitor, tacrolimus or ciclosporin. Biological agents against IL2 receptors such as basiliximab are used in patients with early renal dysfunction to reduce CNI exposure.

The mammalian target of rapamycin (mTOR) pathway is central to control of cell proliferation. mTOR inhibitors are immunosuppressive (sirolimus and everolimus) and theoretically might also have an effect on cancer occurrence in liver transplant recipients. Retrospective analyses suggested an antineoplastic effect of mTOR inhibition in liver transplant recipient. A randomised controlled trial comparing early sirolimus immunosuppression vs. standard immunosuppression in over 500 LT/HCC recipients did not show a significant difference in recurrence-free survival at the study end [22]. In the subgroup analyses, improved 3-year survival was noted at 3 years post-transplant in the sirolimus group, and the greatest improvement was seen in patients who were histologically within Milan criteria.

## Conclusion

Liver transplantation offers the prospect to treat both HCC and cirrhosis with good medium- and long-term survival for patients with HCC. Key areas for research are optimisation of patient selection, achieving good outcome with marginal donors and prevention and treatment of HCC recurrence.

## References

1. Starzl TE, Groth CG, Brettschneider L, Moon JB, Fulginiti VA, Cotton EK, Porter KA. Extended survival in 3 cases of orthotopic homotransplantation of the human liver. Surgery. 1968;63(4):549–63.
2. Mazzaferro V, Regalia E, Doci R, Andreola S, Pulvirenti A, Bozzetti F, Montalto F, Ammatuna M, Morabito A, Gennari L. Liver transplantation for the treatment of small hepatocellular carcinomas in patients with cirrhosis. N Engl J Med. 1996;334(11):693–9.
3. Roayaie S, Blume IN, Thung SN, Guido M, Fiel M, Hiotis S, Labow DM, Llovet JN. Schwartz MEA system of classifying microvascular invasion to predict outcome after resection in patients with hepatocellular carcinoma. Gastroenterology. 2009;137(3):850–5.
4. Yao FY, Ferrell L, Bass NM, Watson JJ, Bacchetti P, Venook A, Ascher NL, Roberts JP. Liver transplantation for hepatocellular carcinoma: expansion of the tumor size limits does not adversely impact survival. Hepatology. 2001;33(6):1394–403.
5. Zheng SS, Xu X, Wu J, Chen J, Wang WL, Zhang M, Liang TB, Wu LM. Liver transplantation for hepatocellular carcinoma: Hangzhou experiences. Transplantation. 2008;85(12):1726–32.
6. Lee SG, Hwang S, Moon DB, Ahn CS, Kim KH, Sung KB, Ko GY, Park KM, Ha TY, Song GW. Expanded indication criteria of living donor liver transplantation for hepatocellular carcinoma at one large-volume center. Liver Transpl. 2008;14(7):935–45.
7. Mazzaferro V, Llovet JM, Miceli R, Bhoori S, Schiavo M, Mariani L, Camerini T, Roayaie S, Schwartz ME, Grazi GL, Adam R, Neuhaus P, Salizzoni M, Bruix J, Forner A, De Carlis L, Cillo U, Burroughs AK, Troisi R, Rossi M, Gerunda GE, Lerut J, Belghiti J, Boin I, Gugenheim J, Rochling F, Van Hoek B, Majno P. Metroticket Investigator Study Group. Predicting survival after liver transplantation in patients with hepatocellular carcinoma beyond the Milan criteria: a retrospective, exploratory analysis. Lancet Oncol. 2009;10(1):35–43.
8. Takada Y, Uemoto S. Liver transplantation for hepatocellular carcinoma: the Kyoto experience. J Hepatobiliary Pancreat Sci. 2010;17(5):527–32.
9. Yao FY, Xiao L, Bass NM, Kerlan R, Ascher NL, Roberts JP. Liver transplantation for hepatocellular carcinoma: validation of the UCSF-expanded criteria based on preoperative imaging. Am J Transplant. 2007;7(11):2587–96.
10. Takada Y, Kaido T, Shirabe K, Nagano H, Egawa H, Sugawara Y, Taketomi A, Takahara T, Wakabayashi G, Nakanishi C, Kawagishi N, Kenjo A, Gotoh M, Toyoki Y, Hakamada K, Ohtsuka M13, Akamatsu N, Kokudo N, Takeda K, Endo I, Takamura H, Okajima H, Wada H, Kubo S, Kuramitsu K, Ku Y, Ishiyama K, Ohdan H, Ito E, Maehara Y, Honda M, Inomata Y, Furukawa H, Uemoto S2, Yamaue H, Miyazaki M, Takada T. LTx-PET study group of the Japanese Society of Hepato-Biliary-Pancreatic Surgery and the Japanese Liver Transplantation Society. Significance of preoperative fluorodeoxyglucose-positron emission tomography in prediction of tumor recurrence after liver transplantation for hepatocellular carcinoma patients: a Japanese multicenter study. J Hepatobiliary Pancreat Sci. 2017;24(1):49–57.

11. Pommergaard HC, Burcharth J, Rosenberg J, Rasmussen A. Serologic and molecular biomarkers for recurrence of hepatocellular carcinoma after liver transplantation: a systematic review and meta-analysis. Transplant Rev. 2016;30:171–7.
12. Han K, Tzimas GN, Barkun JS, Metrakos P, Tchervenkov JI, Hilzenrat N, Wong P, Deschênes M. Preoperative alpha-fetoprotein slope is predictive of hepatocellular carcinoma recurrence after liver transplantation. Can J Gastroenterol. 2007;21:39–45.
13. Viberta E, Azoulay D, Hotia E, Iacopinellia S, Samuel D, Sallouma C, Lemoine A, Bismuth H, Castaing D, Adam R. Progression of alphafetoprotein before liver transplantation for hepatocellular carcinoma in cirrhotic patients: a critical factor. Am J Transplant. 2010;10:129–37.
14. Lai Q, Inostroza M, Rico Juri JM, Goffette P, Lerut J. Delta-slope of alpha-fetoprotein improves the ability to select liver transplant patients with hepatocellular cancer. HPB (Oxford). 2015;17:1085–95.
15. Farid WR, Verhoeven CJ, de Jonge J, Metselaar HJ, Kazemier G, Van der Laan LJW. The ins and outs of microRNAs as biomarkers in liver disease and transplantation. Transpl Int. 2014;27(12):1222–32.
16. Sugimachi K, Matsumura T, Hirata H, Uchi R, Ueda M, Ueo H, Shinden Y, Iguchi T, Eguchi H, Shirabe K, Ochiya T, Maehara Y, Mimori K. Identification of a bona fide microRNA biomarker in serum exosomes that predicts hepatocellular carcinoma recurrence after liver transplantation. Br J Cancer. 2015;112(3):532–8.
17. NHS blood and transplant annual report 2017. https://nhsbtdbe.blob.core.windows.net/umbraco-assets-corp/5007/annual_liver_transplantation_report_2017.pdf.
18. Parikh ND, Waljee AK, Singal AG. Downstaging hepatocellular carcinoma: a systematic review and pooled analysis. Liver Transpl. 2015;21(9):1142–52.
19. Yao FY, Kerlan RK Jr, Hirose R, Davern TJ 3rd, Bass NM, Feng S, Peters M, Terrault N, Freise CE, Ascher NL, Roberts JP. Excellent outcome following down-staging of hepatocellular carcinoma prior to liver transplantation: an intention-to-treat analysis. Hepatology. 2008;48(3):819–27.
20. Duvoux C, Roudot-Thoraval F, Decaens T, Pessione F, Badran H, Piardi T, Francoz C, Compagnon P, Vanlemmens C, Dumortier J, Dharancy S, Gugenheim J, Bernard PH, Adam R, Radenne S, Muscari F, Conti F, Hardwigsen J, Pageaux GP, Chazouillères O, Salame E, Hilleret MN, Lebray P, Abergel A, Debette-Gratien M, Kluger MD, Mallat A, Azoulay D, Cherqui D, Liver Transplantation French Study Group. Liver transplantation for hepatocellular carcinoma: a model including α-fetoprotein improves the performance of Milan criteria. Gastroenterology. 2012;143(4):986–94.
21. Croome KP, Wall W, Chandok N, Beck G, Marotta P, Hernandez-Alejandro R. Inferior survival in liver transplant recipients with hepatocellular carcinoma receiving donation after cardiac death liver allografts. Liver Transpl. 2013;19(11):1214–23.
22. Geissler EK, Schnitzbauer AA, Zülke C, Lamby PE, Proneth A, Duvoux C, Burra P, Jauch KW, Rentsch M, Ganten TM, Schmidt J, Settmacher U, Heise M, Rossi G, Cillo U, Kneteman N, Adam R, van Hoek B, Bachellier P, Wolf P, Rostaing L, Bechstein WO, Rizell M, Powell J, Hidalgo E, Gugenheim J, Wolters H, Brockmann J, Roy A, Mutzbauer I, Schlitt A, Beckebaum S, Graeb C, Nadalin S, Valente U, Turrión VS, Jamieson N, Scholz T, Colledan M, Fändrich F, Becker T, Söderdahl G, Chazouillères O, Mäkisalo H, Pageaux GP, Steininger R, Soliman T, de Jong KP, Pirenne J, Margreiter R, Pratschke J, Pinna AD, Hauss J, Schreiber S, Strasser S, Klempnauer J, Troisi RI, Bhoori S, Lerut J, Bilbao I, Klein CG, Königsrainer A, Mirza DF, Otto G, Mazzaferro V, Neuhaus P, Schlitt HJ. Sirolimus use in liver transplant recipients with hepatocellular carcinoma: a randomized, multicenter, open-label phase 3 trial. Transplantation. 2016;100(1):116–25.

# Chapter 9
# The Role of Interventional Radiology and Image-Guided Ablation in Primary Liver Cancer

**Jen-Jou Wong and Nabil Kibriya**

**Key Learning Points**

1. Percutaneous ablation is a valid curative treatment in patients who meet BCLC stages 0 or A.
2. Ablation should be considered where patients are not candidates for surgery or liver transplantation.
3. There are a range of thermal and nonthermal techniques available, the usage of which is dictated by local availability and expertise.
4. IRE provides an attractive ablation technique for preserving adjacent, heat sensitive structures.
5. Lesions <3 cm, up to maximum of three nodules, are considered for ablation in our institution; however these criteria continue to evolve with experience.

**Areas of Controversy and Uncertainty**

1. There is debate regarding the appropriateness of first-line ablation as preferable to liver resection as a first curative treatment.
2. The role of IRE, while promising, is yet to be fully defined in treatment algorithms.
3. Despite good evidence for effectiveness, treatment availability is variable and affected by funding and a shortage of appropriately trained clinicians.

---

J.-J. Wong (✉)
Department of Interventional Radiology, The Royal Liverpool University Hospital, Liverpool, UK

N. Kibriya
Kings College Hospital, London, UK
e-mail: Nabil.Kibriya@rlbuht.nhs.uk



T. Cross, D. H. Palmer (eds.), *Liver Cancers*,
https://doi.org/10.1007/978-3-319-92216-4_9

## Introduction

Hepatocellular carcinoma is the third most common cause of cancer deaths worldwide and the leading cause of mortality amongst sufferers of cirrhosis and chronic liver disease—the principal cause of death being liver failure. Over 500,000 patients are affected worldwide [1], and the incidence is likely to rise in tandem with the projected increase in the incidence of hepatitis B and C and excessive alcohol ingestion. While surgical resection remains the gold standard curative treatment, less than a third of patients are eligible due to not meeting Milan criteria for liver transplantation (one mass less than 5 cm, or up to three lesions less than 3 cm, without extrahepatic disease or portal hypertension) [2]. Those eligible for liver transplantation are likely to face extended waits given the relative lack of donors—patients are therefore at risk of progression without local disease control, although a period of waiting after loco-regional treatment to assess response can be considered in select patients who may best be served by liver transplantation. Median survival times are 4–6 months without treatment [3].

Percutaneous image-guided liver ablation has become established in the treatment of patients who fall outside of treatment criteria for surgery or poor performance status (PS > 1). Ablation carries a lower risk of complications and mortality due to its minimally invasive nature. Localised ablative treatment also preserves surrounding functional liver parenchyma. A lower procedural cost can be achieved due to shorter inpatient stays compared to surgery. A number of technologies are available, including radiofrequency, microwave, cryoablation and irreversible electroporation to cater for different treatment environments; each of these will be discussed in this chapter.

## Patient Selection

The diagnosis of HCC should be made in line with current guidelines—imaging with either contrast-enhanced CT or dynamic contrast-enhanced MRI and correlation with AFP should be diagnostic in most cases, with liver biopsy reserved for cases where there remains diagnostic uncertainty.

All patients being considered for ablation should be discussed at a multidisciplinary team (MDT) meeting to ensure relevant clinical, biochemical and imaging parameters are discussed and applied to an appropriate staging and treatment algorithm and to ensure other modalities of treatment, in particular surgery and liver transplantation, have been considered.

There are a number of staging and classification systems for HCC. Amongst them, the Barcelona Clinic Liver Cancer staging criteria have been most commonly referred to as the classification system of choice for determining staging, prognosis and guiding treatment (Fig. 9.1) [4]. Percutaneous ablation can be included as part of both curative and disease-control treatment paradigms. In summary, stage 0

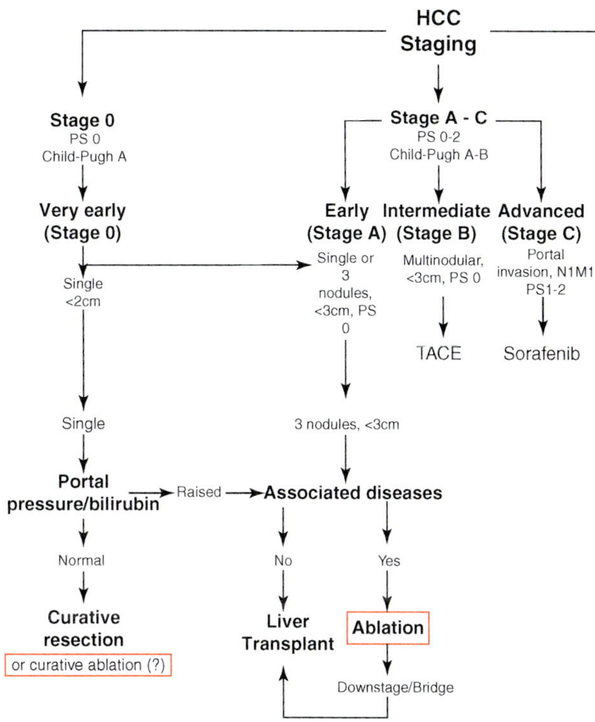


**Fig. 9.1** The roles of ablation in the management of HCC, adapted from the Barcelona Clinic Liver Criteria staging system [4]

patients who are fit and well with very early, single HCC are ideal for surgical resection. Stage A patients, with ≤3 nodules that are less than 3 cm may be suitable for liver transplantation if portal pressure or bilirubin are raised but are otherwise well; those with comorbidities are recommended to undergo ablation. Although not formally included in the guidelines, ablation can also be used to achieve local tumour control and either keep patients within or downgrade previously ineligible patients to meet the Milan criteria for liver transplantation [5]. Ablative treatment can thus provide the prospect of an extended window for waiting list viability given the shortage of donor organs worldwide.

Current evidence points towards surgical resection being superior to RF ablation, even in single small tumours (overall survival HR 0.56; 95% CI 0.40 to 0.78 and 2-year survival HR 0.38; 95% CI 0.17 to 0.84) [6]. Surgical resection should therefore be considered in the first instance, with ablation being reserved for patients who are unsuitable for surgery. It should be noted that many studies have been performed on Asian populations, where patient age and comorbidities are less—directly translating these results into treatment decisions for Western populations should therefore be considered with caution.

## Pre-assessment and Planning

After discussion at specialist MDT, patients should be assessed in a dedicated interventional oncology clinic by an interventional radiologist and hepatologist. The opportunity to meet patients is of paramount importance; assessing the patient's overall health status and suitability as a candidate for ablation can be performed with a direct clinical history and examination, in conjunction with review of the patient notes. An explanation of procedural details can be given, and expectations of the aim of treatment can also be managed (i.e., curative treatment versus disease control). An assessment of the suitability of the target lesion for ultrasound-guided intervention can be performed. Relevant biochemical workup such as full blood count, clotting screen and renal function (at a minimum) can also be arranged.

The potential for complications must be assessed and discussed with the patient (Fig. 9.2). Post-ablation syndrome is a relatively common occurrence, with around a third of patients experiencing flu-like symptoms, including fever, delayed pain, chills and nausea anywhere up to 2-weeks post-procedure. It is thought that ablation leads to the release of cytokines and the resultant inflammatory response as a consequence of necrotic tissue. The likelihood of disease recurrence grows with increasing tumour size and the number of lesions treated in a single sitting. Infection and abscess formation are known to occur post-ablation, and there are varying practices between institutions with regard to the role of prophylactic antibiotics. In our institution, abscess formation is a rare complication and too low in incidence to justify routine antibiotic administration, in line with available evidence [7]. If an abscess does occur, percutaneous drainage maybe necessary in addition to systemic antibiotics. Haemorrhage may occur due to venous bleeding, or more significantly from hepatic artery damage, and thus the possible need for emergency embolization

Potential complications of liver ablation:

- Haemorrhage
  - Intraperitoneal
  - Liver parenchyma
- Biliary damage
  - Biloma
  - Bile duct leak
- Thoracic injury
  - Diaphragmatic perforation
  - Pneumothorax
- Gastrointestinal tract perforation or thermal injury
- Liver abscess
- Portal vein thrombosis
- Tumour seeding
- Skin burns

**Fig. 9.2** Complications of percutaneous ablation

should be discussed with the patient. Non-target organ injury is unusual and not well described in the literature. Thermal damage to surrounding organs (in most cases, the gastrointestinal tract) should be avoided by reviewing previous planning or staging scans. It may be possible to hydro-dissect bowel away from the potential ablation zone, using an 18 g needle and 5% dextrose solution—otherwise reconsidering the appropriateness of thermal ablation against another treatment modality (such as irreversible electroporation, discussed later) may be necessary. Other possible complications include thermal damage to bile ducts, pneumothorax and skin burns.

A further consideration is for lesions adjacent to large vessels where thermal energy at the treatment site can be diminished by a "heat-sink" effect, resulting in less effective treatment and necrosis of the tumour.

Tumour seeding through the ablation tract is a significant possibility if tract ablation is not carried out, as high as 12.5% [8]. However, if tract ablation is performed correctly, tumour seeding incidence is around 1% [9]. If the needle is withdrawn too briskly during tract ablation, or if inappropriately sized or misplaced grounding pads are used in RF ablation, the possibility of superficial thermal burns is increased; second- and third-degree burns have been reported at a rate of 3% [10].

The use of ultrasound or CT-guided techniques is dependent on operator preference, the availability of imaging equipment and the optimum visualisation of the target lesion in the selected imaging modality. Ultrasound is used where possible to minimise radiation dose to both patient and operator and has the advantage of real-time needle guidance into the target lesion. Dual modality imaging can be performed in a dedicated CT intervention scanner enabling placement of the treatment needle with CT fluoroscopy performed during the procedure. An immediate post procedure CT is performed with contrast (if renal function allows) to assess the ablation zone and possible complications.

All available imaging should be reviewed to assess suitability for ablation and to provisionally plan needle entry, route and position. Trans-pleural needle access should be avoided due to patient discomfort and the risk of pneumothorax, haemothorax and pleural seeding. Size should first be assessed—the generally agreed upper limit for ablation is 3 cm. Tumours between 3 and 4.9 cm can still be considered but may require overlapping ablations, while those greater than 5 are at significant risk of incomplete first ablations and recurrence if an appropriately sized treatment margin of 1 cm cannot be achieved [11]. Lesions high in the hepatic dome, while more technically challenging to perform, can still be targeted with an approach starting beneath the thoracic cavity, with appropriate amount of cranial angulation and use of anatomical landmarks.

## Radiofrequency Ablation

Radiofrequency ablation (RFA) utilises the principle of an alternating electrical field to generate radiofrequency waves, which dissipate their energy within the surrounding target tissue as heat. This is achieved by an alternating electric current

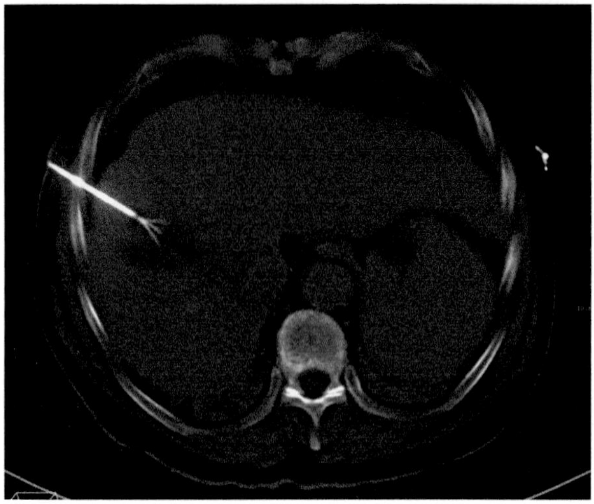

**Fig. 9.3** Radiofrequency ablation of an HCC. The probe is initially inserted with a single tip into the lesion. Once a satisfactory position is achieved, multiple tines can be extended to achieve an appropriately sized ablation zone

causing ionic agitation, generating frictional heat. Eventually, coagulative necrosis of the target tissue is reached. The RFA probe is connected to the generator, which in turn gives basic information such as probe temperature, total ablation time and ablation efficiency. A target temperature of at least 50 °C must be maintained, with the total ablation time dependent on the size of the target lesion and generally dictated by the instructions for use of the machine being used.

Heat dissipates away from the tip of the probe, and heat conductance can be significantly altered by varying impedance characteristics of treated, charred tissue. Depending on the manufacturer, multiple arrays can be extended from within a single delivery needle to achieve target temperatures at each tip within a different portion of the target lesion (Fig. 9.3).

The effectiveness of RFA can be limited where the target area is adjacent to a blood vessel with relatively high flow. A "heat-sink" effect may occur, whereby heat generated is dissipated by adjacent flowing blood, limiting the target temperatures achieved and increasing the risk of incomplete ablation or early recurrence. Caution should therefore be exercised if the intended target lesion is adjacent either to hepatic or portal veins.

When performed under CT fluoroscopy, an immediate assessment of the ablation zone can be performed—low attenuation change and small bubbles of gas can be discerned easily on non-contrast CT. Contrast-enhanced scanning can be performed if complications are suspected. The same cannot be said of ultrasound-guided treatment, where the presence of gas around and at the ablation zone post-treatment makes it an unreliable modality to use in the immediate assessment of the ablation zone.

## Microwave Ablation

Microwave ablation (MWA) aims to achieve coagulative necrosis of target lesions by alternating electromagnetic waves in the spectrum between 900 and 2450 MHz. Taking advantage of the asymmetrical polarity of water molecules, alternating electromagnetic waves cause adjacent water molecules to flip 2–5 billion times a second, resulting in frictional heat that is required to achieve target temperatures [12].

The needle differs significantly from its RFA counterpart—there are no multiple arrays, although systems do exist where several separate probes can be attached and inserted. The ablation zone may be elliptically shaped or spherical depending on the system selected. Additionally, the centre of the ablation zone may be located proximal to the probe tip, or near to it, depending on the way the technology has been implemented (Fig. 9.4). Familiarity with the specific system utilised is therefore of importance. The size of the ablation zone is controlled by the duration of ablation, and also the power delivered to the antennae varied according to each manufacturer's system.

The advantage of MWA over RFA is that the method of heat induction permits target temperatures to be reached more quickly and that there is a reduced susceptibility to heat-sink effects (at least in the immediate ablation zone—the margin may still be susceptible to sub-treatment temperatures) [13, 14]. An upper limit of approximately 4 cm is still generally accepted as the maximum size of a treatable target lesion, although overlapping ablations of larger tumours is feasible. Lesions greater than 5 cm are less likely to achieve initial complete response [11]. A recent meta-analysis suggests that MWA performed similarly to RFA—complete response

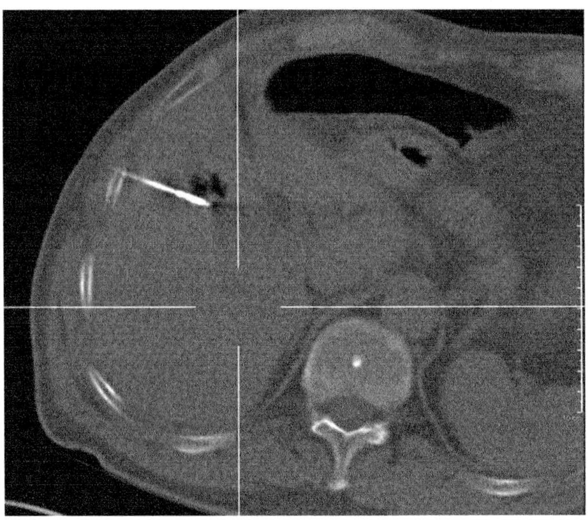

**Fig. 9.4** MWA needle within the liver during treatment. Low attenuation surrounding the tip represents gas generated during thermal coagulative necrosis. The dark band proximal to the needle tip indicates the central point at which the ablation zone will be generated

and recurrence rates were superior on the MWA group though not statistically significant, but MWA outperformed RFA in the sub-analysis of larger lesions ($p = 0.02$) [15].

## Cryoablation

Cryoablation (CA) relies on alternate freezing and thawing to destroy tissues. The technique is based on the Joule-Thomson effect, where compressed argon gas is forced through the tip of the probe, rapidly reducing in pressure and temperature. As a consequence, ice crystals form in intra- and extracellular spaces, drawing water molecules to either side of the cell membrane to form crystals and causing irreparable damage to the membrane and other cellular structures.

Use of CA in comparison to RFA and MWA has been less readily adopted in the UK. The encapsulated structure of HCC has been proposed to lend itself to thermal techniques, because heat is retained within the capsule, and therefore higher temperatures can be achieved and sustained. But some studies suggest that similar complete response and overall survival rates can be achieved with cryoablation as with RFA or MWA [16–18]. A possible advantage over thermal ablation is that the ice ball is more easily identified on CT or US guidance, permitting more reliable assessment of the post-treatment zone and likely effectiveness. However, morbidity and mortality may be slightly higher with this method, as the lack of vessel cauterisation leads to a greater risk of bleeding and a lesser effect on coagulation may predispose necrotic by-products of cryoablation to enter to bloodstream, causing thrombocytopenia and renal dysfunction [18]. The size of the ice ball generated is specific to each needle, making equipment choice and availability more critical than for RFA and MWA, which offer the flexibility of varying ablation zone sizes through adjusting needle or system parameters. Additionally, it is not possible to tract ablate; thus there is a theoretically increased risk of tract seeding.

## Irreversible Electroporation (IRE)

IRE is a new technology that relies on the production of ultrashort but strong electrical fields to create nanopores in cell membranes. Originally developed at a reversible state to deliver DNA and other potential medicinal vectors into a cell, it was realised that increasing the electrical field led to permanency of the open pores in the cell membrane, disrupting cell homeostasis and inducing apoptosis, in contrast to the coagulative necrosis induced by thermal ablation methods. Unlike thermal ablation, IRE spares extracellular matrix and collagenous tissues—e.g., large blood vessels and biliary ducts—making IRE an attractive option for those lesions near sensitive structures, particularly near the liver hilum, colon and gallbladder (Fig. 9.5). Furthermore, the method is not affected by a heat-sink effect of adjacent vessels.

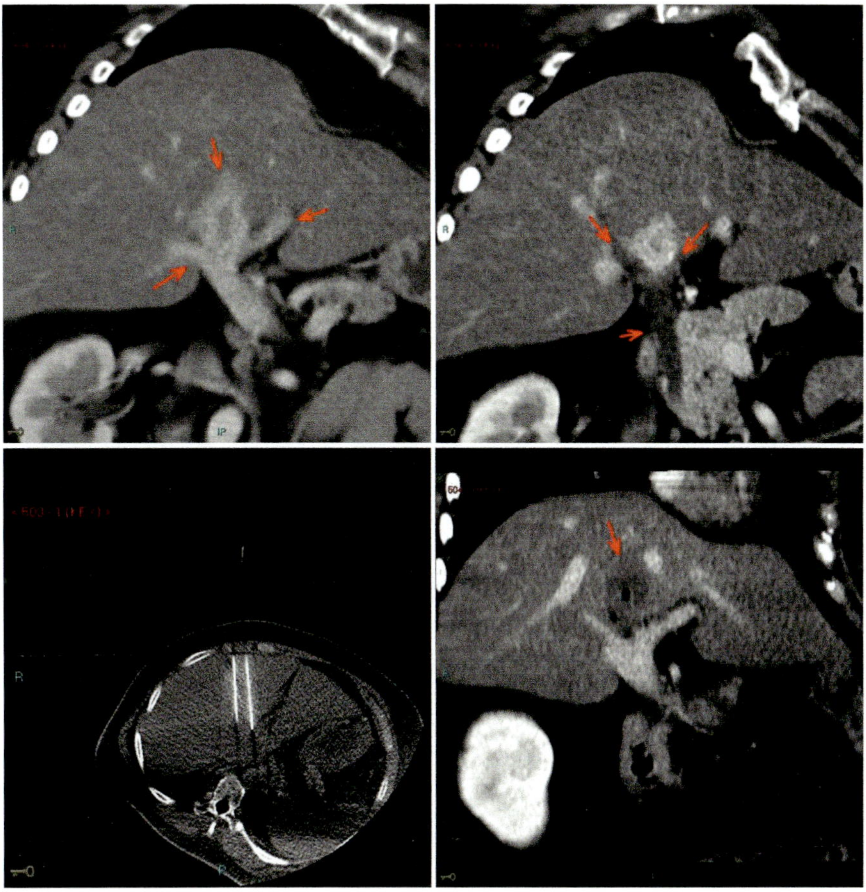

**Fig. 9.5** IRE treatment of a central HCC. The location of this lesion, wrapped by the main portal veins (top left) and also the biliary ducts (top right), raised concern for both heat-sink effect and biliary damage if thermal ablation was chosen. Instead a four-needle IRE treatment was performed, resulting in a successful ablation zone, with no collateral damage (bottom images)

At least two needle placements in parallel are required around the target lesion to form the circuit through which the electrical current is delivered, with an optimised needle distance of 2 cm. Larger lesions require more needles to maintain the 2 cm maximum distance, with a maximum of six needles. Each needle combination is tested to ensure the appropriate current (from 20 to 50 A) and voltages (1500 v/cm) are achieved, before the final pulses between each needle combination are delivered as the final treatment dose. General anaesthesia with muscle paralysis is required, as well as ECG gating. Needle placement can be performed by either CT or ultrasound guidance. Variables such as the voltage and degree of active needle tip exposure can be varied between test pulses to optimise the final treatment dose. The current system on the market is the NanoKnife™ system (Angiodynamics, NY, USA), utilising 19 gauge needles.

IRE is not universally available to the extent thermal ablation and is generally reserved for lesions that are deemed unsuitable for thermal ablation or surgical resection. Its utility and position in treatment algorithms are still not fully determined. Despite ablative damage to surrounding biliary and vascular structures being minimised by IRE itself, damage from needle placement remains a possibility and increased by the fact that at least two separate punctures for the minimum two needles are required. Mortality secondary to cardiac arrhythmias has been reported—this can be greatly reduced with the appropriate cardiac gating.

## Follow-Up and Prognosis

An approximation of the ablation zone can be made whether performed by ultrasound or CT guidance. Thermal ablation methods (i.e., RFA and MWA) when viewed under ultrasound guidance produce gas, which localises the treatment area, before spreading to obscure the field of view. When performed with CT fluoroscopy, the presence of low attenuation change gives an early indication of the ablation zone, although the changes may appear more extensive in the immediate aftermath of treatment compared to the true treatment area as assessed on subsequent follow-up scans.

Most centres treating with ablation techniques do so under general anaesthesia. Use of heavy sedation is possible, but high conversion rates to general anaesthetic have been reported [19]. For IRE, electrical stimulation from the electrodes induces muscles contractions and requires muscle paralysis. Thus, general anaesthesia is mandated followed by an overnight hospital stay that is usually warranted to monitor for possible complications.

At our institution a follow-up scan is performed at 4–6-week post-treatment. This provides sufficient time for post-ablation inflammatory changes to settle, since hyperaemic changes surrounding treated target lesions may otherwise be difficult to differentiate from recurrence. Contrast-enhanced MRI with diffusion-weighted imaging (DWI) is the preferred follow-up modality where there is no contraindication to MRI. Dynamic phase imaging is utilised to assess enhancement of residual tumour. Peripheral hyperaemia may be present in the immediate post-ablation setting; despite similar interpretation difficulties as with CT, DWI is extremely sensitive to detecting recurrence that may not be discernible on CT. Earlier re-intervention can therefore be planned, whether at previous treatment sites or against new target lesions. Triple-phase CT can be performed if MRI is contraindicated or not possible due to patient factors, e.g., the presence of claustrophobia, pacemakers or morbid obesity, although it is less sensitive to early recurrence or new tumours. CT is most useful in the immediate assessment of the macroscopic effects of the ablation zone, evidenced as low attenuation change post-ablation. Peripheral enhancement due to hyperaemic changes can be difficult to differentiate from recurrence or partial ablation. A nodular or eccentric rim enhancement should raise the suspicion of recurrence (Fig. 9.6). Invariably CT is used to assess for complications, e.g., hepatic

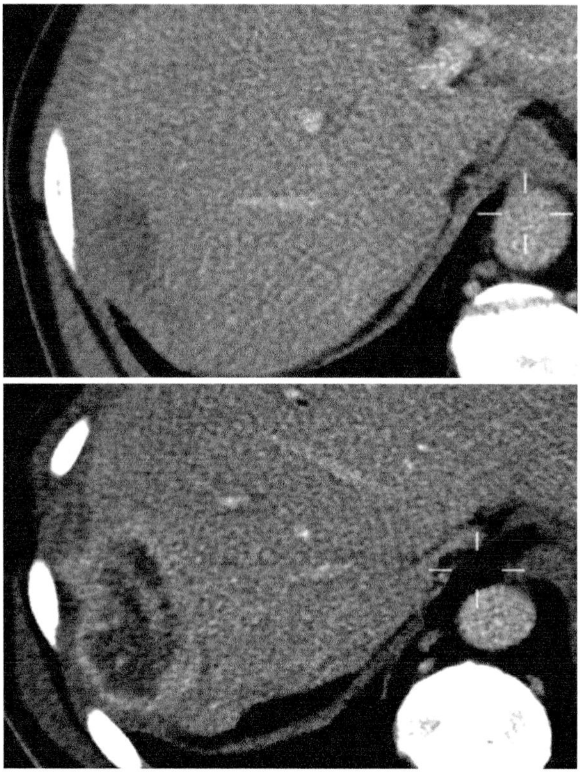

**Fig. 9.6** Initial follow-up scan in a patient treated with MWA, showing smooth, non-enhancing low attenuation change in keeping with matured ablation zone. In the same patient 18 months later, peripheral nodular enhancement surrounds the old ablation site in keeping with recurrence

artery bleed. PET CT has been used where successive CT or MRI follow-up scans have been inconclusive in differentiating post-treatment change from viable tumour. Post-ablation inflammation is FDG avid—delayed imaging by at least 2-month post-procedure allows the initial inflammatory response to resolve, thus making FDG avid abnormalities at this stage sensitive for viable tumour (Fig. 9.7). Yet its cost remains prohibitive in making this the primary follow-up modality, as well as having limited sensitivity to smaller changes that can be discerned only with contrast-enhanced cross axial imaging.

The literature regarding outcomes for liver ablation is significantly skewed towards RFA and MWA as they are the more established modalities compared to CA and IRE. There have been relatively few randomised controlled trials comparing the effectiveness of thermal ablation versus other standards of care. Three RCTs were included in a meta-analysis of randomised and non-randomised controlled trials comparing ablation against hepatic resection. The three non-blinded trials together showed similar recurrence-free survival rates at 1 and 3 years for RFA and resection, but RFA performed less well when pooled 3- and 5-year recurrence-free survival rates were reviewed (RR 1.48, 95% CI 1.14 to 1.94, and RR 1.52, 95% CI 1.18 to 1.97, respectively). Yet, the complication rates were lower in the RFA group (RR 0.18, 95% CI 0.06–0.53, NNT = 3.5) [20]. A later Cochrane meta-analysis

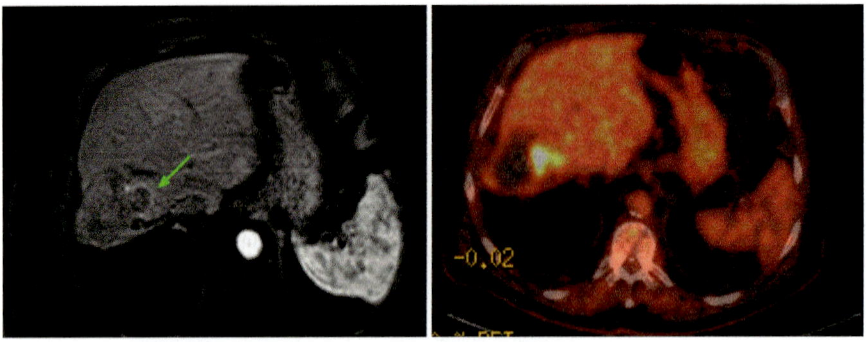


**Fig. 9.7** A thin rind of enhancement on arterial phase MRI typically indicates hyperaemia, but since this appearance was focal and had settled around the rest of the ablation margin, residual disease was suspected, as proven on PET CT

confirmed hepatic resection was more effective than RFA regarding overall survival (hazard ratio (HR) 0.56; 95% CI 0.40–0.78) and 2-year survival (HR 0.38; 95% CI 0.17–0.84) [6]. Surgical resection is considered the gold standard treatment where possible, but where this is not an option [2], ablation is a viable second treatment option. One of the most extensive retrospective reviews of 2982 ablations in 1170 HCC patients reported survival outcomes of 96.6%, 60.2% and 27.3% at 1, 5 and 10 years, respectively, demonstrating the effectiveness of thermal ablation [21].

Xu et al. reviewed 142 HCC patients with 294 treated nodules. Recurrence-free survival rates at 1, 3 and 5 years were reported at 76.1%, 33.1% and 19.5%, respectively [22]. Liang P, while not looking at recurrence-free survival, did report cumulative survival of 93% at 1 year, 82% at 2 years, 72% at 3 years, 63% at 4 years and 51% at 5 years in 288 patients [23]. In a comparative retrospective analysis, Xu et et al. reviewed 301 cases of MWA, reporting recurrence-free survival rates of 94.4%, 71.8% and 46.9% at 1, 3 and 5 years. Compared against 159 cases of RFA (89.9%, 67.3% and 54.9%), no statistical difference was found in local recurrence rates or overall survival [24]. Interestingly, lower rates of local tumour progression in larger treated lesions have been reported in a meta-analysis comparing MWA against RFA [25].

As the role of IRE is generally restricted to situations where tumours are considered to be not amenable to ablation or surgery, reports of effectiveness are restricted to smaller numbers and observational studies. Thomson reported complete ablation in 82% of patients who had HCC ($n = 17$) in an early human study of the effectiveness of IRE. More recently Sutter et al. retrospectively analysed one of the largest cohorts of HCC to date, treating 75 tumours in 58 patients; 6- and 12-month overall local tumour progression-free survival rates were 87% (95% confidence interval [CI] 77%, 93%) and 70% (95% CI 56%, 81%), respectively [26]. Our own unpublished bi-institutional data ($n = 52$, including both HCC and colorectal liver metastases) reports a more modest median time to progression of 8 months. At 12 months, the percentage that was progression free was 49% (95% CI 30%–66%) (N Kibriya - personal communication).

Although multiple small studies have demonstrated the efficacy of IRE as a non-thermal ablative treatment in HCC, these have mostly been part of a mix of aetiologies—further studies are required to further assess the impact of IRE and where it is best used in the treatment armamentarium.

## References


1. Montalto G, Cervello M, Giannitrapani L, Dantona F, Terranova A, Castagnetta LA. Epidemiology, risk factors, and natural history of hepatocellular carcinoma. Ann N Y Acad Sci. 2002;963:13–20.
2. Belghiti J, Kianmanesh R. Surgical treatment of hepatocellular carcinoma. HPB (Oxford). 2005;7(1):42–9.
3. Nagase N, Yuki H, Hamada T, Hirose S, Kawashima R, Inokuchi K. The natural history of hepatocellular carcinoma. A study of 100 untreated cases. Cancer. 1984;54(7):1461–5.
4. Llovet JM, Fuster J, Buix J. The Barcelona approach; diagnosis, staging and treatment of hepatocellular carcinoma. Liver Transpl. 2004;10:115–20.
5. Pompili M, Francica G, Ponziani FR, Iezzi R, Avolio AW. Bridging and downstaging treatments for hepatocellular carcinoma in patients on the waiting list for liver transplantation. World J Gastroenterol. 2013;19(43):7515–30.
6. Weis S, Franke A, Mössner J, Jakobsen JC, Schoppmeyer K. Radiofrequency (thermal) ablation versus no intervention or other interventions for hepatocellular carcinoma. Cochrane Database Syst Rev. 2013;12:CD003046.
7. Bhatia S, et al. Is antibiotic prophylaxis for percutaneous radiofrequency ablation (RFA) of primary liver tumors necessary? Results from a single-center experience. Cardiovasc Intervent Radiol. 2015;38(4):922–8.
8. Llovet JM, Vilana R, Brú C, et al. Barcelona Clínic Liver Cancer (BCLC) Group Increased risk of tumor seeding after percutaneous radiofrequency ablation for single hepatocellular carcinoma. Hepatology. 2001;33(5):1124–9.
9. Stigliano R, Marelli L, Yu D, Davies N, Patch D, Burroughs AK. Seeding following percutaneous diagnostic and therapeutic approaches for hepatocellular carcinoma. What is the risk and the outcome? Seeding risk for percutaneous approach of HCC. Cancer Treat Rev. 2007;33(5):437–47.
10. Mulier S, Mulier P, Ni Y, et al. Complications of radiofrequency coagulation of liver tumours. Br J Surg. 2002;89(10):1206–22.
11. Wang T, et al. Microwave ablation of hepatocellular carcinoma as first-line treatment: long term outcomes and prognostic factors in 221 patients. Sci Rep. 2016;6:32728.
12. Brace C. Microwave ablation technology: What every user should know. Curr Probl Diagn Radiol. 2009;38(2):61–7.
13. Simon CJ, Dupuy DE, Mayo-Smith WW. Microwave ablation: principles and applications. Radiographics. 2005;25(Suppl 1):S69–83.
14. Wright AS, Sampson LA, Warner TF, Mahvi DM, Lee FT Jr. Radiofrequency versus microwave ablation in a hepatic porcine model. Radiology. 2005;236(1):132–9.
15. Facciorusso A, Di Maso M, Muscatiello N. Microwave ablation versus radiofrequency ablation for the treatment of hepatocellular carcinoma: a systematic review and meta-analysis. Int J Hyperth. 2016;32(3):339–44.
16. Wang C, et al. Multicenter randomized controlled trial of percutaneous cryoablation versus radiofrequency ablation in hepatocellular carcinoma. Hepatology. 2015;61(5):1579–90.
17. Rong G, et al. Long-term outcomes of percutaneous cryoablation for patients with hepatocellular carcinoma within Milan criteria. PLoS One. 2015;10(4):e0123065.

18. Wu S, Hou J, Ding Y, Wu F, Hu Y, Jiang Q, Mao P, Yang Y. Cryoablation versus radiofrequency ablation for hepatic malignancies. Medicine (Baltimore). 2015;94(49):e2252.
19. Chakravorty E, et al. Anaesthetic management of radiofrequency tumour ablation: or experience. Indian J Anaesth. 2006;50:123–7.
20. Wang Y, Luo Q, Li Y, Deng S, Wei S, Li X. Radiofrequency ablation versus hepatic resection for small hepatocellular carcinomas: a meta-analysis of randomized and nonrandomized controlled trials. PLoS One. 2014;9(1):e84484.
21. Shiina S, et al. Radiofrequency ablation for hepatocellular carcinoma: 10-year outcome and prognostic factors. Am J Gastroenterol. 2012;107(4):569–77.
22. Xu Y, et al. Microwave ablation for the treatment of hepatocellular carcinoma that met up-to-seven criteria: feasibility, local efficacy and long-term outcomes. Eur Radiol. 2017;27(9):3877–87.
23. Liang P, et al. Prognostic factors for survival in patients with hepatocellular carcinoma after percutaneous microwave ablation. Radiology. 2005;235(1):299–307.
24. Xu Y, et al. Microwave ablation is as effective as radiofrequency ablation for very-early-stage hepatocellular carcinoma. Chin J Cancer. 2017;36(1):14.
25. Chinnaratha MA, Chuang MY, Fraser RJ, Woodman RJ, Wigg AJ. Percutaneous thermal ablation for primary hepatocellular carcinoma: A systematic review and meta-analysis. J Gastroenterol Hepatol. 2016;31(2):294–301.
26. Sutter O, et al. Safety and efficacy of irreversible electroporation for the treatment of hepatocellular carcinoma not amenable to thermal ablation techniques: a retrospective single-center case series. Radiology. 2017;284(3):877–86.

# Chapter 10
# Transarterial Embolization Therapies in Hepatocellular Carcinoma: Principles of Management

**Tim Cross and Jonathan C. Evans**

**Key Learning Points**

1. Transarterial embolization therapies are accepted as effective strategies for patients with intermediate stage HCC (BCLC B).
2. They can be used as a palliative treatment to prolong overall survival, as a bridge to curative treatments in particular liver transplantation or to downstage disease such that curative options including ablative therapies or transplantation might be considered.
3. TACE should not be given where there is complete portal vein occlusion due to the risk of significant liver ischaemia and subsequent liver decompensation and death.
4. The overall fitness of the patient should be considered, and in the main reserved for patients with child-Pugh a cirrhosis and performance status 0.
5. The use of tools such as HAP and ART may help identify patients unlikely to benefit from TACE.

**Areas of Controversy and Uncertainty**

1. None of the embolic techniques (TAE, TACE, DEB-TACE) have been shown to be consistently better than any other in terms of objective response or patient survival. This suggests that it is the embolic component of treatment and not the chemotherapeutic component that is key in determining response.

T. Cross (✉) · J. C. Evans
Department of Hepatology, The Royal Liverpool Hospital, Liverpool, UK

Department of Radiology, The Royal Liverpool Hospital, Liverpool, UK
e-mail: Tim.Cross@rlbuht.nhs.uk



T. Cross, D. H. Palmer (eds.), *Liver Cancers*,
https://doi.org/10.1007/978-3-319-92216-4_10

2. How to treat patients without a radiological response to initial TACE should be reviewed to determine if further TACE is beneficial or an alternative approach should be sought earlier.
3. The practice of giving TAE or SIRT when the patient is more frail and giving alternative forms of TACE in nonresponders, e.g., cisplatin and irinotecan, should be assessed to provide a more robust evidence base.

## Introduction

Hepatocellular carcinoma (HCC) is the sixth commonest cancer worldwide and the third commonest cause of cancer-related death [1, 2]. With a significant proportion of patients presenting at this stage of disease, the use and refinement of transarterial embolic therapies remain an area of interest and research. In the USA, it is estimated that between 1976 and 1980 in comparison with 2011, the incidence of HCC has risen from 1.4/100,0000 cases to 6.2/100,000 cases [1]. The intention of treatment is primarily to prolong survival in comparison with doing nothing, but the risks of toxicity; the potentially detrimental impact on liver function, which may reduce rather than prolong survival; and the impact on quality of life of the patient must be discussed honestly with the patient. Although HCC is seen in non-cirrhotic patients (in particular those with chronic hepatitis B infection), in the UK cirrhosis accounts for the majority of patients with chronic hepatitis C infection (CHC), and non-alcoholic fatty liver disease (NAFLD) accounts for an increasing proportion of HCC cases [3, 4]. The long-term survival is predicated by tumour stage at disease presentation. Patients who have their cancer detected at an early stage have a wider range of therapeutic choices and are more likely to live longer, when compared to those who present late [5–7].

The most commonly used algorithm for the staging and treatment of patients with HCC (as described earlier in the book) is that of the Barcelona Clinic Liver Cancer (BCLC) [8]. In this classification, stages 0–A are considered curable. Stage B is intermediate disease where palliative treatments may slow disease progression or provide a route to curative therapies at a later time, e.g., liver transplantation through downstaging where there is liver-confined disease. Thus, patients with stage B disease at the time of first treatment are considered to be; unresectable, untransplantable and unablatable. TACE is reserved for patients with unresectable and unablatable disease or patients being bridged to liver transplant; thus the majority of patients are BCLC stage B. Even with patients with technically incurable disease, our treatment aim is to elicit a response and downstage the tumour such that a curative option might be considered in the future, e.g., liver transplantation or ablation. In this group of patients, resection is rarely, if ever possible, after TACE. Thus, according to the algorithm, 20% of patients should be found at this stage with a median survival of 20 months (range 14–45 months) [1]. In a UK survey of the provision of ultrasound surveillance for HCC, on a snapshot of 1-month referrals for discussion of HCC multidisciplinary meetings (MDTs), 76 (24%) of 323 patients presented with BCLC stage B disease [9]. Stage C, advanced HCC occurs when there are metastatic deposits (in bone, lymph nodes, lungs, portal vein involvement) but, without liver decompensation, for who systemic therapies might be considered, e.g., sorafenib, lenvatinib, and immunotherapies. Finally, stage D disease occurs in patients with decompensated liver disease in who the prognosis is very poor irrespective of any treatment offered.

## Pathophysiology

The predominant blood supply to the liver parenchyma is from the portal vein. Interestingly, this is not the case for hepatocellular carcinomas. These are predominantly hypervascular tumours that derive their circulation from the hepatic artery. This is, therefore, something that can be exploited when treating patients. The rationale is that by targeting the arterial supply, the healthy "normal" liver tissue is spared from significant liver injury. The analogy is that of a medieval-walled city under siege, where the tumour is the city. The tumour has its "lines of supply" cut off, and so the nutrients sustaining the cancer are removed, and so the tumour dies from ischaemia and subsequently tissue necrosis. Transarterial embolization (TAE) works using this mechanism alone, whereas transarterial chemoembolic therapies (TACE) apply this approach whilst also providing a second hit from directly injecting chemotherapeutic agents or drug-eluting beads laced with toxic drugs. It is postulated that the latter enhance cancer cell death.

## Patient Workup

At our institution once HCC is suspected, the patient is seen in a dedicated liver cancer clinic with a consultant hepatologist and a nurse specialist. A hepatologist explains what has been found and what its implications may be and what the treatment options are. The clinician takes a history and examines the patient to make an assessment of the fitness of the patient as defined by their performance status (measured by the ECOG classification) (Table 10.1) [10]. The diagnostic and staging tests begin with blood tests including full blood count, urea and electrolytes, liver function tests, clotting, alpha-foetoprotein, ca19-9 and carcinoma embryonic antigen (CEA) and a liver screen to try to determine underlying cause, e.g., viral hepatitis (hepatitis B surface antigen, hepatitis B core antibody, hepatitis C antibody), ferritin, alpha-1 antitrypsin and autoimmune liver screen and immunoglobulins. Imaging tests consist of MRI liver, CT chest and, in cases where liver transplantation is the planned treatment, a bone scan to look for bone metastases. In patients unable to tolerate a MRI, a triple-phase CT with intravenous contrast is performed.

**Table 10.1** The ECOG performance status score [10]

| Score | Measures of performance |
|---|---|
| 0 | Fully active, able to carry on all pre-disease performance without restriction |
| 1 | Restricted in physically strenuous activity but ambulatory and able to carry out work of a light or sedentary nature, e.g. light housework and office work |
| 2 | Ambulatory and capable of all self-care but unable to carry out any work activities; up and about more than 50% of waking hours |
| 3 | Capable of only limited self-care; confined to bed or chair more than 50% of waking hours |
| 4 | Completely disabled; cannot carry on any self-care; totally confined to bed or chair |
| 5 | Dead |

Once all the investigations have been performed, the case is discussed at the weekly hepato-biliary cancer multidisciplinary team (MDT) meeting. This meeting is attended by hepatologists, diagnostic radiologists, interventional radiologists, hepatobiliary surgeons, medical oncologists, pathologists, clinical oncologists and nurse specialists. At our institution there is a consultant anaesthetist who attends the meeting. A management decision is made by the group.

If locoregional therapy is planned, including embolic therapies (ET), the patients are reviewed in the interventional radiology clinic. This allows the interventional radiologist to assess the patient and allows the patient to meet the person performing their treatment and provide them with an opportunity to ask questions. It is important to emphasize that this treatment of itself is not curative and the treatment may disrupt liver function and may induce liver decompensation as demonstrated by jaundice, ascites, spontaneous bacterial peritonitis and hepatic encephalopathy.

## Contraindications to Treatment

### *Absolute Contraindications*

Complete main branch portal vein thrombosis
Metastatic hepatocellular carcinoma
Ascites
Hepatic encephalopathy

### *Relative Contraindications (Applied in Our Unit)*

Non-occlusive bland thrombus
Portal vein (tumour) thrombus of second-order branches
Bilirubin >30
Albumin <34
ECOG performance status ≥1

Treatment should be delivered within 4 weeks of the imaging to guide therapy to ensure that the disease has not progressed to a level where ET would not deliver any benefit to the patient. Further blood tests are performed no more than 1 week prior to the treatment and should include full blood count, clotting studies (prothrombin time (PT) and activated partial thromboplastin time (APTT), as well as repeat urea and electrolytes (U&Es) and liver function tests (LFTs). The interventional radiologist performs the procedure using aseptic technique and at our centre blood product replacement, if the platelets are $<50 \times 10^9$, haemoglobin is <9 g/dl, the prothrombin time is >18 s (INR > 1.5), and the fibrinogen level is <1.0. The eGFR should be >30 ml/Kg/min. The patient is admitted on the morning of the procedure or the night before if they have a time travel period of >1 h.

## *Assessing the Risk of Doing Harm*

Although ET targets the arterial supply and hence should not incur any significant parenchymal damage, in reality, this is a risk, and ET may lead to a deterioration in liver synthetic function leading to liver failure and death. This constitutes a catastrophic outcome. To avoid this clinicians have been seeking tools that will help identify those patients in who treatment may do more harm. Kadalayil and colleagues performed an assessment of outcomes of patients treated by TACE or TAE at the Royal Free Hospital in London and the Queen Elizabeth Hospital in Birmingham, UK [11]. Patients were assigned one point if albumin <36 g/dl, bilirubin >17 μmol/l, AFP >400 ng/ml or size of dominant tumour >7 cm. The hepatoma arterial embolization prognostic (HAP) score was calculated by summing these points. Patients were divided into four risk groups based on their HAP scores; HAP A, B, C and D (scores 0, 1, 2 and >2, respectively). The median survival for the groups A, B, C and D was 27.6, 18.5, 9.0 and 3.6 months, respectively. Thus, patients with HAP C fared no better than patients with BCLC C disease, and patients with HAP D performed no better than patients with BCLC D disease in who would normally be offered best supportive care only [11]. A raised serum bilirubin which has been persistent for months or years would be less concerning than a recent sudden sharp rise, and this should always prompt further investigation and perhaps restaging of the disease. In our unit, TACE is rarely offered to patients with HAP ≥ C, and alternative treatments such as systemic therapies or SIRT should be considered where clinical intervention and performance status allow.

## Selection of Transarterial Embolic Therapy

Once the decision has been made that embolic therapy (ET) is indicated, it is the decision of the interventional radiologist, in conjunction with the MDT or their hepatologist to decide what ET should be chosen. This is an area of considerable discussion and controversy. The treatment options include conventional TACE (cTACE) where chemotherapic agents such as doxorubicin, cisplatin or mitomycin C are delivered by a feeding hepatic artery into the tumour and then the lesion is embolized with foam or sponge particles. Another option is to embolize the feeding vessel without the additional delivery of a chemotherapeutic agent by way of foam or embolizing microspheres called transarterial embolization (TAE). The final option is to deliver drug and embolization at the same time using microscopic beads laced with drug-eluting beads—DEB-TACE. Some of the key studies assessing the different modalities are summarized in Table 10.2 [12–21].

Since the introduction of embolic therapy, there have been ongoing studies to try to demonstrate the superiority of one method over another. A previously published meta-analysis did not demonstrate support of the use of either TAE or TACE in patients with unresectable liver-confined HCC. This meta-analysis consisted of 9 trials with 645 participants. Six trials compared TACE with control, and three trials compared TAE with control. The authors concluded that there was insufficient evidence to support its use until further studies were available [22].

## TACE Procedure

The procedure is performed with local anaesthesia at our institution. We use drug-eluting beads which are very well tolerated and rarely cause side effects. Patients receive 1 g of intravenous paracetamol upon entering the intervention room.

Arterial access is achieved using a Seldinger technique. Most commonly the femoral artery is used, but some centres prefer the brachial approach which allows for quicker patient mobilization post-procedure. Following local anaesthesia, a 4 or 5 French sheath is inserted into the femoral artery. Coeliac axis and superior mesenteric arteriography is performed to evaluate liver supply and give a roadmap for guiding more selective catheterization.

A microcatheter is then used to identify the tumour-feeding vessels, which may be many and may have an extrahepatic source, especially when larger tumours are close to the liver capsule or are exophytic. The internal mammary artery or inferior phrenic artery may supply tumours close to the diaphragmatic surface, whereas renal capsular branches or mesenteric branches may supply tumours near the inferior surface of the liver.

Cone-beam CT fluoroscopy allows easier identification of all feeding vessels and indicates how much liver parenchyma is going to be exposed to embolic material. If there are many feeding branches of the right or left hepatic artery, then it may be more practical to deliver the treatment in a lobar fashion rather than individually select all of the individual feeding arteries. We try to be as selective as possible to reduce the risk of post-embolization syndrome (PES), but it is important to ensure that all of the tumour has been treated. Figure 10.1 shows an arteriogram used for a chemoembolization.

We give a small bolus of intra-arterial nitrate before bead delivery to reduce the risk of spasm, which could adversely affect treatment delivery. The prepared drug-eluting beads are delivered from a 2 ml luer lock syringe in a pulsatile fashion

**Table 10.2** Summary of evidence for trials for transarterial chemoembolization, DEB-TACE and bland embolization

| Treatment | Authors | Number | Summary |
|---|---|---|---|
| TACE (conventional) | Solomon et al. [12] | 38 | Cisplatin, doxorubicin, |
| | | | Mitomycin C, ethiodol |
| | | | Polyvinyl alcohol |
| | | | Biologic response 70% partial, |
| | | | 15% minor, 15% stable |
| | Lo et al. [13] | 40 | Cisplatin, lipiodol, gelatin sponge |
| | | | Particles vs symptomatic treatment |
| | | | Treatment group: 1 and 3 year |
| | | | Survival 57% and 26% versus 32% |
| | | | And 3% (p0.002) |
| | Marelli et al. [14] | 175 | Meta-analysis with 1, 3, 5 year |
| | | | Survival of 62%, 30%, 19% |
| | | | Median survival 18 months |
| | Llovet et al. [15] | 545 | Meta-analysis TACE vs tamoxifen |
| | | | No benefit bland embolization |
| | | | Benefit TACE with cisplatin or |
| | | | Doxorubicin OR 0.42 (95% CI 0.2–0.88) |
| DEB–TACE | Lammer et al. [16] | 212 | CR 27% vs 22%, disease control |
| | | | 63% vs 42% ($p = 0.11$) |
| | | | Reduced liver toxicity and side |
| | | | Effects ($p < 0.001$) |
| | Golfieri et al. [17] | 177 | DEB-TACE vs cTACE. No difference |
| | | | Survival, tumour response or time |
| | | | To progression |
| | | | Less pain DEB-TACE. ECOG, albumin |
| | | | And tumour number predict survival |
| | Facciorusso et al. [18] | 676 | Meta-analysis TACE vs TAE. No |
| | | | Difference 1, 2, or 3 year survival |
| | | | No difference response or |
| | | | Progression-free survival. Less |
| | | | Toxicity with TAE |
| TAE | Kluger et al. [19] | 25 | TACE vs TAE pre-OLT |
| | | | TAE less procedures. Necrosis of |
| | | | Explant 36% TAE vs 26% TACE |
| | | | No difference 3-year recurrence and |
| | | | Overall survival |
| | Masarweh et al. [20] | 405 | TAE vs TACE. No difference in mean |
| | | | Survival. 72% vs 74% ($p = 0.66$) |
| | Brown et al. [21] | 101 | Microspheres vs DEB-TACE |
| | | | No difference RECIST response or |
| | | | Progression or overall survival |

Abbreviations: TACE; DEB, TAE, OLT, RECIST

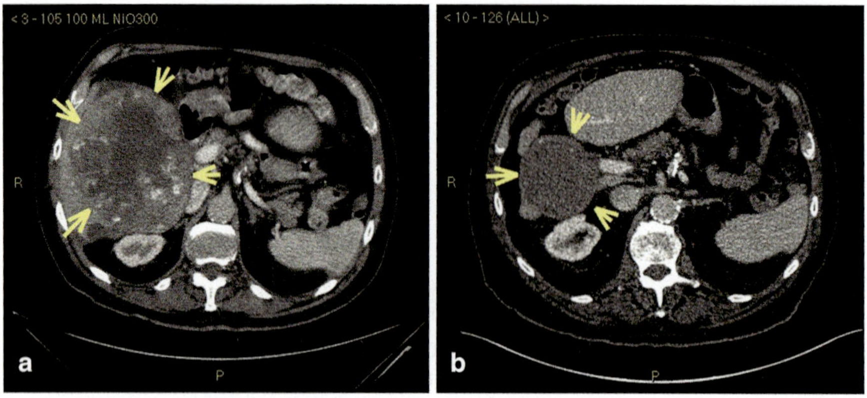


**Fig. 10.1** (**a**) MRI scan shows a large hypervascular right-sided liver lesion. This demonstrated wash-out on the portal-venous phase of dynamic imaging. (**b**) The same patient scanned 10 years later. There has been a marked reduction in size of the lesion

until there is "near stasis". This means the contrast that is delivered with the beads takes four to five heartbeats to clear the tip of the microcatheter. It is important to use a microcatheter as it is less likely to cause arterial spasm, allows for a more controlled delivery and does not significantly affect the laminar flow required to carry the beads along the feeding artery.

When all planned treatment has been delivered the catheters are removed and placed in a cytotoxic waste bin. We prefer not to perform post-treatment arteriography as there is a risk of flushing out beads that may still be hovering in the delivered vessel. A vessel closure device is used to seal the arterial puncture site. Figure 10.2 shows a pre- and post-treatment response to transarterial chemoembolization (Fig. 10.2).

Patients are encouraged to drink plenty of fluid over the ensuing 24 h. Occasionally intravenous fluids are required if the patient feels nauseous. The majority of patients can be discharged the following morning.

## Evidence Supporting Embolic Therapies

Despite concerns, ET has been pursued with enthusiasm by some clinicians. A Bayesian network meta-analysis of 55 randomized controlled trials (12 with direct comparisons) including 5763 patients with preserved liver function and unresectable HCC showed that all embolization strategies (TAE, TACE, DEB-TACE and TARE) showed a significant survival gain when compared with a control group of no treatment intervention. The median survival for controls was 13.9 months (11–11.7), TACE 18.1 months (15.6–21.6), DEB-TACE 20.6 months (14.5–29.4), TAE 20.8 months (16.2–27.1), TARE 24.3 (16.8–37.3), TAC E + radiotherapy 30.1 months (24.6–37.3) and finally TACE + ablation 33.3 months (26.4–42.5) [23].

There is known to be a correlation between a radiological response to treatment and survival. This is the supposition upon which assessing treatments with imaging

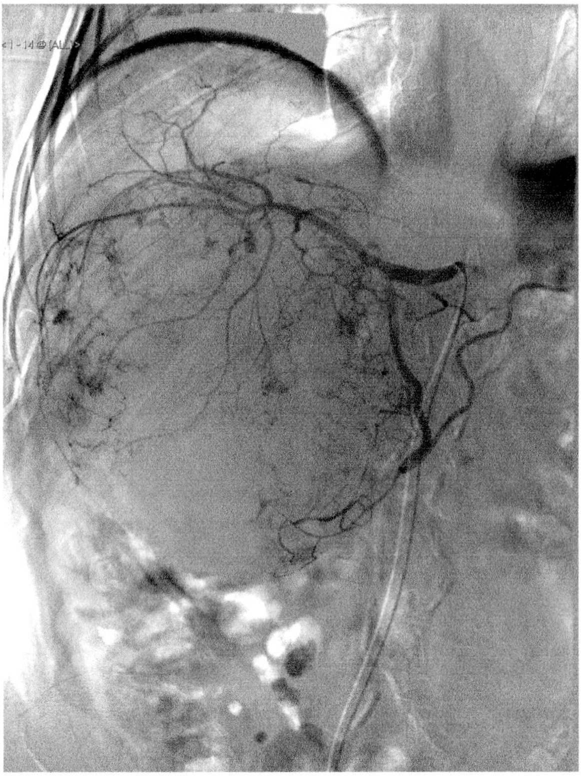

**Fig. 10.2** Hepatic arteriogram pre-TACE shows a large vascular lesion with feeding arteries and smaller tumour blushes within the main body of the tumour. The main outline of the tumour can be clearly delineated. The images are from the same patient from Fig. 10.1

is based. Objective response is the sum of complete response and partial response. In the study by Lammer and colleagues comparing DEB-TACE with conventional TACE, there was an objective response of 52% versus 44%. In the Katsanos study, the most profound objective response was witnessed when patients had both TACE with either an ablation technique or with external radiotherapy. The hierarchy of effectiveness as defined by the surface area under the cumulative rankogram (SUCRA) from least to most effective was TACE odds ratio (OR) (95% confidence interval, CI) 13.9 (6.91–31.9), SUCRA 21%; TAE OR 16.2 (CI 7.78–38.8) SUCRA 35%; DEB-TACE OR 17.4 (CI 7.59–45.5), SUCRA 40%; TACE + adjuvant OR 18.7 (95% CI 8.25–49.3), SUCRA 47%; DEB-TACE + adjuvant OR 24.8 (7.78–90), SUCRA 59%; TARE OR 26.9 (95% CI 8.44–93.8), SUCRA 62%; TACE + radiotherapy OR 52.4 (95% CI 23.6–128.9) SUCRA 85%; and TACE + ablation OR 142 (95%CI 55.9–395.4), SUCRA 99%. DEB-TACE and TACE with adjuvant treatment or radiotherapy gave rise to the greatest number of adverse events [23]. In terms of overall survival, the most effective treatment was TACE with ablation or radiotherapy. The meta-analysis can be criticized because the studies took place over two decades and the management of chronic liver disease may have improved over that time, e.g., hepatitis C treatment. A recurring challenge is that the majority of these studies contain heterogeneous populations and may contain mixed tumour types, with different disease aetiologies with different patient and tumour characteristics, so clinicians should resist the temptation to infer too much from some of the data. Moreover, the fact that TACE and ablation/radiotherapy had the best objective response and overall survival may be indicative of greater tumour responsiveness, and if this is a surrogate of survival, it is logical that they live longer.

## Adverse Effects Associated with Embolic TACE

After TACE some patients experience pain. This is due to the localized liver ischaemia induced following treatment. This often settles with analgesia and tends to be worst in the first 24 h after treatment. Many centres manage these patients within the hospital for 24 h after their treatment. Some patients experience the post-embolization syndrome (PES). This arises when there is fever without sepsis together with pain, nausea and sometimes vomiting. This often settles on its own but can be very debilitating for patients and make them averse to future interventions. Several strategies to mitigate its severity have been suggested, but none are universally followed. They can include antibiotics, intra-arterial lidocaine, acupuncture and administration of $5\text{-HT}^3$ receptor antagonists [24].

Other complications of ET include:

- Bruising or bleeding at the skin puncture site
- Hair loss
- Immunosuppression and increased risk of infections
- Abnormal liver function and liver decompensation, e.g., jaundice and ascites
- Pulmonary embolism and deep vein thrombosis
- Inflammation of the gallbladder
- Liver abscess formation at the site of tumour necrosis
- Tumour lysis syndrome

## Assessing Response to Treatment

At our centre, a contrast MRI liver (or dual-phase CT) is performed 4–6 weeks after treatment. The images are reviewed by a multidisciplinary team meeting with interventional radiology, hepatology and oncology. The tumour nodules are compared with their pretreatment scans and the area of arterialization and washout assessed. Viable tumour shows arterialization in the arterial phase and then washout in the portal venous phase. The radiologist assesses this, and a tumour with a complete response will lose all arterialization, and a hypodense region will be observed on the scan. Historically, response evaluation criteria in solid tumours (RECIST) guideline criteria were used which were as follows [25].

*RECIST to assess radiological response to treatment of hepatocellular carcinoma*

- Complete response (CR) is the disappearance of all target lesions.
- Partial response (PR) is defined as a minimum of a 30% decrease in the sum of the longest diameter of target lesions, taking as reference the baseline sum longest diameter.
- Progressive disease (PD) occurs when there is at least a 20% increase in the sum of the longest diameter of target lesions, taking as reference the smallest sum longest diameter recorded since when treatment started or the appearance of one or more new lesions.
- Stable disease (SD) is neither sufficient shrinkage to qualify for partial response nor sufficient increase to qualify for progressive disease, taking as reference the smallest sum longest diameter since the treatment started.

Tumours may respond but often show no size reduction 6 weeks after treatment. This would be recorded as stable disease using the RECIST criteria when, in fact, there may have been a complete response. Therefore the RECIST criteria have been updated and are now termed the mRECIST criteria [25]. This is now the preferred tool to determine a radiological response to treatment. They are summarized as follows:

*mRECIST to assess radiological response to treatment of hepatocellular carcinoma*

- Complete response (CR): the disappearance of any intra-tumoural arterial enhancement in all target lesions.
- Partial response (PR): at least a 30% decrease in the sum of diameters of viable (contrast enhancement in the arterial phase) target lesions, taking as reference the baseline sum of the diameters of target lesions.
- Progressive disease (PD): an increase of at least 20% in the sum of the diameters of viable (enhancing) target lesions, taking as reference the smallest sum of the diameters of viable (enhancing) target lesions recorded since the treatment started.
- Stable disease (SD): any cases that do not qualify for either partial response or progressive disease.

Additional terms which are used when assessing response to treatment include:

*Target lesion*: this is the lesion to which the locoregional therapy has been applied.

*Non-target lesion*: this can include the development of markers of progressive disease or hepatic decompensation and include portal vein thrombosis, local pathological lymph.

nodes, lung and bone metastases and also new ascites or pulmonary effusions.

*New lesion*: a new HCC developing in a region separate to where HCC therapy has been applied.

Overcalling of equivocal lesions as new HCC should be discouraged since it has a major impact on the outcome of studies with a radiologic endpoint, such as tumour response or time to progression [25]. More importantly, it could impact on patient treatment and therapeutic options leading to incorrect choices becoming made for the patient, e.g., palliative and not curative treatments being offered.

## Decisionmaking for Further Treatments

If there has been a complete response to treatment, then no further treatment may be necessary. If the lesion has reduced in size but remains greater than 3 cm at its maximal diameter, in the absence of features of liver decompensation or patient factors, further TACE/TAE could be considered. If the dominant lesion reduces in size to 3 cm or less, it may be possible to use an ablation technique (radiofrequency ablation, microwave ablation, cryoablation). There is evidence that combined therapies such as TACE with ablation offer better survival than TACE alone, but this may just be due to case selection and bias [23]. At our centre if there are a maximum of three lesions post-TACE <3 cm, we would attempt to ablate those lesions pending discussions of other therapies such as liver transplantation where appropriate. If there are more than three lesions or one of the lesions is still >3 cm, TACE would be the first choice of therapy. If there has been a partial response or no apparent response to TACE, many centres, including our own, would consider a further attempt at TACE. It would be useful to quantify what proportion of patients who do not respond to a first TACE respond to a second treatment. If this response is low, the early adoption of a different strategy might be beneficial to the patient. This is a research question that should be addressed.

For lesions that do not respond despite a second treatment, the options include offering a different embolic therapeutic approach such as selective internal radiotherapy (SIRT) or using a different embolic approach, e.g., a different therapeutic agent such as cisplatin or irinotecan beads or conventional TACE. There is no evidence to support the use of the latter approach, and studies to evaluate this are needed. The role of stereotactic body radiotherapy (SBRT) could be a useful alternative to TACE refractory liver-confined disease, for patients remaining within the intermediate stage of HCC (BCLC B), and its role demands further evaluation in this setting or perhaps in the long term as an alternative to TACE [26].

## Patient Assessment Before Further Transarterial Embolic Therapy

If a further TACE is planned, it is important to ensure there has been no significant impact on the patient's liver function. The appearance of ascites, of any volume, is a contraindication to TACE in our unit, as is the onset of clinically detectable jaundice. An assessment of the patient and biochemical variables is necessary before any further treatment is undertaken. The HAP score [11] has not been validated in sequential embolic therapies but is used in our centre as a guide. The ART strategy has been validated in this setting and is a useful tool to use when considering further ET [27]. In short, if the ART score before a second treatment is >2.5, that will identify patients who will not benefit from further TACE. This is summarized in Table 10.3. Discussion with the patient is important. In the face of a post-TACE

**Table 10.3** Models to predict risk of liver decompensation post-TACE

| | | |
|---|---|---|
| Kadalayil et al. [11] | The HAP score | AFP > 400 ng/mL = 1 |
| | | Tumour >7 cm = 1 |
| | | Albumin <36 g/dL = 1 |
| | | Bilirubin >17 μmol/L = 1 |
| Sum of scores | | |
| HAP A = 0 | Median survival 27.6 months | |
| HAP B = 1 | Median survival 18.5 months | |
| HAP C = 2 | Median survival 9 months | |
| HAP D > 2 | Median survival 3.8 months | |
| Permits identification at risk of liver decompensation after TACE | | |
| Hucke et al. [27] | The ART strategy | Radiologic tumour response |
| | | Present = 0, absent = 1 point |
| | | AST rise >25% |
| | | Present =4 points, absent = 0 |
| | | Child-Pugh score increase |
| | | 1 point rise = 1.5 points |
| | | ≥2 points = 3 points |
| | | Absent = 0 points |
| A score of >2.5 identifies patients who do not benefit from further TACE | | |

syndrome, some patients may not wish to have further treatment, although bland embolization or SIRT may be a more "gentle" treatment that could be considered. The balance between treating tumour and maintaining satisfactory liver synthetic function and patient performance status is paramount. Our centre does not give ET to patients with a performance status ≥2 and will be selective about patients with a performance status of 1. Under the BCLC staging, these patients would be classified as BCLC C (advanced disease) irrespective of the tumour disease burden. A new rise in bilirubin >30 μmol/L, a drop in albumin to <34 g/DL, a rising AFP or increase in tumour or new disease would prompt restaging prior to any treatment decision as locoregional therapy may no longer be indicated and systemic therapies or best supportive treatments might need to be considered.

## TACE Plus Treatments

There has been much interest in a combined approach with TACE/TAE plus other therapies. The network meta-analysis performed by Katsanos and colleagues showed the best responses were to be achieved in patients able to receive TACE with either an ablative technique or an external radiotherapy technique [23]. The additions of adjuvant chemotherapies to TACE, including sorafenib, have offered no survival advantage and cannot be supported at this time [23, 28]. But this strategy remains an area of interest, and the evolving role of immune therapies such as the checkpoint inhibitor, nivolumab, has sparked further interest, and a trial of DEB-TACE with nivolumab or placebo is recruiting in the USA (NCT03143270), and a similar phase III study is planned in the UK.

## Conclusions

Transarterial embolization therapies are accepted as effective strategies for patients with intermediate stage HCC (BCLC B). They can be used as a palliative treatment to prolong overall survival, as a bridge to curative treatments in particular liver transplantation or to downstage disease such that curative options including ablative therapies or transplantation might be considered. TACE should not be given where there is complete portal vein occlusion due to the risk of significant liver ischaemia and subsequent liver decompensation and death. It should be used with caution with partial main branch portal vein thrombosis and where there is branch occlusion. The overall fitness of the patient should be considered and in the main reserved for patients with Child-Pugh A cirrhosis. Some centres might consider treatment for patients with low Child-Pugh B, B7 disease, but the use of the HAP score and the ART strategy has shown that even with liver-confined disease, the impact of liver function as well as the tumour characteristics can have a significant impact in survival. The choice of ET may be determined by access and clinician preference; despite each therapy being effective when compared to no intervention, none of the embolic techniques have been shown to be consistently better than any other [23]. The adverse effects must be clearly explained to patients. Follow-up scan 4–6 weeks after treatment is mandated to guide therapy, and the current consensus is that if a lesion does not respond to two treatment cycles, alternatives should be considered, e.g., alternative form of TACE, SIRT, SBRT or systemic therapy.

## References

1. European Association for the Study of the Liver. EASL-EORTC clinical practice guidelines: management of hepatocellular carcinoma. J Hepatol. 2012;56(4):908–43.
2. El-Serag HB. Epidemiology of viral hepatitis and hepatocellular carcinoma. Gastroenterology. 2012;142(6):1264–73 e1.
3. Njei B, Rotman Y, Ditah I, Lim JK. Emerging trends in hepatocellular carcinoma incidence and mortality. Hepatology. 2015;61:191–9.
4. Dyson J, Jaques B, Chattopadyhay D, Lochan R, Graham J, Das D, et al. Hepatocellular cancer: the impact of obesity, type 2 diabetes and a multidisciplinary team. J Hepatol. 2014;60(1):110–7.
5. Llovet JM, Bustamante J, Castells A, Vilana R, Ayuso Mdel C, Sala M, et al. Natural history of untreated nonsurgical hepatocellular carcinoma: rationale for the design and evaluation of therapeutic trials. Hepatology. 1999;29(1):62–7.
6. El-Serag HB. Hepatocellular carcinoma. N Engl J Med. 2011;365(12):1118–27.

7. Padhya KT, Marrero JA, Singal AG. Recent advances in the treatment of hepatocellular carcinoma. Curr Opin Gastroenterol. 2013;29(3):285–92.
8. Llovet JM, Brú C, Bruix J. Prognosis of hepatocellular carcinoma: the BCLC staging classification. Semin Liver Dis. 1999;19(3):329–38.
9. Cross TJ, Villaneuva A, Shetty S, Wilkes E, Reeves H, et al. A national survey of the provision of ultrasound surveillance for the detection of hepatocellular carcinoma. Frontline Gastroenterol. 2016;7:82–9.
10. Oken M, Creech R, Tormey D, et al. Toxicity and response criteria of the Eastern Cooperative Oncology Group. Am J Clin Oncol. 1982;5:649–55.
11. Kadalayil L, Benini R, Pallan L, O'Beirne J, Marelli L, et al. A simple prognostic scoring system for patients receiving transarterial embolisation for hepatocellular cancer. Ann Oncol. 2013;24(10):2565–70.
12. Solomon B, Soulen MC, Baum RA, Haskal ZJ, Shlansky-Goldberg RD, Cope C. Chemoembolization of hepatocellular carcinoma with cisplatin, doxorubicin, mitomycin-C, ethiodol, and polyvinyl alcohol: prospective evaluation of response and survival in a U.S. population. J Vasc Interv Radiol. 1999;10(6):793–8.
13. Lo CM, Ngan H, Tso WK, Liu CL, Lam CM, Poon RT, Fan ST, Wong J. Randomized controlled trial of transarterial lipiodol chemoembolization for unresectable hepatocellular carcinoma. Hepatology. 2002;35(5):1164–71.
14. Marelli L, Stigliano R, Triantos C, Senzolo M, Cholongitas E, Davies N, Tibballs J, Meyer T, Patch DW, Burroughs AK. Transarterial therapy for hepatocellular carcinoma: which technique is more effective? A systematic review of cohort and randomized studies. Cardiovasc Intervent Radiol. 2007;30(1):6–25. Review
15. Llovet JM, Bruix J. Systematic review of randomized trials for unresectable hepatocellular carcinoma: chemoembolization improves survival. Hepatology. 2003;37(2):429–42. Review
16. Lammer J, Malagari K, Vogl T, Pilleul F, Denys A, et al. Prospective randomized study of doxorubicin-eluting-bead embolization in the treatment of hepatocellular carcinoma: results of the PRECISION V study. Cardiovasc Intervent Radiol. 2010;33(1):41–52.
17. Golfieri R, Giampalma E, Renzulli M, Cioni R, Bargellini I, et al. Randomised controlled trial of doxorubicin-eluting beads vs conventional chemoembolisation for hepatocellular carcinoma. Br J Cancer. 2014;111(2):255–64.
18. Facciorusso A, Di Maso M, Muscatiello N. Drug-eluting beads versus conventional chemoembolization for the treatment of unresectable hepatocellular carcinoma: a meta-analysis. Dig Liver Dis. 2016;48(6):571–7.
19. Kluger MD, Halazun KJ, Barroso RT, Fox AN, Olsen SK, et al. Bland embolization versus chemoembolization of hepatocellular carcinoma before transplantation. Liver Transpl. 2014;20(5):536–43.
20. Massarweh NN, Davila JA, El-Serag HB, Duan Z, Temple S, et al. Transarterial bland versus chemoembolization for hepatocellular carcinoma: rethinking a gold standard. J Surg Res. 2016;200(2):552–9.
21. Brown KT, Do RK, Gonen M, Covey AM, Getrajdman GI, et al. Randomized trial of hepatic artery embolization for hepatocellular carcinoma using doxorubicin-eluting microspheres compared with embolization with microspheres alone. J Clin Oncol. 2016;34(17):2046–53.
22. Oliveri RS, Wetterslev J, Gluud C. Transarterial (chemo)embolization for unresectable hepatocellular carcinoma. Cochrane Database Syst Rev. 2011;Issue 3:Art. No CD004787.
23. Katsanos K, Kitrou P, Spiliopoulos S, Maroulis I, Petsas T, Karnabatidis D. Comparative effectiveness of different transarterial embolization therapies alone or in combination with local ablative or adjuvant systemic treatments for unresectable hepatocellular carcinoma: a network meta-analysis of randomized controlled trials. PLoS One. 2017;12(9):e0184597.
24. Blackburn H, West S. Management of postembolization syndrome following hepatic transarterial chemoembolization for primary or metastatic liver cancer. Cancer Nurs. 2016;39(5):E1–E18.

25. Lencioni R, Llovet JM. Modified RECIST (mRECIST) assessment for hepatocellular carcinoma. Semin Liver Dis. 2010;30(1):52–60.
26. Hasan S, Thai N, Uemura T, Kudithipudi V, Renz P, et al. Hepatocellular carcinoma with child Pugh-a cirrhosis treated with stereotactic body radiotherapy. World J Gastrointest Surg. 2017;9(12):256–63.
27. Hucke F, Sieghart W, Pinter M, Graziadei I, Vogel W, Muller C, et al. The ART-strategy: sequential assessment of the ART score predicts outcome of patients with hepatocellular carcinoma re-treated with TACE. J Hepatol. 2014;60(1):118–26.
28. Meyer T, Fox R, Ma YT, Ross PJ, James MW, Sturgess R, et al. Sorafenib in combination with transarterial chemoembolisation in patients with unresectable hepatocellular carcinoma (TACE 2): a randomised placebo-controlled, double-blind, phase 3 trial. Lancet Gastroenterol Hepatol. 2017;2(8):565–75.

# Chapter 11
# Radioembolisation in Hepatocellular Carcinoma: Principles of Management

**Bruno Sangro and Andrea Casadei Gardini**

**Key Learning Points**

1. RE is currently used for the treatment of HCC patients when transarterial chemoembolisation has failed to produce a tumour response or is not indicated because the tumours are too large or too numerous or have invaded the portal vein branches.
2. In the advanced HCC, RE can be an alternative to the systemic agent sorafenib particularly when the drug is contraindicated or patients show poor tolerability.
3. Additionally, RE can be used to induce hypertrophy of the contralateral lobe to the tumour and rescue for surgery those patients that are unresectable due to small future liver remnant or to induce complete tumour ablation in 'radiation segmentectomy'.
4. Although radioembolisation is well tolerated, attention should be given during the first 3 months to complications arising from excessive radiation of the lungs, the liver or the GI tract, for which specific recommendation about diagnostic workup and management are available.
5. A multidisciplinary team involving all relevant therapeutic disciplines such as hepatologists, medical and radiation oncologists, interventional radiologists and liver surgeons is key to a successful radioembolisation program.

---

B. Sangro (✉)
Liver Unit and HPB Oncology Area, Clinica Universidad de Navarra,
IDISNA and CIBEREHD, Pamplona, Spain
e-mail: bsangro@unav.es

A. C. Gardini
Department of Medical Oncology, Istituto Scientifico Romagnolo per Lo Studio e Cura Dei Tumori (IRST) IRCCS, Meldola, Italy
e-mail: andrea.casadei@irst.emr.it



T. Cross, D. H. Palmer (eds.), *Liver Cancers*,
https://doi.org/10.1007/978-3-319-92216-4_11

**Areas of Controversy and Uncertainty**

1. A standardised, validated dosimetric approach in which prescribed activity is calculated on the basis of a target amount of radiation delivered to the tumour and non-tumour liver volumes is lacking.
2. The role of RE as an alternative to sorafenib in the first-line treatment of HCC patients with portal vein invasion is debatable.

## Radioembolisation

Radioembolisation (RE), also called transarterial radioembolisation (TARE) or selective internal radiotherapy therapy (SIRT), is an invasive, image-guided procedure that delivers intra-arterial brachytherapy to cancer in the liver. RE is based on the injection of microspheres loaded or labelled with yttrium-90 (Y90) into the hepatic arterial circulation.

Contrary to healthy liver, 80–100% of the blood flow of hepatocellular carcinoma (HCC) is supplied by branches of the hepatic arteries [1]. Besides, the vascular resistance of HCC vessels is low, and this increases the chances of particles injected into a hepatic artery to reach the tumour vasculature [2]. RE takes advantage of this situation to deliver most of the radiation emitted by Y90 inside liver tumours, although a contributing therapeutic role of the embolisation of tumour microvascularisation by millions of non-biodegradable particles cannot be ruled out. Much experience has been obtained from two devices are approved for clinical use in the EU including SIR-Spheres resin microspheres (Sirtex Medical) and TheraSphere glass microspheres (BTG). QuiremSpheres is a new device that consists in microparticles loaded with holmium 166 (Terumo), but there is very little experience, and the consistent results observed with resin and glass microspheres should not be extrapolated. The first two devices are loaded with Y90, a pure beta emitter with a short half-life of 2.67 days and a short tissue penetration of 2.5 mm as an average [3]. Their main differences are shown in Table 11.1.

RE and transarterial chemoembolisation (TACE) are both delivered through catheterisation of the tumour-feeding vessels. However, they differ considerably in the mechanism of action and procedural issues related to the requirement of superselective catheterisation. TACE works mainly by inducing tumour ischemia.

**Table 11.1** Main differences between devices available for liver radioembolisation

| | SIR-Spheres | TheraSphere |
|---|---|---|
| Material | Resin | Glass |
| Average size per particle | 22 ± 10 μm | 32 ± 10 μm |
| Average activity per particle | 50 Bq | 2500 Bq |
| Amount of microspheres in a typical treatment | 40–80 million | 1–5 million |

TACE particles are in fact 3–10 times larger than RE microspheres (100–500 μm vs. 25–35 μm in diameter). A greater particle diameter results in occlusion of medium to large arteries, and the radiological aim of TACE is indeed blood flow stagnation or interruption. Contrary, RE is not followed by significant reduction in arterial blood flow. The lack of significant ischemic effect allows lobar or even whole-liver RE to be performed safely without inducing acute liver decompensation [4]. Otherwise, RE anti-tumour activity is based in delivering a tumouricidal dose of radiation to tumour nodules while largely sparing non-tumoural liver from the effect of radiation. Therefore, the therapeutic effect of RE largely depends on factors such as hepatic arterial flow distribution, arterial vascularisation of the target tumour, functional integrity of the uninvolved liver and relative radiosensitivities of tumour and non-tumour tissues.

## Patient Selection

### *Current Indications*

RE is currently used in several situations where intra-arterial therapies could offer potential benefits that will be discussed later in detail, including but not limited to:

- Single or multiple tumours with portal vein invasion (PVI).
- Multiple tumours that cannot be treated by superselective TACE.
- Tumours that show incomplete response after one or two sessions of TACE.
- Single large tumours, particularly when resection is contraindicated due to a small future liver remnant.
- Small tumours in patients waiting for liver transplantation.

RE should be indicated after thorough discussion of alternative treatment options in the setting of a multidisciplinary team involving all relevant therapeutic disciplines such as hepatologists, medical and radiation oncologists, interventional radiologists and liver surgeons [3]. Particular attention should be paid to the relative benefit of RE versus TACE for any specific patient condition. In this regard, there is not much oncologic sense in using locoregional therapies such as RE to treat patients with extrahepatic disease including those with regional lymph nodes. These patients are likely better served by systemic therapies.

### *Contraindications*

RE should be contraindicated in the presence of the following scenarios (although specific contraindications have been developed by the manufacturers) summarised in Table 11.2.

**Table 11.2** Absolute and relative contraindications to radioembolisation

| |
|---|
| *Absolute contraindications* |
| A significant risk of microsphere deposition in the GI tract based on vascular anatomy and MAA scan results |
| Lung shunt >20% (for resin microspheres) or estimated radiation to lung tissue >30 Gy (resin or glass microspheres) |
| Decompensated cirrhosis (jaundice, ascites, encephalopathy, recent variceal haemorrhage) |
| Any technical contraindications to intra-arterial treatment including renal failure (serum creatinine >2 mg/dl, glomerular filtration rate <30 ml/min) |
| *Relative contraindications* |
| Massive tumour involving both lobes (especially if tumour involvement >50%) |
| Bile duct occlusion or incompetent papilla due to stent or surgery |
| Lung shunt 10–20%, particularly if associated with reduced intra-tumoural MAA uptake |
| Lack of significant intra-tumoural uptake of MAA (also in the tumour thrombus) |
| Portal vein invasion involving the main trunk |

A significant risk of radioactive *microsphere deposition in the gastrointestinal tract*. Nowadays, injection of Y90 microspheres into the common hepatic artery is formally contraindicated, while a double injection into the right and left hepatic arteries is preferred to a single injection into the proper hepatic artery. If a single injection into the proper hepatic artery is decided, the tip of the catheter should be placed distally to the origin of the gastroduodenal artery, and/or this artery should be coil embolised. Special attention should be paid if the left hepatic artery is involved in the treatment plan to potential collaterals connecting this artery to the GI tract. GI ulcerations are a frightful complication of RE that may impair patient quality of life for weeks or months [5]. Therefore, RE is better contraindicated when an unequivocal GI uptake is observed in the MAA scan (particularly if SPECT-CT is used). Contraindication is the best option even if no obvious collaterals are observed during angiography since hemodynamic conditions under power contrast injection may change blood flow patterns.

An excessive *lung shunting* that could result in the lungs absorbing a dose of radiation that could cause pneumonitis. Glass and resin microspheres manufacturers consider that any lung shunt fraction (LSF, as estimated by the MAA scan) that could result in the delivery of 30 Gy to the lungs should be considered an absolute contraindication to RE. With resin microspheres, any LSF > 20% should also contraindicate RE irrespective of the resulting dose of radiation absorbed by the lungs, while a 50% reduction in prescribed activity has to be implemented for LSF between 10% and 20%. This additional precaution is likely beneficial since radiation pneumonitis can rarely also occur in patients in which the 30 Gy threshold was supposedly not reached [6]. High LSF is usually observed in large primary liver tumours with vascular invasion. RE indication should be carefully individualised in these patients since trans-tumoural shunt usually results in a lower delivery of radiation to the tumour that may compromise treatment efficacy. A history of chronic obstructive pulmonary disease does not contraindicate RE unless severe pulmonary insufficiency is present.

*Significant liver dysfunction* is an obvious contraindication for RE. However, defining significant in this setting is not an easy task. Radioembolisation-induced liver disease (REILD) is at the basis of this contraindication. Even in superselective RE, some non-tumoural liver tissue absorbs a certain amount of radiation. This may lead to clinical liver decompensation or not depending on several factors including the severity of the damage induced (mostly related to the amount of radiation delivered), volume of non-tumoural tissue involved and hepatic functional reserve at baseline. The usual presentation of liver decompensation after RE is REILD, which consists in the occurrence of ascites and jaundice 4–8 weeks after RE in the absence of tumour progression or bile duct occlusion [7]. A conservative approach to patient selection and activity calculation is much warranted in HCC patients. Ascites or a total bilirubin >2 mg/dl at the time of evaluation should be considered an absolute contraindication. Since the risk of REILD is higher in patients with a small liver volume (<1.5 l) or an abnormal total bilirubin (>1.2 mg/dl), additional precautions could be considered in these patients. An albumin level <3 g/dl and AST/ALT levels >5 times the upper limit of normal also increase the risk of liver toxicity. The ALBI grade [8] is a good indicator of liver functional reserve and patients in ALBI grade 3 are likely poor candidates for RE.

A high tumour burden can make RE both ineffective due to reduced relative amount of radiation for any given injected activity and dangerous due to compromised functional reserve. RE is at least discouraged when tumour volume is >50% of the total liver volume.

A high arterial blood flow to tumours provides the best chance of success after RE. Arterial blood flow and vessel density may be heterogeneous, particularly in large tumours. While dose estimates indicate the average dose per volume, different parts of the tumour may absorb from massive to sublethal doses of radiation. Lesions that achieve an objective response are those that absorb higher average doses of radiation measured using intraoperative probes or estimated from pretreatment MAA planar scintigraphy. More importantly, higher doses of tumour-absorbed radiation are associated with improved survival in HCC patients and lack of significant MAA uptake can be considered an argument against RE [9].

The use of RE for the treatment of HCC patients with portal vein thrombosis (PVT) has been hindered by concerns about the risk of liver failure. Since Y90 is a microembolic procedure causing no occlusion of large hepatic arteries, it can be safely used in the setting of PVT, even when it involves the main portal trunk [10]. However, the low median survival observed after RE in patients with main trunk portal vein invasion (<6 months) makes these patients poor candidates for RE. If RE is nevertheless considered, lack of MAA uptake in the tumour thrombus should be considered a contraindication to RE.

Other contraindications include any contraindication to angiography (bleeding diathesis, vascular abnormalities, renal insufficiency), pregnancy or lactation. A proposed algorithm for patient selection based on the results of the pretreatment evaluation is shown on Fig. 11.1.

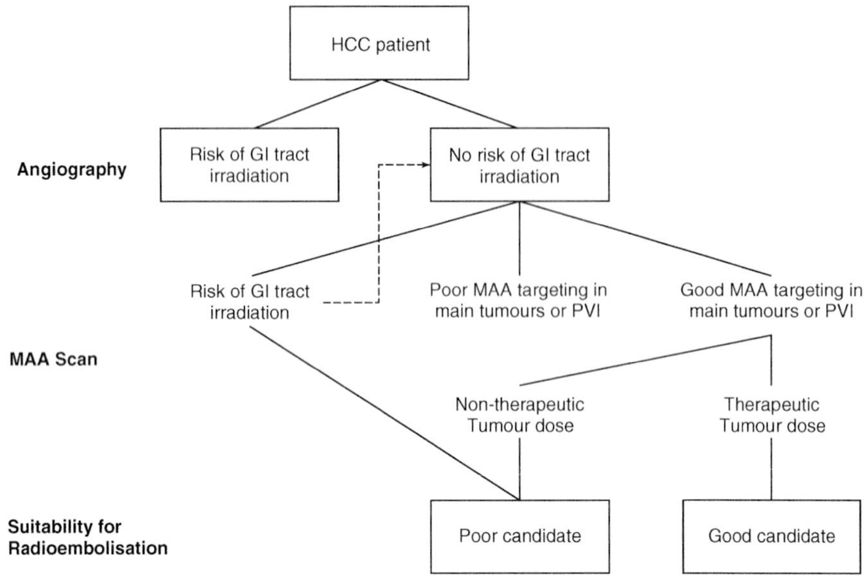


**Fig. 11.1** Algorithm for selecting the optimal candidates for radioembolisation based on the results of the pretreatment evaluation

## Pretreatment Evaluation and Treatment

The main purpose of RE is to reduce tumour burden as much as possible while preserving the functional capacity of the non-tumoural liver. As mentioned before, subclinical liver damage occurs as a result of the deployment of radioactive microparticles in non-tumoural areas of the liver. REILD ensues only when the extension and intensity of such damage is large enough to produce a clinically relevant liver decompensation. Contrary to patients with metastatic liver disease from colorectal or neuroendocrine tumours, those with HCC may develop REILD after lobar RE or in the absence of prior chemotherapy. But this occurs rarely if a personalised approach to treatment planning and activity calculation is used [7].

One strategy is to spare as much liver volume as possible from liver damage. If the lesion is located in a segment of the liver provided by a major arterial branch without significant leakage, a high Y90 activity can be injected superselectively safely in what has been called radiation segmentectomy [11]. Radiation absorbed by the tumour in this approach can be as high as 1000 Gy, way above the tumouricidal dose for epithelial tumours. Likewise, radiation lobectomy is an option when there is extensive involvement of a single lobe. Radiation absorbed by the lobe is not as high as in radiation segmentectomy, but it is high enough to frequently produce liver atrophy and compensatory hypertrophy in the contralateral lobe [12]. Hypertrophy is usually less intense in cirrhotic patients. When treating bilateral tumours, a single-session bilobar treatment can be safely performed at least using resin microspheres [4] particularly if a conservative activity calculation is used [7]. Alternatively, some centres prefer to treat both lobes in a sequential fashion although this practice is derived from a single retrospective study [13] and increases the cost significantly. In any case, a multidisciplinary team discussion is crucial in the evaluation of these patients to select the treatment design that is more appropriate to the individual treatment aim.

Technically, RE consists of a two-step procedure. A pre-SIRT evaluation involving angiography and macroaggregated albumin (MAA) scan is completed prior to the RE procedure. Although they are typically performed in two sessions separated 1–2 weeks, they can be performed as a sequential single-day procedure. In the pre-RE evaluation, the abdominal arterial anatomy is explored, and any potentially problematic collateral vessel is embolised to allow a full coverage of the tumour volume and prevent extrahepatic microsphere deposition. Celiac and superior mesenteric artery angiograms allow recognition of variants such as aberrant or accessory hepatic arteries and the identification of parasitic vessels that supply hepatic tumours. High-power contrast injection is used to recognise small vessels and to provide a supraphysiological flow that helps in detecting reflux that may occur during the therapeutic procedure. All blood vessels that may be at risk of reflux are embolised permanently using steel coils. Cystic artery embolisation is evaluated case by case as the risk of cholecystitis from radiation is very low. Once the vascular map is established, the planning procedure is completed by injecting MAA and performing planar or preferably SPECT-CT MAA scan imaging. The size of MAA is comparable to Y90 microspheres, and the MAA scan therefore enables to estimate the LSF and the dose of radiation that will be absorbed by the lungs, any extrahepatic uptake due to unnoticed collateral vessels, intrahepatic distribution of Y90 microspheres and the dose of radiation that will be absorbed by the tumour and the non-tumoural compartments [14]. Pre-RE evaluation minimises the potential for non-target clinical toxicities, including gastric ulceration, pancreatitis, skin irritation and radiation pneumonitis.

The optimal 90Y activity is calculated differently for resin and glass microspheres. For resin beads, it can be calculated using the body surface area (BSA) formula or a partition model [15]. The BSA activity planning is the standard method and is particularly suited for bilobar RE in metastatic disease. However, the activity prescribed is usually considered too high for patients with metastatic tumours previously exposed to anticancer chemotherapy or those with primary tumours in the setting of cirrhosis [16]. A more conservative approach with reduced prescribed activities can be based on BSA tables used in pivotal clinical trials [17] or by reducing the activity provided by the formula by 10–20% depending on the perceived potential frailty of the liver [7]. The partition model can be used as an alternative to the BSA formula in tumours with a neat MAA uptake particularly when a lobar or segmental approach is decided. In the partition model, the average doses of radiation likely to be absorbed by the lungs, the non-tumoural liver and the tumours are estimated from the activity of MAA measured in these compartments after MAA injection. It is therefore essential to inject MAA at the same location where Y90 microspheres will be later injected if the partition model will be used for activity calculation. The target is the dose of radiation absorbed by any given compartment depending on treatment aim and patient condition. If both lobes are involved, the target is to keep the dose absorbed by the non-tumoural liver below 40 Gy. If the

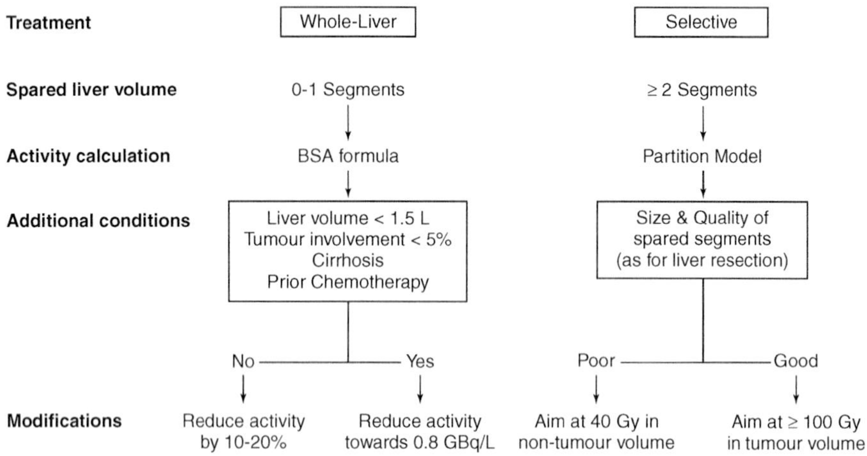


**Fig. 11.2** Activity calculation algorithm used at Clinica Universidad de Navarra (Modified from Ref. [7])

amount of non-tumoural liver that can be spared from radiation is large and healthy enough, the target is to keep the dose absorbed by the tumours above 120 Gy (Fig. 11.1). As mentioned earlier, the dose absorbed by the lungs should be always kept below 30 Gy. For glass beads, the volume of the targeted liver (segment, lobe or entire liver) is calculated, and teams have to select the prescribed activity within a range of 80–150 Gy of radiation absorbed by this volume irrespective of tumour involvement. Attempts to use a dosimetric approach in which a specific target dose to the tumour is calculated have been proposed and await validation. A proposed algorithm for patient selection based on the results of the pretreatment evaluation is show on Fig. 11.2.

Treatment should be performed within 2–4 weeks after the workup but can also be on the same day. Collateral vessel patency and identification of new collaterals should be explored before injection Y90 microspheres, especially when collaterals have been embolised since changes in local haemodynamics may reverse flow in previously unnoticed vessels. The location of the tip of the catheter close to a bifurcation increases the chances of mismatch between MAA and Y90 microspheres distribution[2] and should be avoided. Slow infusions are recommended. Analgesics and anti-emetics should be given only to patients that experience symptoms during or after the procedure.

## Post-treatment Follow-Up

Although RE is by and large well tolerated, attention should be given during the first 3 months to signs and symptoms of complications. A summary of the current recommendations for the prevention, workup and treatment of such events is provided

**Table 11.3** Summary of recommendations for the prevention and treatment of complications of RE (for a more detailed report see Ref. [6])

| Prevention | Workup | Treatment |
|---|---|---|
| *Pneumonitis* | | |
| Reduce prescribed activity or contraindicate if lung shunt >10% (if ≥15%, strongly consider an alternative treatment)<br>Keep dose of radiation to lung tissue <30 Gy | Chest CT scan if hypoxemia, cough or dyspnoea within the first 2 months post-SIRT<br>Functional tests to confirm restrictive pattern and altered carbon monoxide diffusion level | Steroids on a very empiric basis<br>Oxygen supply as needed |
| *GI ulcerations* | | |
| Avoid access of microspheres to GI tract by coil embolization, a more distal injection or flow redistribution<br>If a false-positive GI uptake of MAA is suspected, consider repeating angiography and MAA | Upper endoscopy if upper abdominal pain 4–8 weeks after SIRT, particularly if associated with nausea, loss of appetite or anaemia<br>Presumptive diagnosis based on gross morphology | High-dose proton pump inhibitors, sucralfate, anti-emetics, analgesics and gastric promotility agents<br>If severe, consider total parenteral nutrition or jejunostomy |
| *REILD* | | |
| Contraindicate RE if total bilirubin >2 mg/dL or non-tumoural ascites<br>Consider reducing prescribed activity for patients with steatohepatitis or cirrhosis, where the liver is <1.5 L, and in patients with intense exposure to chemotherapy<br>Spare as many liver segments as possible | Suspect REILD in any patient that develops jaundice and ascites within the first 3 months after SIRT<br>US-Doppler to check for bile duct obstruction, ascites and portal/hepatic vein patency. If bile duct obstruction is discarded, liver CT or MRI to rule out tumour progression<br>Blood test to measure liver damage and function | Diuretics and monitor liver function<br>If liver function starts to decline, consider defibrotide<br>If liver failure develops, consider transjugular intra-hepatic portosystemic stent-shunt (TIPS) placement |
| *Cholecystitis* | | |
| If necessary, place the catheter distal to the cystic artery. If not feasible, perform temporary occlusion of the cystic artery during the treatment procedure (vasospasm or Gelfoam) | Suspect radiation cholecystitis in any patient with persistent right upper quadrant tenderness 4–6 weeks following SIRT. Liver US, CT or MRI to check for a thickened wall, pericholecystic fluid, intramural gas or hydrops | Provide IV hydration and analgesics on demand<br>Symptomatic therapy with analgesics and anti-emetics<br>Consider cholecystostomy (preferred) or cholecystectomy if with fever, intense pain or signs of wall necrosis or rupture |

in Table 11.3. The indiscriminate use of proton pump inhibitors, ursodeoxycholic acid or even heparin and low-dose steroids is not supported by strong evidence although it is common practice in many centres.

Assessing response to radioembolisation can be complex. As opposed to systemic treatments where all tumours are simultaneously and homogeneously exposed to the agent, in intra-arterial therapies tumours can be treated at different time points and in a heterogeneous way. Size criteria such as those recommended by the Response Evaluation Criteria in Solid Tumours (RECIST) guidelines are the most common reporting standards. Criteria that take into account the volume of a tumour that lacks contrast enhancement in the arterial phase of contrast-enhanced imaging because of treatment-induced necrosis have been developed and are commonly used after TACE and also serve well to RE. However, it usually takes longer to see changes in contrast enhancement or tumour shrinkage after RE than it does after TACE. A minimum of 3 months is recommended before lack of response is declared after RE.

## Specific Indications and Expected Outcomes

Most of the published experience with RE is focused on patients that were not considered appropriate candidates to TACE [1]. Since there were no effective systemic anticancer agents until 2007, this group includes patients who failed TACE, had tumours that were considered too large or too numerous to be treated by TACE or showed vascular invasion into the portal or hepatic veins. Outcomes are consistent depending on tumour stage at baseline and across devices as shown in Table 11.4.

In the largest multicentre study of 325 patients, median OS was 12.8 months, varying by stage: 24.4 months for BCLC-A, 16.9 months for BCLC-B and 10.0 months for BCLC-C [4]. Independent prognostic factors were worse performance status, higher tumour burden, worse liver function and extrahepatic disease. The treatment was well tolerated, and there were very few treatment-emergent CTCAE grade 3 events. For patients that were potential candidates for sorafenib therapy as from the inclusion criteria in the pivotal SHARP trial, survival was quite comparable [1]. Two recent phase 3 multicentre clinical trials conducted in France [24] and the Asia-Pacific region [25] randomised patients to sorafenib or RE using resin microspheres. There were no differences in the primary endpoint of overall survival, but RE was associated with fewer adverse events and better quality of life. In SARAH, RE resulted in delayed progression in the liver and a higher response rate (19.0% vs. 11.6%) that were not translated into better overall survival (median 8.0 vs. 9.9 months) or PFS (4.1 vs. 3.7 months). In SIRveNIB, RE resulted in delayed TTP at any site (6.41 vs 5.39 months, but only in the per-protocol analysis) and higher RR (16.5% vs. 1.7%) that were not transferred into better OS. In both studies around 20% of patients were randomised to RE but could not get the treatment. This numbers are well above the 5–10% rate of contraindications due to findings during the RE workup reported in most series from experienced centres. Furthermore, the lack of differences in the pre-planned subgroup analysis of patients with portal vein invasion was unexpected. In a previous retrospective study, RE was associated with a longer OS than sorafenib (8.8 vs. 5.4 months) [26]. Two other trials are exploring if combining RE with sorafenib can result in a better survival than sorafenib alone (NCT01126645 and NCT01556490).

Most guidelines recommend TACE as first-line therapy for the intermediate stage [27]. Expanding from the high rate of objective, durable remissions in advanced

**Table 11.4** Patient characteristics and long-term outcomes of large mixed-case series of HCC patients treated with radioembolisation

| | | Staging | Liver function | Tumour burden | Performance status | Response rate | Response duration | Survival | Survival by BCLC stage |
|---|---|---|---|---|---|---|---|---|---|
| Author, year | N | BCLC (A/B/C/D) | Child-Pugh (A/B) | Single tumours | ECOG >0 | EASL criteria | TTP (months) | Median (months) | Median (months) |
| Salem [18][a] | 291 | 17/28/52 | 45/52 | 27% | 44% | 57% | 7.9 | | A: 26.9<br>B: 17.2<br>C: 7.3 |
| Hilgard [19] | 108 | 2/51/55 | 77/22 | Nr | 49% | 40% | 10 | 16.4 | B: 16.4<br>C: NR |
| Mazzaferro [20] | 52 | 0/33/67 | 83/17 | 3% | 40% | 40% | 11 | 15 | B: 18<br>C: 13 |
| Sangro [21] | 325 | 16/27/56 | 268/57 | 24% | 46% | NR | NR | 12.8 | A: 24.4<br>B: 16.9<br>C: 10 |
| Vilgrain [22][b] | 174 | 7/53/114 | 153/20 | 46% | 37% | 19.5%[c] | NR | 9.9 | NR |
| Chow [23][b] | 130 | 0/83/46 | 117/12 | NR | 18% | 23.1%[c] | 6.41 | 11.2 | B: 13.5<br>C: 9.2 |

[a]Data are for patients with no extrahepatic disease
[b]Data are for the per-protocol population
[c]By RECIST 1.1 criteria
*NR* not reported

tumours, most experienced centres started exploring the use of RE in less advanced cases. A number of retrospective series comparing TACE and RE showed similar efficacy and suggested that a randomised trial with OS as primary endpoint should recruit more than a thousand patients. Three small randomised trials have been reported. The first one was a pilot trial with no statistical assumptions that randomised 24 patients and observed no difference in OS (592 days for RE vs. 788 days for TACE) or TTP (371 days for RE versus 336 days for TACE) [28]. The second one had quality of life as primary endpoint and randomised 28 patients [29]. No difference was observed in quality of life, frequency of adverse events, PFS (3.6 months for RE and 3.7 months for TACE) or OS. A third study had time to progression as primary endpoint [30]. It was prematurely closed due to slow accrual after having randomised 45 patients. Patients treated with RE had a significantly longer TTP (HR, 0.122; 95% CI, 0.027–0.557) although no difference was found in OS (17.7 months for RE vs. 18.6 months for SIRT). These three randomised trials differed in the patient population. In the two first studies, patients were mostly in the intermediate stage with bilobar tumours, while in the third most were in the early stage and unilobar.

Besides providing tumour control, SIRT can be used to induce hypertrophy of the contralateral lobe to the tumour, which generally occurs within the first 3–6 months following RE [12]. A systematic review showed that the percentage of hypertrophy after SIRT ranges from 29% to 47%. This effect may allow to bring patients to surgery with good final outcomes. The safety of RE before surgery was analysed in a retrospective study that showed how RE was not associated with worsened safety outcomes after resection or transplantation [31].

Finally, RE can induce complete necrosis in small (<3 cm) tumours particularly when a high Y90 activity is injected into a segmental tumour-feeding artery and tumour-absorbed radiation is increased over 200 Gy in 'radiation segmentectomy' [32]. Local tumour ablation can therefore be the aim of RE for early tumours that cannot be ablated due to their location in the dome or near the large vessels in patients that are otherwise not candidates for resection or transplantation due to age, cirrhosis or comorbidities (Fig. 11.3) [32].

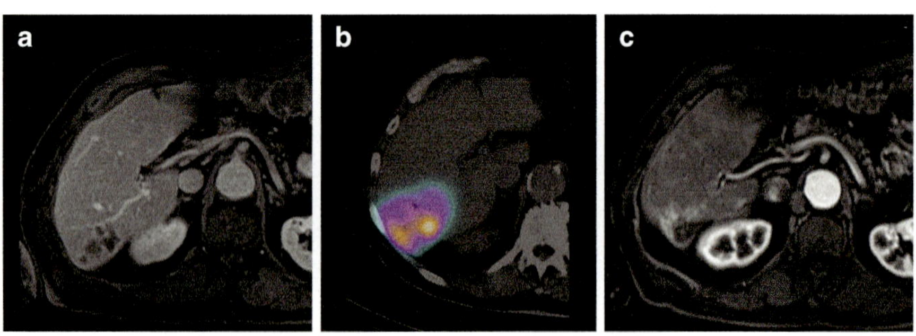


**Fig. 11.3** Superselective segmental radioembolisation or radiation segmentectomy. (**a**) CT scan before treatment showing a multinodular tumour in segment VI. (**b**) PET scan showing intense radiation in segment VI after superselective injection of Y90 resin microspheres into the segmental artery. (**c**) Significant atrophy of segment VI and lack of tumour activity 1 year after treatment

## References


1. Sangro B, Iñarrairaegui M, Bilbao JI. Radioembolization for hepatocellular carcinoma. J Hepatol. 2012 Feb;56(2):464–73.
2. Aramburu J, Antón R, Rivas A, Ramos JC, Sangro B, Bilbao JI, et al. Liver cancer arterial perfusion modelling and CFD boundary conditions methodology: a case study of the haemodynamics of a patient-specific hepatic artery in literature-based healthy and tumour-bearing liver scenarios. Int J Numer Method Biomed Eng. 2016;32(11) https://doi.org/10.1002/cnm.2764.
3. Kennedy A, Coldwell D, Sangro B. Radioembolization for the treatment of liver tumours: general principles. Am J Clin Oncol. 2012;35(1):91–9.
4. Sangro B, Carpanese L, Cianni R, Golfieri R, Gasparini D, Ezziddin S, et al. Survival after yttrium-90 resin microsphere radioembolization of hepatocellular carcinoma across Barcelona clinic liver cancer stages: a European evaluation. Hepatology. 2011;54(3):868–78.
5. Rodríguez-Lago I, Carretero C, Herráiz M, Subtil JC, Betés M, Rodríguez-Fraile M, et al. Long-term follow-up study of gastroduodenal lesions after radioembolization of hepatic tumors. World J Gastroenterol. 2013;19(19):2935–40.
6. Sangro B, Martínez-Urbistondo D, Bester L, Bilbao JI, Coldwell DM, Flamen P, et al. Prevention and treatment of complications of selective internal radiation therapy: expert guidance and systematic review. Hepatology. 2017 Sep;66(3):969–82.
7. Gil-Alzugaray B, Chopitea A, Iñarrairaegui M, Bilbao JI, Rodriguez-Fraile M, Rodriguez J, et al. Prognostic factors and prevention of radioembolization-induced liver disease. Hepatology. 2013 Mar;57(3):1078–87.
8. Johnson PJ, Berhane S, Kagebayashi C, Satomura S, Teng M, Reeve HL, et al. Assessment of liver function in patients with hepatocellular carcinoma: a new evidence-based approach—the ALBI grade. J Clin Oncol. 2015;33(6):550–8.
9. Sangro B, Rodriguez M. Radioembolization for hepatocellular carcinoma: gaining insight on a personalized approach. Liver Int. 2017;37(1):32–4.
10. Iñarrairaegui M, Thurston KG, Bilbao JI, D'Avola D, Rodriguez M, Arbizu J, et al. Radioembolization with use of Yttrium-90 resin microspheres in patients with hepatocellular carcinoma and portal vein thrombosis. J Vasc Interv Radiol. 2010;21(8):1205–12.
11. Riaz A, Gates VL, Atassi B, Lewandowski RJ, Mulcahy MF, Ryu RK, et al. Radiation segmentectomy: a novel approach to increase safety and efficacy of radioembolization. Int J Radiat Oncol Biol Phys. 2011;79(1):163–71.
12. Fernández-Ros N, Silva N, Bilbao JI, Iñarrairaegui M, Benito A, Davola D, et al. Partial liver volume radioembolization induces hypertrophy in the spared hemiliver and no major signs of portal hypertension. HPB (Oxford). 2014;16(3):243–9.
13. Seidensticker R, Seidensticker M, Damm R, Mohnike K, Schütte K, Malfertheiner P, et al. Hepatic toxicity after radioembolization of the liver using 90Y-microspheres: sequential lobar versus whole liver approach. Cardiovasc Intervent Radiol. 2012;35(5):1109–18.
14. Sancho L, Rodriguez-Fraile M, Bilbao JI, Beorlegui Arteta C, Iñarrairaegui M, Moran V, et al. Is a technetium-99m macroaggregated albumin scan essential in the workup for selective internal radiation therapy with yttrium-90? An analysis of 532 patients. J Vasc Interv Radiol. 2017;28(11):1536–42.
15. Lau WY, Kennedy AS, Kim YH, Lai HK, Lee RC, Leung TW, et al. Patient selection and activity planning guide for selective internal radiotherapy with yttrium-90 resin microspheres. Int J Radiat Oncol Biol Phys. 2012;82(1):401–7.
16. Kennedy AS, Ball D, Cohen SJ, Cohn M, Coldwell DM, Drooz A, et al. Multicenter evaluation of the safety and efficacy of radioembolization in patients with unresectable colorectal liver metastases selected as candidates for (90)Y resin microspheres. J Gastrointest Oncol. 2015;6(2):134–42.
17. van Hazel GA, Heinemann V, Sharma NK, Findlay MP, Ricke J, Peeters M, et al. SIRFLOX: randomized phase III trial comparing first-line mfolfox6 (plus or minus Bevacizumab) versus

mFOLFOX6 (plus or minus Bevacizumab) plus selective internal radiation therapy in patients with metastatic colorectal cancer. J Clin Oncol. 2016;34(15):1723–31.
18. Salem R, Lewandowski RJ, Mulcahy MF, et al. Radioembolization for hepatocellular carcinoma using Yttrium-90 microspheres: a comprehensive report of long-term outcomes. Gastroenterology. 2010;138:52–64.
19. Hilgard P, Hamami M, Fouly AE, et al. Radioembolization with yttrium- 90 glass microspheres in hepatocellular carcinoma: European experience on safety and long-term survival. Hepatology. 2010;52:1741–9.
20. Mazzaferro V, Sposito C, Bhoori S, et al. Yttrium90 radioembolization for intermediate-advanced hepatocarcinoma: a phase II study. Hepatology. https://doi.org/10.1002/hep.26014.
21. Sangro B, Carpanese L, Cianni R, European Network on Radioembolization with Yttrium-90 Resin Microspheres (ENRY). Survival after Yttrium-90 resin microsphere radioembolization of hepatocellular carcinoma across Barcelona clinic liver cancer stages: a European evaluation. Hepatology. 2011;54:868–78.
22. Vilgrain V, Pereira H, Assenat E, et al. Efficacy and safety of selective internal radiotherapy with yttrium-90 resin microspheres compared with sorafenib in locally advanced and inoperable hepatocellular carcinoma (SARAH): an open-label randomised controlled phase 3 trial. Lancet Oncol. 2017;18(12):1624–36. https://doi.org/10.1016/S1470-2045(17)30683-6.
23. Chow PKH, Gandhi M, Tan SB, et al. SIRveNIB: Selective Internal Radiation Therapy Versus Sorafenib in Asia- Pacific Patients With Hepatocellular Carcinoma. J Clin Oncol. 2018;36(19):1913–21. https://doi.org/10.1200/JCO.2017.76.0892.
24. Vilgrain V, Pereira H, Assenat E, Guiu B, Ilonca AD, Pageaux GP, et al. Efficacy and safety of selective internal radiotherapy with yttrium-90 resin microspheres compared with sorafenib in locally advanced and inoperable hepatocellular carcinoma (SARAH): an open-label randomised controlled phase 3 trial. Lancet Oncol. 2017;18(12):1624–36.
25. Pierce H, Chow W, Gandhi M, Asia-Paciifc Hepatocellular Carcinoma Trials Group. Phase III multi-Centre open-label randomized controlled trial of selective internal radiation therapy (SIRT) versus sorafenib in locally advanced hepatocellular carcinoma: the SIRveNIB study. J Clin Oncol. 2017;35(15_suppl):4002.
26. de la Torre MA, Buades-Mateu J, de la Rosa PA, Lué A, Bustamante FJ, Serrano MT, et al. A comparison of survival in patients with hepatocellular carcinoma and portal vein invasion treated by radioembolization or sorafenib. Liver Int. 2016;36(8):1206–12.
27. European Association for the Study of the Liver. EASL–EORTC clinical practice guidelines: management of hepatocellular carcinoma. Eur J Cancer. 2012;48(5):599–641.
28. Pitton MB, Kloeckner R, Ruckes C, Wirth GM, Eichhorn W, Wörns MA, et al. Randomized comparison of selective internal radiotherapy (SIRT) versus drug-eluting bead transarterial chemoembolization (DEB-TACE) for the treatment of hepatocellular carcinoma. Cardiovasc Intervent Radiol. 2015;38(2):352–60.
29. Kolligs FT, Bilbao JI, Jakobs T, Iñarrairaegui M, Nagel JM, Rodriguez M, et al. Pilot randomized trial of selective internal radiation therapy vs. chemoembolization in unresectable hepatocellular carcinoma. Liver Int. 2015;35(6):1715–21.
30. Salem R, Gordon AC, Mouli S, Hickey R, Kallini J, Gabr A, et al. Y90 Radioembolization significantly prolongs time to progression compared with chemoembolization in patients with hepatocellular carcinoma. Gastroenterology. 2016;151(6):1155–63.
31. Pardo F, Sangro B, Lee RC, Manas D, Jeyarajah R, Donckier V, et al. The post-sir-spheres surgery study (p4s): retrospective analysis of safety following hepatic resection or transplantation in patients previously treated with selective internal radiation therapy with yttrium-90 resin microspheres. Ann Surg Oncol. 2017;24(9):2465–73.
32. Salem R, Mazzaferro V, Sangro B. Yttrium 90 radioembolization for the treatment of hepatocellular carcinoma: biological lessons, current challenges, and clinical perspectives. Hepatology. 2013;58(6):2188–97.

# Chapter 12
# Oncotherapies for HCC

**Alexa Childs and Tim Meyer**

**Key Learning Points**

1. Forty percent of patients diagnosed with hepatocellular carcinoma (HCC) are currently candidates for systemic therapy.
2. Sorafenib is a multi-targeted tyrosine kinase inhibitor and has been for standard of care for advanced BCLC stage C disease since 2007.
3. Sorafenib improves median survival by nearly 3 months versus placebo (10.7 vs 7.9 months) but has little benefit with patients beyond Child-Pugh A cirrhosis.
4. There is currently no benefit from adjuvant or combination systemic and surgical/locoregional therapies.
5. Lenvatinib could be used as an alternative to sorafenib as a first-line therapy.
6. Regorafenib is the first approved second-line treatment for patients who progress on first-line therapy.
7. The role of immune therapy is being explored, and outcomes for these trials may significantly change the management of patients with advanced HCC.

A. Childs · T. Meyer (✉)
Department of Oncology, UCL Cancer Institute, University College London, London, UK

Department of Oncology, Royal Free Hospital, London, UK
e-mail: t.meyer@ucl.ac.uk



T. Cross, D. H. Palmer (eds.), *Liver Cancers*,
https://doi.org/10.1007/978-3-319-92216-4_12

**Areas of Controversy and Uncertainty**

1. The role of adjuvant and combination therapies has been an active area of research, but the results of trials have been disappointing.
2. Immune therapy has revolutionized outcomes in patients with advanced malignant melanoma and non-small cell lung cancer, but how and when it might be used in patients with HCC has yet to be fully determined.
3. The ability to individualize treatment against specific tumour targets remains an aspiration for clinicians managing HCC.

## Introduction

Liver cancer is the second leading cause of cancer-related mortality worldwide and accounted for 745,000 deaths in 2012, of which 50% occurred in China alone [1]. The incidence closely matches the prevalence reflecting the lethal nature of this disease and very low rates of cure. Around 30% cases are eligible for curative interventions such as transplantation, resection or ablation, and a further 20% may be suitable for transarterial therapy. Of the remaining 50%, 10% require symptomatic supportive care, leaving 40% who are candidates for systemic therapy [2]. For the last decade, the standard of care for advanced HCC has been sorafenib, an oral multi-targeted tyrosine kinase inhibitor which is associated with a median survival of around 11 months representing a 3-month improvement over placebo [3]. Numerous trials in the first- and second-line setting have failed, but in the past year, there has finally been progress that will improve outcomes in patients with advanced disease and has the potential to also improve outcomes in earlier-stage disease.

## Chemotherapy

Chemotherapy has been used in the treatment of HCC for over 40 years, although the evidence base for efficacy remains weak. Doxorubicin has historically been regarded as the standard chemotherapy agent for HCC on the basis of an initial single-arm study performed in 14 patients, which reported a response rate of 79% [4]. Studies conducted subsequently were limited by the absence of an appropriate control arm and the use of surrogate markers of response such as hepatomegaly and AFP. Despite this, they still failed to reproduce the results seen in the initial study, with reported response rates varying between 1 and 35% [5]. Only 1 randomized trial of 106 patients has compared doxorubicin to best supportive care (BSC) and reported a small benefit in median survival, despite lower-than-expected survival in both arms (2.7 months for doxorubicin vs 1.9 months in those receiving BSC) [6]. Response rates were only 3% in the context of a 25% treatment-related mortality rate, which is significantly higher than that seen in subsequent studies, where mortality rates have been in the region of 3% or less [7].

There has been interest in alternative chemotherapeutic regimens, and four randomized controlled trials have been performed in different patient populations using doxorubicin as the control arm. The PIAF regimen (cisplatin, interferon, doxorubicin and fluorouracil) was investigated after a promising response rate of 26% was reported in an initial phase II study [8]. In a trial performed in Hong Kong, 188 patients were randomized to receive either PIAF or doxorubicin, and whilst the superior response rate of PIAF was confirmed (10.5% vs 20.9%), there was no significant difference seen in (OS) [7]. Nolatrexed, a thymidylate synthase inhibitor, has been compared to doxorubicin in a study conducted across 445 patients recruited from a Western population and shown to have a significantly worse OS (5.1 months vs 7.4 months [HR 0.753 $p = 0.0068$]), along with increased toxicity [9]. A global study of 339 patients investigating the microtubule inhibitor T138067 was also negative and failed to demonstrate any improvement in survival when compared to doxorubicin (5.7 vs 5.6 months, respectively) [10]. The FOLFOX regime (fluorouracil and oxaliplatin) has been compared to doxorubicin in 371 patients recruited from Asian countries of which 70% were from mainland China [11]. Response rates were higher with FOLFOX (8.2% vs 2.7%, $p = 0.0233$), and a small benefit in median survival was also seen on long-term follow-up (6.4 months vs 5.0 months, $p = 0.0425$).

In summary, the available evidence suggests that chemotherapy may provide a modest survival benefit, but patient selection remains of key importance to limit toxicity. The current data support the use of FOLFOX over doxorubicin.

## Sorafenib

Sorafenib, an oral multi-targeted tyrosine kinase inhibitor against Raf, VEGFR, PDGFR and c-Kit [12], was the first systemic treatment proven to have a survival benefit in advanced HCC. It was approved in 2007 on the basis of two large multicentre, randomized, placebo-controlled studies. The phase III Sorafenib HCC Assessment Randomized Protocol (SHARP) trial was performed in a predominantly Western population recruited from Europe, North America, South America and Australasia and demonstrated a significantly improved OS in patients with advanced HCC and well-preserved liver function (>95% Child-Pugh A) [3]. Investigators reported a median OS benefit of nearly 3 months with sorafenib therapy (10.7 vs 7.9 months; HR 0.69, [95% CI 0.55–0.87], $p < 0.001$) and improved time to progression (TTP) 5.5 months for sorafenib versus 2.8 months for placebo (0.58, [95% CI 0.45–0.74] $p < 0.001$). This was despite an objective response rate of only 2% according to response evaluation in solid tumours criteria (RECIST). The overall incidence of treatment-related adverse events was 80% in the sorafenib arm compared to 52% in the placebo group, with grade 3 adverse events in the sorafenib arm consisting predominantly of diarrhoea (8% vs 2%, $p < 0.001$), hand-foot skin reaction (8% vs 1%, $p < 0.001$), hypertension (2% vs <1%, $p = 0.28$) and abdominal pain (2% vs <1%, $p = 0.17$). The positive effect of sorafenib on OS and TTP was confirmed by the results of the phase III Sorafenib Asia-Pacific trial [13], performed in China, South Korea and Taiwan, thereby establishing sorafenib as the standard of care in patients with advanced HCC. Child-Pugh class A was an entry criteria for both the SHARP trial and the Asia-Pacific study, but data regarding sorafenib in Child-Pugh B patients is now available from post-marketing studies and field of practice audits. The GIDEON study is the largest prospective study to date and has evaluated the impact of liver function in a cohort of >3000 patients treated with sorafenib, including 666 with Child-Pugh class B [14]. In the final analysis, overall adverse events were similarly observed in both Child A and B patients, but the rate of sorafenib discontinuation in Child-Pugh B patients was higher as compared to Child-Pugh A (40% vs 25%). More importantly, the median survival of patients with a Child-Pugh class beyond A treated with sorafenib is extremely poor at around 3.6 months [15] suggesting that it is not cost effective to offer such patients therapy. Similar findings were reported in a UK audit in which patients with Child-Pugh B disease treated with sorafenib had a survival of only 4.6 months [16].

To establish if some subgroups benefit more than others, Bruix et al. conducted an exploratory subgroup analysis of the SHARP data and found that sorafenib consistently improved OS across HCC patients, irrespective of disease aetiology, baseline tumour burden, performance status and prior therapy [17]. OS in the sorafenib arm appeared higher in those patients with HCV compared to those with HBV (HBV sorafenib OS 9.7 months vs placebo 6.1 months; HCV sorafenib OS 14 months vs placebo 7.4 months), leading to the suggestion that patients with HCV-related HCC may derive more clinical benefit from sorafenib treatment than patients with HBV-related HCC. A subsequent pooled analysis of the SHARP and Asia-Pacific trial confirmed that the greatest benefit for sorafenib was observed in the patients with hepatitis C but also in those with no extrahepatic spread and a low neutrophil-to-lymphocyte ratio [18].

Another study examined circulating biomarkers from SHARP study cohort and found that high baseline plasma angiopoietin 2 (Ang2) and vascular endothelial growth factor (VEGF) were independently associated with worse prognosis but had no predictive value, whilst high c-KIT and low hepatocyte growth factor showed a trend towards enhanced survival benefit from sorafenib [19]. Numerous other potential biomarkers have also been evaluated, including interleukin 6 and interleukin 8 [20], insulin-like growth factor (IGF) [21, 22], transforming growth factor (TGF-β1) [22] and hepatocyte growth factor (HGF) [19, 23], but their role remains unproven.

The positive outcomes in advanced disease prompted the evaluation of sorafenib in earlier-stage disease. The STORM trial randomized patients who had undergone surgical resection or ablation to sorafenib 400 mg twice daily or match placebo for a maximum of 4 years. There was neither difference in recurrence free survival between the two arms at 33.3 and 33.7 months, respectively, nor was there evidence of an improvement in OS [24]. Combining sorafenib with transarterial chemoembolization has been similarly disappointing. Two trials, the global SPACE trial and the UK TACE 2 trial, randomized patients receiving TACE, performed with doxorubicin eluting beads, to combined therapy with sorafenib or matched placebo [25, 26]. Both trials were negative with no improvement in their respective primary endpoints, time to progression or progression-free survival. Hence, there remains a significant unmet need for systemic therapy that is effective in the adjuvant setting or in combination with locoregional therapy.

Sorafenib-based drug combinations have also been disappointing to date. Initially encouraging data were reported by Abou-Alfa et al. who compared doxorubicin alone with the combination of doxorubicin and sorafenib in 97 patients recruited across North and South America and Europe [27]. OS was improved in the combination group as compared to doxorubicin alone (13.7 vs 6.5 months), but the absence of a comparative sorafenib group precluded any assessment of synergism between doxorubicin and sorafenib. A subsequent phase III trial comparing sorafenib with sorafenib plus doxorubicin was conducted with the primary endpoint of OS [28]. The study was discontinued early at planned interim analysis when median OS was found to be 9.3 months (95% CI 7.1–12.9) for combination therapy and 10.5 months (95% CI 7.4–14.3) for sorafenib monotherapy [HR 1.06 (95% CI 0.8–1.4)] in the context of increased toxicity in the combination arm. The SEARCH trial compared the combination of sorafenib and the EGFR antagonist erlotinib with sorafenib and placebo in a randomized, double-blind, placebo-controlled trial. There was no significant difference in median OS at 9.5 months and 8.5 months, respectively [29].

In summary, sorafenib has been the only approved systemic therapy for the treatment of advanced HCC for the past 10 years. The survival benefit is modest, and response rate is negligible. It has no role as an adjuvant therapy and, to date, has not demonstrated improvement when used in combination with locoregional therapy or other systemic agents.

## *First-Line Phase III Trials*

Since the approval of sorafenib in 2007, large randomized trials have sought to improve the survival benefit seen with sorafenib monotherapy in the first-line setting. Several have evaluated antiangiogenic therapies with limited success. Sunitinib [30], linifanib [31] and brivanib [32] have all been compared with sorafenib in the recently reported negative phase III studies. However, the impasse was broken by the recently reported REFLECT trial in which lenvatinib was evaluated in the first-line setting. Lenvatinib is an orally active, tyrosine kinase inhibitor with multiple targets, including VEGFR 1–3, FGFR 1–4, PDGFRα, RET and KIT. It was initially evaluated in both phase I and II studies, the latter of which enrolled 46 advanced HCC patients who had previously received treatment with sorafenib [33, 34]. The primary endpoint of time to progression (TTP) was 7.4 months, 37% of patients achieved a response, and the median OS was 18.7 months. In light of these results, a phase III non-inferiority trial (REFLECT study) was conducted comparing lenvatinib with sorafenib as first-line treatment in 954 patients with unresectable HCC and preserved liver function (Child-Pugh A). The study met its primary endpoint demonstrating that the median OS with lenvatinib was non-inferior to sorafenib (13.6 vs 12.3 months; HR 0.92 95% CI 0.79–1.06) [35]. The study also showed statistically significant improvements for secondary endpoints, including progression-free survival (7.4 vs 3.7 months; HR 0.66 95% CI 0.57–0.77 $p < 0.00001$), time to progression (8.9 vs 3.7 months; HR 0.63 95% CI 0.53–0.73 $p < 0.00001$) and objective response rate (24.1 vs 9.2% $p < 0.00001$). These findings may lead to the approval of lenvatinib as a first-line agent for unresectable HCC, in which case strategies for the differential use of lenvatinib and sorafenib in the clinical setting will need to be determined.

On the basis of the currently available evidence, sorafenib remains the first-line standard of care for patients with advanced HCC pending approval of lenvatinib.

## *Second-Line Phase III Trials*

Several trials assessing targeted agents after progression on sorafenib have produced disappointing results. Brivanib, a selective inhibitor of VEGFR and FGFR, was compared to placebo in a randomized phase III study recruiting HCC patients who were refractory or intolerant to first-line treatment with sorafenib [36]. Although TTP was significantly longer in the brivanib arm, the primary endpoint of OS was not met. The REACH trial randomized patients to receive ramucirumab, a VEGFR-2 monoclonal antibody, or best supportive care following sorafenib, and again, no significant difference in OS was reported (HR 0.87 [95% CI 0.72–1.05]; $p = 0.14$) [37]. Interestingly, however, a prespecified subgroup of patients with a baseline AFP concentration of 400 ng/mL or greater exhibited a significantly improved OS compared to placebo (7.8 months vs 4.2 months, respectively). The hypothesis that ramucirumab is more effective in patients with a high AFP is being tested in the ongoing REACH-2 trial (NCT02435433).

The mTOR pathway is activated in up to 45% of HCC [38] and is associated with poorly differentiated tumours, early recurrence and worse prognosis [39, 40]. In view of this, the mTOR inhibitor everolimus was evaluated in the second-line phase III EVOLVE-1 trial which recruited a total of 546 HCC patients [41]. Unfortunately, no significant difference was seen in OS, reported as 7.6 months in the experimental arm compared to 7.3 months with placebo (HR 1.05; $p = 0.67$). Tuberous sclerosis complex 2 (TSC2) functions as a negative regulator of the mTOR pathway, and subsequent preclinical studies have suggested that tumours with loss of TSC2 expression may have enhanced sensitivity to mTOR inhibition. In a retrospective analysis of the EVOLVE-1 data, investigators assessed patient TSC2 status by immunohistochemistry and found that TSC2-null/low patients treated with everolimus tended to have longer OS than those who received placebo or those patients with high TSC2 expression who received everolimus [42]. This preliminary data may justify further investigation of TSC2 as a potential predictive biomarker for everolimus treatment. Arginine depletion has also been explored in HCC based on the observation that HCC is auxotrophic for this semi-essential amino acid. Patients who had failed or were intolerant to sorafenib were randomized 2:1 to PEGylated arginine deiminase (PEG-ADI 20) by weekly IM injection or matched placebo. The trial was negative with a median OS of 7.8 and 7.4 months, respectively (HR = 1.022 (95% CI, 0.847, 1.233) $p = 0.884$) [43]. However, patients with arginine depletion beyond 8 weeks had better survival than those with less than or equal to 4 weeks (12.3 vs 7.3 months), suggesting that strategies to prolong arginine depletion could be pursued.

Most recently, a phase III trial of regorafenib, a multi-kinase inhibitor of VEGFR, PDGFR, FGFR, TIE2, KIT, RET and RAF, has reported positive results in the second-line setting. An initial open-label phase II study assessed 36 patients pre-treated with sorafenib and demonstrated an acceptable safety profile with median OS of 13.8 months and disease control rate of 72% [44]. Following this, the phase III RESORCE study recruited 573 patients with advanced HCC who had progressed on sorafenib. Patients were required to have received sorafenib for at least 20 days at a dose of at least 400 mg/day. Median OS, the primary endpoint of the study, was significantly greater in patients who received regorafenib than placebo (10.6 vs 7.8 months; HR 0.63 95% CI 0.50–0.79; $p < 0.0001$) [45]. This phase III trial of regorafenib is the first to show an OS benefit compared with placebo in patients who have failed sorafenib treatment and has established a new standard of care for second-line therapy in HCC.

## Molecularly Stratified Trials

The hepatocyte growth factor (HGF)-MET axis has been implicated in hepatocarcinogenesis, and high levels of c-MET expression have been associated with vascular invasion, tumour recurrence and reduced survival in several studies [46]. Overexpression of c-MET is reported in 20–80% of HCC tumours, making it a valid potential target for therapy. Tivantinib, a selective c-MET receptor tyrosine kinase inhibitor, has been investigated in advanced HCC as part of a randomized, placebo-controlled phase II trial, where patients were stratified according to level of c-MET expression [47]. Patients with high c-MET expression treated with tivantinib had significantly improved OS compared to those treated with placebo (median OS 7.2 months for tivantinib vs 3.8 months for placebo (HR 0.38; 95% CI 0.18–0.81). For patients with c-MET low tumours, there were no differences in mTTP, mOS or DCR. Disappointingly, a large second-line, placebo-controlled phase III study of tivantinib in patients selected for high c-MET expression did not improve OS which was 8.4 and 9.1 months for tivantinib and placebo, respectively [48]. There are several other c-MET inhibitors of differing specificity in various stages of clinical development for HCC at the current time, including cabozantinib, foretinib, capmatinib and tepotinib. Only the ongoing phase II study of tepotinib is actively recruiting patients according to levels of c-MET expression (NCT02115373).

The RAS/RAF/MEK/ERK pathway has a pivotal role in cellular proliferation, and a small subset of HCC patients have tumour growth which is driven by constitutive activation of a mutant RAS [49, 50] which can be targeted by the selective inhibition of downstream targets such as MEK. In an initial phase II study evaluating refametinib in combination with sorafenib, only 5% of patients had evidence of RAS mutations; however, three of these four patients went on to achieve a partial response [51]. The combination therapy had a pronounced toxicity profile, however, with an 80% rate of grade 3 and 4 adverse events and four treatment-related patient deaths on study. In light of this, a phase II study is currently underway to explore the efficacy and safety of refametinib monotherapy in advanced RAS-mutated HCC (NCT01915589).

Whilst stratified trials have been disappointing to date, several studies have defined molecular subclassifications in hepatocellular carcinoma, and these will need to be carefully incorporated into future trial design [52].

## Immunotherapy

Many different immunotherapeutic approaches have been investigated in HCC to date; these include vaccine platforms based on RNA and dendritic cells, adoptive T-cell therapy, cytokines and gene therapy [53]. The presence of tumour-infiltrating lymphocytes in HCC [54] confirms the immunogenicity of this tumour type and further rationale for this therapy can be found in the fact that relapse rates post transplantation and resection are reduced in patients with dense lymphocytic infiltration [55, 56]. Recently, the remarkable success of checkpoint inhibitors in tumour types such as melanoma and non-small cell lung cancer [57–60] has stimulated great interest in their potential role in HCC.

Tremelimumab, an anti-CTLA-4 monoclonal antibody, was the first checkpoint inhibitor to be tested in patients with HCC and chronic HCV infection. In a phase II study of 21 patients, it achieved a response rate of 17%, disease control rate of 76% and a median time to progression of 6.5 months [61]. Interestingly, a significant drop in viral load was also seen on treatment. Local tumour destruction during ablation or chemoembolization could potentially enhance tumour-specific antigen presentation, and in view of this tremelimumab has also been evaluated in combination with TACE/RFA in a pilot study of 32 patients which confirmed the feasibility of the approach [62]. Again, a significant antiviral effect was observed with 12 out of 14 patients experiencing reduction in HCV viral load. Together, these studies demonstrate that tremelimumab can be administered safely to a cirrhotic patient population and has a potential antitumour and antiviral effect warranting further investigation.

Targeting the PD-1/PD-L1 has also been explored. Nivolumab is a fully human IgG4 anti-PD-1 monoclonal antibody and has been evaluated in an HCC-specific multicentre phase I/phase II trial which recruited a total of 262 patients [63]. In the dose expansion cohort, an overall response rate of 20% by RECIST 1.1 was reported, and the survival rate at 9 months was 74%, with some patients achieving durable responses exceeding 12 months. The response rate was similar across the hepatitis B and C infected and the uninfected cohorts. Prior sorafenib did not affect response rate, and there was no clear relationship between response and tumour PD-L1 expression. With extended follow-up, the median survival of patients treated second-lines was 15.6 months which compares favourably with previously reported second-line trials [64]. A first-line phase III study comparing nivolumab with sorafenib has completed recruitment, and results are expected in 2018 (NCT02576509).

Many ongoing trials are evaluating other checkpoint-targeting molecules and combinations thereof. A key priority is the identification of biomarkers to define the responsive subpopulation.

## Conclusion

Sorafenib represented a modest but important step forward in the treatment of advanced HCC, but it has taken 10 years to make further meaningful advances. In the first-line setting, the REFLECT study has demonstrated that lenvatinib has a non-inferior OS to sorafenib and has clinically significant antitumour effects. The improved ORR with lenvatinib may favour its use over sorafenib in patients who remain symptomatic due to heavy disease burden and potentially allow downstaging of disease, but the optimum sequence of these therapies remains unknown. In the second-line setting, the RESORCE trial has proven the activity of regorafenib with a manageable safety profile and provides a treatment option to those patients who remain fit enough for further therapy after progression on sorafenib. There is an increasing interest in the role of immunotherapy in advanced HCC, and phase III evidence on the role of nivolumab is expected within the next year which might further change the care of patients with advanced HCC.

## References

1. Ferlay J, Soerjomataram I, Dikshit R, Eser S, Mathers C, Rebelo M, et al. Cancer incidence and mortality worldwide: sources, methods and major patterns in GLOBOCAN 2012. Int J Cancer. 2015;136(5):E359–86.
2. European Association for the Study of the L, European Organisation for R, Treatment of C. EASL-EORTC clinical practice guidelines: management of hepatocellular carcinoma. J Hepatol. 2012;56(4):908–43.
3. Llovet JM, Ricci S, Mazzaferro V, Hilgard P, Gane E, Blanc JF, et al. Sorafenib in advanced hepatocellular carcinoma. N Engl J Med. 2008;359(4):378–90.
4. Olweny CL, Toya T, Katongole-Mbidde E, Mugerwa J, Kyalwazi SK, Cohen H. Treatment of hepatocellular carcinoma with adriamycin. Preliminary communication. Cancer. 1975;36(4):1250–7.
5. Burroughs A, Hochhauser D, Meyer T. Systemic treatment and liver transplantation for hepatocellular carcinoma: two ends of the therapeutic spectrum. Lancet Oncol. 2004;5(7):409–18.

6. Lai CL, Wu PC, Chan GC, Lok AS, Lin HJ. Doxorubicin versus no antitumor therapy in inoperable hepatocellular carcinoma. A prospective randomized trial. Cancer. 1988;62(3):479–83.
7. Yeo W, Mok TS, Zee B, Leung TW, Lai PB, Lau WY, et al. A randomized phase III study of doxorubicin versus cisplatin/interferon alpha-2b/doxorubicin/fluorouracil (PIAF) combination chemotherapy for unresectable hepatocellular carcinoma. J Natl Cancer Inst. 2005;97(20):1532–8.
8. Leung TW, Patt YZ, Lau WY, Ho SK, Yu SC, Chan AT, et al. Complete pathological remission is possible with systemic combination chemotherapy for inoperable hepatocellular carcinoma. Clin Cancer Res. 1999;5(7):1676–81.
9. Gish RG, Porta C, Lazar L, Ruff P, Feld R, Croitoru A, et al. Phase III randomized controlled trial comparing the survival of patients with unresectable hepatocellular carcinoma treated with nolatrexed or doxorubicin. J Clin Oncol. 2007;25(21):3069–75.
10. Posey J, Johnson P, Mok T, Hirmand M, Dahlberg S, Kwei L, et al. Results of a phase 2/3 open-label, randomized trial of T138067 versus doxorubicin (DOX) in chemotherapy-naïve, unresectable hepatocellular carcinoma (HCC). J Clin Oncol. 2005;23(90160):4035.
11. Qin S, Bai Y, Lim HY, Thongprasert S, Chao Y, Fan J, et al. Randomized, multicenter, open-label study of oxaliplatin plus fluorouracil/leucovorin versus doxorubicin as palliative chemotherapy in patients with advanced hepatocellular carcinoma from Asia. J Clin Oncol. 2013;31(28):3501–8.
12. Wilhelm SM, Adnane L, Newell P, Villanueva A, Llovet JM, Lynch M. Preclinical overview of sorafenib, a multikinase inhibitor that targets both Raf and VEGF and PDGF receptor tyrosine kinase signaling. Mol Cancer Ther. 2008;7(10):3129–40.
13. Cheng AL, Kang YK, Chen Z, Tsao CJ, Qin S, Kim JS, et al. Efficacy and safety of sorafenib in patients in the Asia-Pacific region with advanced hepatocellular carcinoma: a phase III randomised, double-blind, placebo-controlled trial. Lancet Oncol. 2009;10(1):25–34.
14. Lencioni R, Kudo M, Ye SL, Bronowicki JP, Chen XP, Dagher L, et al. GIDEON (Global Investigation of therapeutic DEcisions in hepatocellular carcinoma and Of its treatment with sorafeNib): second interim analysis. Int J Clin Pract. 2014;68(5):609–17.
15. Edeline J, Blanc JF, Johnson P, Campillo-Gimenez B, Ross P, Ma YT, et al. A multicentre comparison between Child Pugh and Albumin-Bilirubin scores in patients treated with sorafenib for Hepatocellular Carcinoma. Liver Int. 2016;36(12):1821–8.
16. King J, Palmer DH, Johnson P, Ross P, Hubner RA, Sumpter K, et al. Sorafenib for the treatment of advanced hepatocellular cancer–a UK audit. Clin Oncol (R Coll Radiol). 2017;29(4):256–62.
17. Bruix J, Raoul JL, Sherman M, Mazzaferro V, Bolondi L, Craxi A, et al. Efficacy and safety of sorafenib in patients with advanced hepatocellular carcinoma: subanalyses of a phase III trial. J Hepatol. 2012;57(4):821–9.
18. Bruix J, Cheng AL, Meinhardt G, Nakajima K, De Sanctis Y, Llovet J. Prognostic factors and predictors of sorafenib benefit in patients with hepatocellular carcinoma: analysis of two phase III studies. J Hepatol. 2017;67(5):999–1008.
19. Llovet JM, Pena CE, Lathia CD, Shan M, Meinhardt G, Bruix J, et al. Plasma biomarkers as predictors of outcome in patients with advanced hepatocellular carcinoma. Clin Cancer Res. 2012;18(8):2290–300.
20. Shao Y, Hsu C, Huang C, Cheng A. Use of plasma angiogenesis-related factors to investigate the association of interleukin 8 and interleukin 6 levels with efficacy of sorafenib-based antiangiogenic therapy in patients with advanced hepatocellular carcinoma (HCC). J Clin Oncol. 2011;29(4_suppl):199.
21. Shao YY, Huang CC, Lin SD, Hsu CH, Cheng AL. Serum insulin-like growth factor-1 levels predict outcomes of patients with advanced hepatocellular carcinoma receiving antiangiogenic therapy. Clin Cancer Res. 2012;18(14):3992–7.
22. Lin TH, Shao YY, Chan SY, Huang CY, Hsu CH, Cheng AL. High serum transforming growth factor-beta1 levels predict outcome in hepatocellular carcinoma patients treated with sorafenib. Clin Cancer Res. 2015;21(16):3678–84.

23. Miyahara K, Nouso K, Tomoda T, Kobayashi S, Hagihara H, Kuwaki K, et al. Predicting the treatment effect of sorafenib using serum angiogenesis markers in patients with hepatocellular carcinoma. J Gastroenterol Hepatol. 2011;26(11):1604–11.
24. Bruix J, Takayama T, Mazzaferro V, Chau GY, Yang J, Kudo M, et al. Adjuvant sorafenib for hepatocellular carcinoma after resection or ablation (STORM): a phase 3, randomised, double-blind, placebo-controlled trial. Lancet Oncol. 2015;16(13):1344–54.
25. Lencioni R, Llovet JM, Han G, Tak WY, Yang J, Guglielmi A, et al. Sorafenib or placebo plus TACE with doxorubicin-eluting beads for intermediate stage HCC: the SPACE trial. J Hepatol. 2016;64(5):1090–8.
26. Meyer T, Fox R, Ma YT, Ross PJ, James MW, Sturgess R, et al. Sorafenib in combination with transarterial chemoembolisation in patients with unresectable hepatocellular carcinoma (TACE 2): a randomised placebo-controlled, double-blind, phase 3 trial. Lancet Gastroenterol Hepatol. 2017;2(8):565–75.
27. Abou-Alfa GK, Johnson P, Knox JJ, Capanu M, Davidenko I, Lacava J, et al. Doxorubicin plus sorafenib vs doxorubicin alone in patients with advanced hepatocellular carcinoma: a randomized trial. JAMA. 2010;304(19):2154–60.
28. Abou-Alfa GK, Niedzwieski D, Knox JJ, Kaubisch A, Posey J, Tan BR, Kavan P, Goel R, Murray JJ, Bekaii-Saab TS, Tam VC, Rajdev L, Kelley RK, Siegel A, Balletti J, Harding JJ, Schwartz LH, Goldberg RM, Bertagnolli MM, Venook AP. Phase III randomized study of sorafenib plus doxorubicin versus sorafenib in patients with advanced hepatocellular carcinoma (HCC): CALGB 80802 (Alliance). J Clin Oncol. 2016;34(suppl 4S):Abstr 192.
29. Zhu AX, Rosmorduc O, Evans TR, Ross PJ, Santoro A, Carrilho FJ, et al. SEARCH: a phase III, randomized, double-blind, placebo-controlled trial of sorafenib plus erlotinib in patients with advanced hepatocellular carcinoma. J Clin Oncol. 2015;33(6):559–66.
30. Cheng AL, Kang YK, Lin DY, Park JW, Kudo M, Qin S, et al. Sunitinib versus sorafenib in advanced hepatocellular cancer: results of a randomized phase III trial. J Clin Oncol. 2013;31(32):4067–75.
31. Cainap C, Qin S, Huang WT, Chung IJ, Pan H, Cheng Y, et al. Linifanib versus Sorafenib in patients with advanced hepatocellular carcinoma: results of a randomized phase III trial. J Clin Oncol. 2015;33(2):172–9.
32. Johnson PJ, Qin S, Park JW, Poon RT, Raoul JL, Philip PA, et al. Brivanib versus sorafenib as first-line therapy in patients with unresectable, advanced hepatocellular carcinoma: results from the randomized phase III BRISK-FL study. J Clin Oncol. 2013;31(28):3517–24.
33. Ikeda M, Okusaka T, Mitsunaga S, Ueno H, Tamai T, Suzuki T, et al. Safety and pharmacokinetics of lenvatinib in patients with advanced hepatocellular carcinoma. Clin Cancer Res. 2016;22(6):1385–94.
34. Ikeda K, Kudo M, Kawazoe S, Osaki Y, Ikeda M, Okusaka T, et al. Phase 2 study of lenvatinib in patients with advanced hepatocellular carcinoma. J Gastroenterol. 2017;52(4):512–9.
35. Cheng A-L, Finn RS, Qin S, Han K-H, Ikeda K, Piscaglia F, et al. Phase III trial of lenvatinib (LEN) vs sorafenib (SOR) in first-line treatment of patients (pts) with unresectable hepatocellular carcinoma (uHCC). J Clin Oncol. 2017;35(15_suppl):4001.
36. Llovet JM, Decaens T, Raoul JL, Boucher E, Kudo M, Chang C, et al. Brivanib in patients with advanced hepatocellular carcinoma who were intolerant to sorafenib or for whom sorafenib failed: results from the randomized phase III BRISK-PS study. J Clin Oncol. 2013;31(28):3509–16.
37. Zhu AX, Park JO, Ryoo BY, Yen CJ, Poon R, Pastorelli D, et al. Ramucirumab versus placebo as second-line treatment in patients with advanced hepatocellular carcinoma following first-line therapy with sorafenib (REACH): a randomised, double-blind, multicentre, phase 3 trial. Lancet Oncol. 2015;16(7):859–70.
38. Sahin F, Kannangai R, Adegbola O, Wang J, Su G, Torbenson M. mTOR and P70 S6 kinase expression in primary liver neoplasms. Clin Cancer Res. 2004;10(24):8421–5.
39. Zhou L, Huang Y, Li J, Wang Z. The mTOR pathway is associated with the poor prognosis of human hepatocellular carcinoma. Med Oncol. 2010;27(2):255–61.

40. Villanueva A, Chiang DY, Newell P, Peix J, Thung S, Alsinet C, et al. Pivotal role of mTOR signaling in hepatocellular carcinoma. Gastroenterology. 2008;135(6):1972–83, 83 e1-11.
41. Zhu AX, Kudo M, Assenat E, Cattan S, Kang YK, Lim HY, et al. Effect of everolimus on survival in advanced hepatocellular carcinoma after failure of sorafenib: the EVOLVE-1 randomized clinical trial. JAMA. 2014;312(1):57–67.
42. Huynh H, Hao HX, Chan SL, Chen D, Ong R, Soo KC, et al. Loss of tuberous sclerosis complex 2 (TSC2) is frequent in hepatocellular carcinoma and predicts response to mTORC1 inhibitor everolimus. Mol Cancer Ther. 2015;14(5):1224–35.
43. Abou-Alfa GK, Qin S, Ryoo B-Y, Lu S-N, Yen C-J, Feng Y-H, et al. Phase III randomized study of second line ADI-peg 20 (A) plus best supportive care versus placebo (P) plus best supportive care in patients (pts) with advanced hepatocellular carcinoma (HCC). J Clin Oncol. 2016;34(15_suppl):4017.
44. Bruix J, Tak WY, Gasbarrini A, Santoro A, Colombo M, Lim HY, et al. Regorafenib as second-line therapy for intermediate or advanced hepatocellular carcinoma: multicentre, open-label, phase II safety study. Eur J Cancer. 2013;49(16):3412–9.
45. Bruix J, Qin S, Merle P, Granito A, Huang YH, Bodoky G, et al. Regorafenib for patients with hepatocellular carcinoma who progressed on sorafenib treatment (RESORCE): a randomised, double-blind, placebo-controlled, phase 3 trial. Lancet. 2017;389(10064):56–66.
46. Gherardi E, Birchmeier W, Birchmeier C, Vande Woude G. Targeting MET in cancer: rationale and progress. Nat Rev Cancer. 2012;12(2):89–103.
47. Santoro A, Rimassa L, Borbath I, Daniele B, Salvagni S, Van Laethem JL, et al. Tivantinib for second-line treatment of advanced hepatocellular carcinoma: a randomised, placebo-controlled phase 2 study. Lancet Oncol. 2013;14(1):55–63.
48. Rimassa L, Assenat E, Peck-Radosavljevic M, Zagonel V, Pracht M, Caremoli ER, et al. Second-line tivantinib (ARQ 197) vs placebo in patients (Pts) with MET-high hepatocellular carcinoma (HCC): results of the METIV-HCC phase III trial. J Clin Oncol. 2017;35(15_suppl):4000.
49. Yea S, Narla G, Zhao X, Garg R, Tal-Kremer S, Hod E, et al. Ras promotes growth by alternative splicing-mediated inactivation of the KLF6 tumor suppressor in hepatocellular carcinoma. Gastroenterology. 2008;134(5):1521–31.
50. Challen C, Guo K, Collier JD, Cavanagh D, Bassendine MF. Infrequent point mutations in codons 12 and 61 of ras oncogenes in human hepatocellular carcinomas. J Hepatol. 1992;14(2–3):342–6.
51. Lim HY, Heo J, Choi HJ, Lin CY, Yoon JH, Hsu C, et al. A phase II study of the efficacy and safety of the combination therapy of the MEK inhibitor refametinib (BAY 86-9766) plus sorafenib for Asian patients with unresectable hepatocellular carcinoma. Clin Cancer Res. 2014;20(23):5976–85.
52. Zucman-Rossi J, Villanueva A, Nault JC, Llovet JM. Genetic landscape and biomarkers of hepatocellular carcinoma. Gastroenterology. 2015;149(5):1226–39 e4.
53. Prieto J, Melero I, Sangro B. Immunological landscape and immunotherapy of hepatocellular carcinoma. Nat Rev Gastroenterol Hepatol. 2015;12(12):681–700.
54. Unitt E, Rushbrook SM, Marshall A, Davies S, Gibbs P, Morris LS, et al. Compromised lymphocytes infiltrate hepatocellular carcinoma: the role of T-regulatory cells. Hepatology. 2005;41(4):722–30.
55. Unitt E, Marshall A, Gelson W, Rushbrook SM, Davies S, Vowler SL, et al. Tumour lymphocytic infiltrate and recurrence of hepatocellular carcinoma following liver transplantation. J Hepatol. 2006;45(2):246–53.
56. Wada Y, Nakashima O, Kutami R, Yamamoto O, Kojiro M. Clinicopathological study on hepatocellular carcinoma with lymphocytic infiltration. Hepatology. 1998;27(2):407–14.
57. Brahmer J, Reckamp KL, Baas P, Crino L, Eberhardt WE, Poddubskaya E, et al. Nivolumab versus docetaxel in advanced squamous-cell non-small-cell lung cancer. N Engl J Med. 2015;373(2):123–35.
58. Larkin J, Hodi FS, Wolchok JD. Combined nivolumab and ipilimumab or monotherapy in untreated melanoma. N Engl J Med. 2015;373(13):1270–1.

59. Robert C, Long GV, Brady B, Dutriaux C, Maio M, Mortier L, et al. Nivolumab in previously untreated melanoma without BRAF mutation. N Engl J Med. 2015;372(4):320–30.
60. Hodi FS, O'Day SJ, McDermott DF, Weber RW, Sosman JA, Haanen JB, et al. Improved survival with ipilimumab in patients with metastatic melanoma. N Engl J Med. 2010;363(8):711–23.
61. Sangro B, Gomez-Martin C, de la Mata M, Inarrairaegui M, Garralda E, Barrera P, et al. A clinical trial of CTLA-4 blockade with tremelimumab in patients with hepatocellular carcinoma and chronic hepatitis C. J Hepatol. 2013;59(1):81–8.
62. Duffy AG, Ulahannan SV, Makorova-Rusher O, Rahma O, Wedemeyer H, Pratt D, et al. Tremelimumab in combination with ablation in patients with advanced hepatocellular carcinoma. J Hepatol. 2016;66(3):545–51.
63. Sangro B, Melero I, Yau TC, Hsu C, Kudo M, Crocenzi TS, Kim T-Y, Choo S, Trojan J, Meyer T, Kang Y-K, Anderson J, Dela Cruz CM, Lang L, Neely J, El-Khoueiry AB. Safety and antitumor activity of nivolumab (nivo) in patients (pts) with advanced hepatocellular carcinoma (HCC): Interim analysis of dose-expansion cohorts from the phase 1/2 CheckMate-040 study. J Clin Oncol. 2016;34(Suppl):Abstract 4078.
64. Crocenzi TS, El-Khoueiry AB, Yau TC, Melero I, Sangro B, Kudo M, et al. Nivolumab (nivo) in sorafenib (sor)-naive and -experienced pts with advanced hepatocellular carcinoma (HCC): CheckMate 040 study. J Clin Oncol. 2017;35(15_Suppl):4013.

# Part II
# Cholangiocarcinoma

# Chapter 13
# Mixed Hepatocellular/ Cholangiocarcinomas: Current Perspectives and Management

**Ray Tan, Alberto Quaglia, and Paul J. Ross**

**Key Learning Points**

1. cHCC-CC accounts for 0.4–14% of primary liver tumours.
2. Diagnosis is based on histology. This uses a combination of morphology, immunohistochemistry, in situ hybridization and molecular biology.
3. Diagnosis is optimally established on whole tumours.
4. Tumours are classified according to 2010 WHO classification.
5. Genetics reflect those of classical HCC and cholangiocarcinoma.
6. Hepatic resection with hilar nodal dissection is the optimal management resulting in 5-year survival of approximately 28%.

R. Tan
Department of Medical Oncology, Guy's Cancer, Guy's and St Thomas' NHS Foundation Trust, London, UK
e-mail: ray.tan@nhs.net

A. Quaglia
The Institute of Liver Studies, King's College Hospital, London, UK
e-mail: alberto.quaglia@nhs.net

P. J. Ross (✉)
Department of Medical Oncology, Guy's Cancer, Guy's and St Thomas' NHS Foundation Trust, London, UK

Department of Oncology, King's College Hospital NHS Foundation Trust, London, UK
e-mail: Paul.Ross@gstt.nhs.uk


T. Cross, D. H. Palmer (eds.), *Liver Cancers*,
https://doi.org/10.1007/978-3-319-92216-4_13

**Areas of Controversy and Uncertainty**

1. Incidence of the tumour is poorly understood due to the management of HCC based on imaging and AFP.
2. Aetiological factors are poorly defined; the current view is that these are similar to other primary liver tumours.
3. Growing understanding of the complexity of the spectrum of these tumours. However, much to be learnt as molecular biology is studied that will influence classification and management.
4. Can cHCC-CC be distinguished from classical HCC by imaging?
5. In advanced disease can diagnosis be established using needle biopsy?
6. Is there a need for repeat biopsy as disease progresses?
7. Data from liver transplantation are low in volume. Is there a role for liver transplantation?
8. What are the optimal locoregional and systemic therapies for advanced disease?

## Pathology

The term combined or mixed hepatocellular-cholangiocarcinoma (cHCC-CC) refers to a rare variant of primary malignant epithelial liver tumours in which both hepatocellular carcinoma and cholangiocarcinoma are present in the same lesion. It accounts for 0.4–14% of all primary liver tumours. The diagnosis is currently histological and is based on tumour cell morphology and immunohistochemistry.

The first known description of tumours with both hepatocellular and cholangiocellular differentiation is in the paper by Wells in 1903 [1]. The histological classification of cHCC-CC has evolved considerably over the years and has included the occurrence of hepatocellular and cholangiocellular differentiation in separate lesions in the same liver, in separate lesions coming into contact with each other and within a single tumour mass [2–4]. Early studies were based purely on morphological observations. The resemblance of tumour cells to hepatocytes or cholangiocytes or their conventional neoplastic counterparts would define the tumour phenotype. More recent studies have used a combination of morphology and techniques such as immunohistochemistry, in situ hybridization, electron microscopy and molecular biology to demonstrate lineage-specific markers. New concepts in liver embryology, observations in animal models of liver carcinogenesis and regeneration, the characterisation of the hepatic progenitor/stem cell compartment and advances in the understanding of cell plasticity led to the concept that at least a proportion of these tumours may derive from progenitor/stem cells with the potential of dual hepatocellular and cholangiocellular differentiation. The current understanding is that the spectrum of primary liver carcinoma has pure (by morphological and immunohistochemical criteria) hepatocellular carcinoma and cholangiocellular carcinoma at its two ends and a plethora of tumours exhibiting various combinations of hepatocellular, biliary and progenitor cell morphological and immunohistochemical

**Table 13.1.** 2010 WHO classification

| | | |
|---|---|---|
| Classical cHCC-CC | | Histologically typical areas of HCC together with those of CC in the same tumour |
| cHCC-CC with stem cell features | | |
| | Typical | Nests of mature hepatocyte-like tumour cells surrounded by small cells exhibiting IHC markers of progenitor cells |
| | Intermediate | Small homogeneous cells comprising most of the tumour that are intermediate between hepatocytes and cholangiocytes and showing immunohistochemical markers of both |
| | Cholangiocellular | Small cells with a high nuclear/cytoplasmic ratio and hyperchromatic oval-shaped nuclei arranged in a tubular anastomosing (antler-like) pattern within a dense, sclerotic stroma and also expressing progenitor/stem cell markers |

phenotypes in between. The reader is referred to the comprehensive review by Brunt and colleagues, where a detailed description of the immunomarkers commonly used in the interpretation of cHCC-CC is given [5]. Whether cHCC-CC derives from transformed hepatocytes or cholangiocytes acquiring stem cell features, transformed progenitor/stem cell maintaining dual differentiation potential, or even hepatoblasts, remains to be proven. cHCC-CC occurs often in tumour previously treated by local ablation therapy and in particular transarterial chemoembolization [6–8]. This observation raises the possibility that tumour progenitor/stem cells resistant to chemotherapy and hypoxia may gain a selective growth advantage and cause tumour progression.

The currently used WHO 2010 classification (Table 13.1.) encapsulates this complexity. It classifies cHCC-CCs into two main categories: classical cHCC-CC and cHCC-CC with stem cell features.

Of note, coexistence of hepatocellular and cholangiocellular carcinoma as two separate lesions in the same liver is not considered as cHCC-CC. Fibrolamellar carcinoma and hepatoblastoma are not included in the currently accepted definition of cHCC-CC.

## Genetics

Genetic studies looking into the genetic signature and molecular biology of cHCC-CCs are currently few in number. Further studies are needed in order to help better understand the pathogenesis and clinical presentation of cHCC-CCs. Genomic and genetic analyses of cHCC-CC have similar molecular characteristics with both intrahepatic cholangiocarcinoma and classic HCC. Frequent alterations in primary liver cancers include genes such as *TP53*, *WNT*, *CTNNB1* and cell cycle-related genes such as *CCND1* and *CDKN2A* [9]. Recently, *IDH1*/*IDH2* mutations have been observed in four different HCC tumours [10]. An additional 11 tumours with gene expression patterns similar to the *IDH1-/IDH2*-mutated samples were observed. These tumours histopathologically resemble HCC but have clinical and genetic features of cholangiocarcinomas and HCCs suggestive of a possible biphenotypic stem cell origin. This observation is supportive of the concept that HCC and iCCA represent two ends of a spectrum, and the presence of *IDH1/IDH2* mutations shifts a tumour towards a biliary phenotype.

## Clinical Features

The rarity of this cancer has made it difficult to define epidemiologically. A population-level analysis using the Surveillance, Epidemiology and End Results (SEER) database for the period 1988–2009 included 465 patients with cHCC-CC [11]. This occurred more frequently in patients who were white, male and older than 65 years. In a US population of patients undergoing liver transplantation for cHCC-CC, hepatitis C and alcoholic cirrhosis were the most frequent secondary diagnoses, similar to patients with HCC [12]. cHCC-CC is considered an aggressive tumour with poor long-term survival. Good quality clinical data remains limited. cHCC-CC, similarly to both HCC and CC, usually develops asymptomatically until it becomes more advanced, at which point it may cause symptoms such as right upper quadrant abdominal pain, weight loss, pruritus, fever and fatigue. Clinical signs may include hepatomegaly or abdominal distension due to ascites.

## Diagnosis

The majority of series have found no major differences in the presentation of cHCC-CC with those of classical HCC or iCCA. The tumour markers alpha-fetoprotein (AFP) and carbohydrate antigen 19-9 (Ca 19-9) have been found to be serum markers for HCC and CC, respectively. Both may also be elevated in cHCC-CC, and a simultaneous increase in both along with clinical and radiological suspicion of malignancy should make one consider cHCC-CC as a potential diagnosis. It is worth noting that AFP is elevated less frequently and also tends to be lower in cHCC-CC compared to HCC.

The accepted dogma has been that preoperative non-invasive diagnosis of cHCC-CC with conventional imaging is almost impossible. The majority based on imaging resemble classical HCC. However, Potretzke and colleagues reviewed imaging of 61 patients with histologically confirmed cHCC-CC according to the diagnostic imaging criteria recommenced by the American College of Radiology Liver Imaging Reporting and Data System (Li-RADS) (Table 13.2) [13]. Multiphasic contrast-enhanced MRI scans (48 patients) and CT scans (13 patients) were obtained pretreatment. According to Li-RADS major features in 33 (54%) patients met major criteria for HCC. However, 29 of 33 had at least 1 ancillary feature

**Table 13.2** Li-RADS ancillary features favouring malignancy and features favouring non-hepatocellular (HCC) malignancy over HCC

| Ancillary features favouring malignancy | Features favouring non-HCC malignancy over HCC |
|---|---|
| Midmoderate T2 hyperintensity | Rim or peripheral arterial phase hyperenhancement |
| Restricted diffusion | Portal venous and delayed phase progressive central enhancement |
| Distinctive rim[a] | Peripheral washout appearance |
| Corona enhancement[a] | Marked diffusion restriction |
| Mosaic architecture[a] | Liver surface retraction |
| Nodule-in-nodule architecture[a] | Biliary obstruction disproportionate to that expected on basis of size of mass |
| Intralesional fat[a] | |
| Lesional iron sparing | |
| Lesional fat sparing | |
| Hepatobiliary phase hypointensity | |

[a]Feature specifically favours HCC over malignancy in general

favouring non-HCC malignancy. Overall 54 of 61 (88%) of cHCC-CC in this study could be categorised as non-HCC malignancy indicating the importance of an algorithm such as Li-RADS for assessment of liver lesions.

Although definitive diagnosis of cHCC-CC based on tumour markers and imaging alone is challenging, certain findings should prompt strong consideration of cHCC-CC pre-biopsy. These would be imaging features of both HCC and CC, raised AFP as well as Ca 19-9 and imaging appearances which contradict the tumour marker (e.g. CC features on imaging but a raised AFP).

The definitive diagnosis of cHCC-CC requires histological examination. Extensive sampling of surgically resected tumours is necessary to ensure that the microscopy examination is carried out on a sufficient amount of tissue and that areas of divergent differentiation are not missed. Sampling error remains a major concern when interpreting core needle biopsy specimens, particularly with small and/or single pass samples as they may not be representative. Multiple biopsies from different areas of the tumour mass would be necessary to minimise sampling error.

## Management

Surgical resection and liver transplantation are the only curative options. Hepatic resection with hilar lymph node dissection is the recommended treatment for cHCC-CC in non-cirrhotic patients. In common with all surgery, this is dependent on the general medical condition of the patient, tumour extent and local anatomical conditions. The aim should be complete excision with negative margins and minimal impact on liver function. For patients with liver cirrhosis, hepatic resection should be carefully considered based on their functional reserve.

cHCC-CC tends to behave like HCC with respect to portal and hepatic venous infiltration and like CC with respect to lymph node metastasis. In fact, lymph node metastasis is a more significant problem in cHCC-CC than in either HCC or CC. The Liver Cancer Study Group of Japan studied the frequency of distant metastasis in autopsied patients with primary liver cancer and found that lymph node metastasis was observed in 30.3% of patients with HCC, 68.6% of patients with CC and 76.2% of patients with cHCC-CC [14]. However, despite this it remains controversial with regards to whether lymph node dissection improves prognosis.

The role of liver transplantation in cHCC-CC, unlike in HCC, is not well-defined. Outcomes following liver transplantation are difficult to interpret because of the low number of reported cases. Most of the available data is based on patients who were initially misdiagnosed with HCC.

Groeschl et al. performed a retrospective comparative cohort study of surgical treatment using the SEER database for the period 1973–2008 [15]. Fifty-four patients diagnosed with cHCC-CC were included, 19 (35%) underwent liver transplantation and 35 (65%) hepatic resection. One-year overall survival was 89% following transplantation compared to 71% with hepatic resection; 3-year overall survivals were 48% and 46%, respectively. Median overall survival for all the patients with cHCC-CC was 36 months. (95% CI, 19–89, $P = 0.01$). A more recent analysis of patients using the United Network for Organ Sharing (UNOS) database between 1994 and 2013 included 94 patients with cHCC-CC [12]. Overall survival rates following liver transplantation for cHCC-CC at 1, 3 and 5 years were 82%, 47% and 40%. These were significantly inferior to those observed for classical HCC but similar to those for cholangiocarcinoma.

In the population-level analysis, Garacini et al. observed that most patients had no interventional treatment, 13.1% liver transplantation, 10.0% major hepatectomy, 7.6% minor hepatectomy and 4% ablative therapy [11]. Five-year overall survival rates were 41.1% with liver transplantation, 28.1% with major hepatectomy, 27.1% with minor hepatectomy and 0 for those treated with ablative therapies or without interventional treatment. Whilst a univariate analysis demonstrated a better 5-year survival for patients treated with liver transplantation compared to hepatectomy, this was not confirmed in a multivariate analysis.

This data clearly demonstrates that patients with tumours amenable to surgical intervention have superior survival to those treated with local ablative therapy or non-interventional therapy. However, the outcomes from liver transplantation are inferior to those of patients with HCC. Indeed, two retrospective studies have observed no definitive survival advantage for liver transplantation compared to resection. It remains to be seen with better selection criteria to these studies whether there is a role for liver transplantation in cHCC-CC. Currently, major hepatic resection remains the best option for those with tumours amenable to same.

Patients treated with liver resection or transplantation with curative intent management of recurrence need to be informed by histology from the recurrence. Our group have described the histological pattern of surgically resected primary and metastatic classic cHCC-CC in four patients [16]. This emphasised the heterogeneous presentation and unpredictable behaviours of these tumours. The first case had a primary tumour and subsequent bilateral adrenal metastases demonstrating a similar combined phenotype. Further metastases had a purely HCC component. A second case demonstrated that only one component metastasised with a histological pattern similar to the predominant and less-differentiated HCC component (Fig. 13.1). In another cases it was the minor cholangiocellular component that recurred. In the fourth case, the two components showed a different tropism, with HCC metastasising to paravertebral tissue and brain and cholangiocarcinoma to the lung. Consequently, when considering systemic therapy, it is important to have an understanding of which component is predominant. Indeed, systemic therapies could give a selective advantage of one component on the other over time.

Data on non-surgical treatment of cHCC-CC is extremely limited, and no clinical trial data is available. Non-surgical options include transarterial chemoembolization (TACE), radioembolisation, hepatic arterial infusion chemotherapy, ablative therapies and systemic chemotherapy. One of the few studies reporting on outcomes

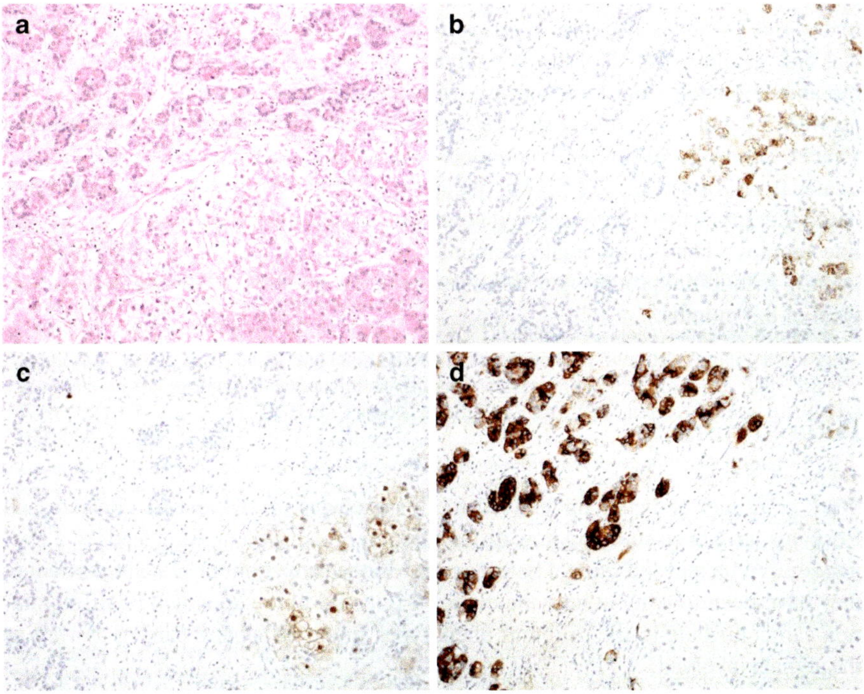


**Fig. 13.1** Sixty-eight year old female patient. Surgical resection specimen containing a 50 mm diameter mixed hepatocellular-cholangiocellular caracinoma, classic-type. (**a**) Haematoxylin and eosin (H&E) stain show an area of cholangiocellular differentiation in the top left corner, adjacent to an area of hepatocellular differentiation with clear cell changes in the lower part of the field. This is supported by immunohistochemistry which shows that the hepatoid tumour cells stain for Hep-Par-1 (**b**) and arginase-1 (**c**), whereas the tubulo-glandular structures do not stain for these markers but stain instead for CA 19-9 (**d**). Magnification: 200× in each picture

10. Cancer Genome Atlas Research Network. Comprehensive and integrative genomic characterization of hepatocellular carcinoma. Cell. 2017;169(7):1327–1341.e23. https://doi.org/10.1016/j.cell.2017.05.046.
11. Garancini M, Goffredo P, Pagni F, Romano F, Roman S, Sosa JA, Giardini V. Combined hepatocellular-cholangiocarcinoma: a population-level analysis of an uncommon primary liver tumor. Liver Transpl. 2014;20(8):952–9. https://doi.org/10.1002/lt.23897.
12. Vilchez V, Shah MB, Daily MF, Pena L, Tzeng CW, Davenport D, Hosein PJ, Gedaly R, Maynard E. Long-term outcome of patients undergoing liver transplantation for mixed hepatocellular carcinoma and cholangiocarcinoma: an analysis of the UNOS database. HPB (Oxford). 2016;18(1):29–34. https://doi.org/10.1016/j.hpb.2015.10.001.
13. Potretzke TA, Tan BR, Doyle MB, Brunt EM, Heiken JP, Fowler KJ. Imaging features of biphenotypic primary liver carcinoma (Hepatocholangiocarcinoma) and the potential to mimic hepatocellular carcinoma: LI-RADS analysis of CT and MRI features in 61 cases. AJR Am J Roentgenol. 2016;207(1):25–31. https://doi.org/10.2214/AJR.15.14997.
14. The Liver Cancer Study Group of Japan. Primary liver cancer in Japan: clinicopathologic features and results of surgical treatment. Ann Surg. 1990;211:277–87.
15. Groeschl RT, Turaga KK, Clark Gamblin T. Transplantation versus resection for patients with combined hepatocellular carcinoma-cholangiocarcinoma. J Surg Oncol. 2013;107(6):608–12. https://doi.org/10.1002/jso.23289.
16. De Vito C, Sarker D, Ross P, Heaton N, Quaglia A. Histological heterogeneity in primary and metastatic classic combined hepatocellular-cholangiocarcinoma: a case series. Virchows Arch. 2017; https://doi.org/10.1007/s00428-017-2196-x.
17. Fowler K, Saad NE, Brunt E, Doyle MB, Amin M, Vachharajani N, Tan B, Chapman WC. Biphenotypic primary liver carcinomas: assessing outcomes of hepatic directed therapy. Ann Surg Oncol. 2015;22(13):4130–7. https://doi.org/10.1245/s10434-015-4774-y.
18. Rogers JE, Bolonesi RM, Rashid A, Elsayes KM, Elbanan MG, Law L, Kaseb A, Shroff RT. Systemic therapy for unresectable, mixed hepatocellular-cholangiocarcinoma: treatment of a rare malignancy. J Gastrointest Oncol. 2017;8(2):347–51. https://doi.org/10.21037/jgo.2017.03.03.
19. Govaere O, Roskams T. Pathogenesis and prognosis of hepatocellular carcinoma at the cellular and molecular levels. Clin Liver Dis. 2015;19(2):261–76. https://doi.org/10.1016/j.cld.2015.01.002.

# Chapter 14
# Epidemiology and Pathogenesis of Cholangiocarcinoma

**Stephen McClements and Shahid A. Khan**

## Introduction

Cholangiocarcinoma is the second most common primary liver cancer after hepatocellular carcinoma and is associated with a high mortality, often attributed to late diagnosis when the opportunity for curative therapies has passed. Cholangiocarcinoma accounts for approximately 3% of all gastrointestinal cancers worldwide, with a prevalence in autopsy studies of 0.01–0.46% [1].

## Clinical Anatomy and Classification

The term cholangiocarcinoma (CCA) refers to cancers arising in the intrahepatic, perihilar or extrahepatic (distal) biliary tree and excludes cancers of the gallbladder and ampulla (Fig. 14.1) [2]. Intrahepatic cholangiocarcinoma (iCCA) originates in the peripheral ductules or large ducts within the liver; this represents less than 10% overall. Extrahepatic cancers are classified as either perihilar cholangiocarcinoma (pCCA) representing 50% or distal cholangiocarcinoma (dCCA) representing 40% [3]. The transition zone between perihilar and distal disease is the insertion point of the cystic duct.

Cancers arising in the perihilar region, also referred to as Klatskin tumours in the International Classification of Diseases (ICD), have been further classified according to their patterns of involvement of the hepatic ducts (the Bismuth-Corlette classification) (Fig. 14.2):

- Type I: tumours below the confluence of the left and right hepatic ducts.
- Type II: tumours reaching the confluence but not involving left or right hepatic ducts.

S. McClements · S. A. Khan (✉)
Liver Unit, St Mary's Hospital Campus, Imperial College London, London, UK
e-mail: Shahid.khan@imperial.ac.uk



T. Cross, D. H. Palmer (eds.), *Liver Cancers*,
https://doi.org/10.1007/978-3-319-92216-4_14

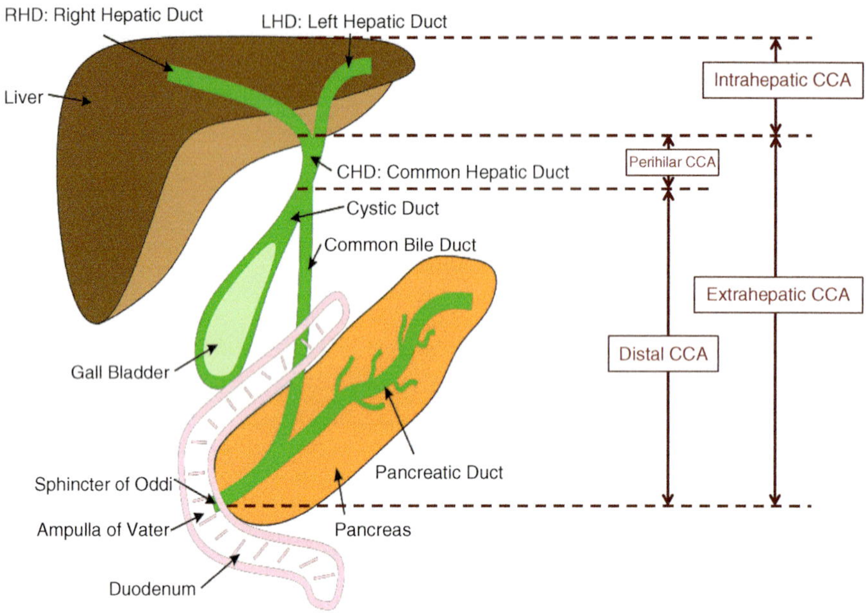


**Fig. 14.1** Sites of the different sub-types of cholangiocarcinoma (CCA)

**Fig. 14.2** Bismuth classification of biliary strictures [4]

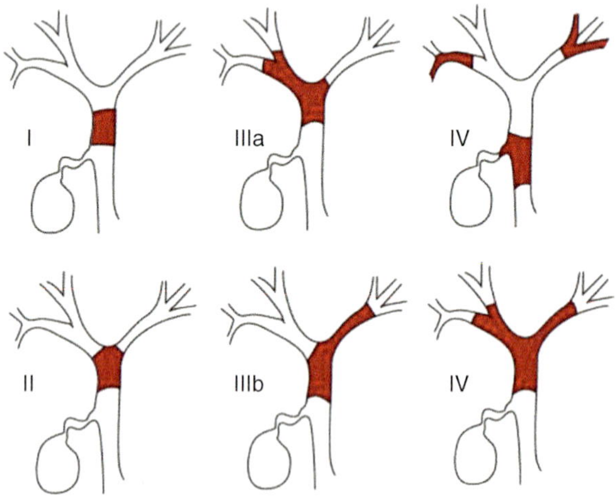


- Type III: tumours occluding the common hepatic duct and either the right (IIIa) or the left (IIIb) hepatic duct.
- Type IV: tumours that are multicentric or involving both right and left hepatic ducts.

## Epidemiology

The incidence of cholangiocarcinoma (CCA) increases with age and typically presents in the fifth or sixth decade; the noteworthy exceptions to this trend are the tumours presenting in patients with primary sclerosing cholangitis (PSC) and choledochal cysts which can present much earlier (see section "Risk Factors" below). There is a slight male predominance, which appears to reflect the higher incidence of risk factors (particularly PSC) in men.

The emerging concept is that the three anatomical groups (iCCA, pCCA and dCCA) differ significantly in their tumour biology, clinical characteristics, and epidemiology. Overall rates of cholangiocarcinoma diagnoses appear to be rising globally; however, there is not a balanced distribution between the subtypes.

Many countries including North America, Japan, Europe and Australia have reported an increased incidence of intrahepatic disease (iCCA) coupled by a decreasing incidence of extrahepatic disease (pCCA and dCCA); however, the data are inconsistent and must be viewed cautiously, and actually this trend is seemingly reversed in other countries.

There is clearly some geographical variation in incidence largely attributed to the distribution of risk factors in different countries; for instance, South East Asia has an increased incidence of iCCA related to endemic liver fluke infection (see below).

The distribution of risk factors, however, does not fully explain the global variability in incidence, and several confounding factors have been identified that contribute to the data inconsistencies.

Although biologically these three subsets of CCA appear to represent distinct clinical entities, International classifications have not consistently distinguished between pCCA and dCCA and instead distinguish only intrahepatic disease (iCCA) and extrahepatic disease (where pCCA and dCCA are combined).

Additionally the nomenclature of periductal disease (pCCA) (previously referred to as Klatskin tumours) has evolved in sequential editions of the International Classification of Diseases (ICD); initially they were considered as a distinct entity (within the intrahepatic spectrum), then laterally could be placed within either the intrahepatic or extrahepatic classification dependant on tumour margins. This phenomenon means that pCCAs are classified differently, according to which edition of ICD is applied and as different countries adopt the updated editions of the ICD at different times (often over long time periods). True representation of incidence based on retrospective international data is extremely challenging.

The apparent rise in iCCA may also be artefactual when historic misclassification is taken into account; as diagnostic tests have become more sophisticated and widely available, the risk of CCA being misclassified has been reduced. The distinction between iCCA and HCC requires detailed investigations, and the importance of making this distinction is now clinically more relevant as treatment modalities and outcomes have advanced. This change has undoubtedly altered the rates of accurate iCCA diagnosis. There has also been an observed dichotomy of increased rates of iCCA diagnosis coupled with a decreased incidence of 'cancer of unknown primary', and this again adds weight to the argument that much of the apparent increase incidence of iCCA may in fact reflect more accurate diagnosis rather than a greater number of total cancers per se.

The summary of current epidemiological data therefore is difficult to reconcile given the heterogeneity of recording and classification practices employed internationally, and the apparent rise in incidence needs to be interpreted with caution until more consistent and uniform data recording practices are adopted.

## Risk Factors

Although the majority of cases of cholangiocarcinoma are sporadic with no clear predisposing factors, several risk factors have been identified which share the common property of precipitating chronic inflammation of the biliary tree [5].

## Primary Sclerosing Cholangitis

Primary sclerosing cholangitis is the commonest known predisposing condition for cholangiocarcinoma in the west. It tends to present earlier in PSC patients than in sporadic cases, typically affecting the 30–50-year age group. About a third of patients with primary sclerosing cholangitis who develop cholangiocarcinoma do so within 2 years of diagnosis, and the risk of cholangiocarcinogenesis seems unrelated to the duration of the inflammatory disease. Two-thirds of patients with primary sclerosing cholangitis have associated inflammatory bowel disease, especially ulcerative colitis. No association has been shown between the risk of cholangiocarcinoma and the presence, severity, and extent of inflammatory bowel disease in this group of patients [6].

## Parasitic Infection

A large body of experimental and epidemiological data suggests a pathogenic association between liver fluke infestation, especially *Opisthorchis viverrini* (and less definitively *Clonorchis sinensis*), and cholangiocarcinoma [7]. Eating undercooked fish infects humans with adult worms inhabiting and laying eggs in the biliary system. These parasites are endemic in parts of South East Asia and are largely attributed to the marked increase in iCCA observed in countries such as Thailand.

## Fibropolycystic Liver Disease

Caroli's syndrome (congenital biliary cysts), congenital fibrosis and choledocal cysts (cystic dilatations of the biliary tree) carry a 15% risk of malignant change after the second decade, at an average age of 34 years [8]. The mechanism of carcinogenesis is unclear but could be related to biliary stasis, reflux of pancreatic juice causing chronic inflammation or activation of bile acids and deconjugation of carcinogens [9]. Bile duct adenomas and biliary papillomatosis are also associated with the development of cholangiocarcinoma.

## Intrahepatic Biliary Stones

Hepatolithiasis is rare in the west, but relatively common in parts of Asia, and is associated particularly with peripheral intrahepatic cholangiocarcinoma. Up to 10% of patients with hepatolithiasis develop cholangiocarcinoma [10]. In Taiwan, up to 70% of patients with cholangiocarcinoma undergoing resection reportedly have intrahepatic biliary stones, and in Japan this figure is 6–18% [11]. Biliary stones are thought to cause bile stasis, predisposing to recurrent bacterial infections and subsequent inflammation, a potential cofactor for cholangiocarcinogenesis.

## Chemical Carcinogen Exposure

Several chemical toxins have been associated with cholangiocarcinoma. Promutagenic DNA adducts have been identified in cholangiocarcinoma tissue, indicating exposure to DNA-damaging agents [12]. Thorotrast, a radiological contrast agent banned in the 1960s for its carcinogenic properties, has been strongly associated with the development of cholangiocarcinoma many years after exposure, increasing the risk to 300 times that of the general population [13]. Associations have also been made with exposure to by-products from the rubber and chemical industries, including dioxins and nitrosamines [14], as well as with alcohol and smoking [15].

## Viral Hepatitis

Cirrhosis, of any cause, has also been associated with cholangiocarcinoma; a large cohort study of over 11,000 patients with cirrhosis, followed up over 6 years, showed a tenfold risk compared with the general population [15]. More specifically, hepatitis B and C viruses have been linked to the cancer. A case-control study from Korea reported that 12.5% of patients with cholangiocarcinoma tested positive for hepatitis C virus and 13.8% for hepatitis B virus surface antigen (HBsAg), compared with 3.5% and 2.3% of controls [15]. In a second case-control study from Italy, 23% of patients with cholangiocarcinoma were positive for antihepatitis C virus, and 11.5% were HbsAg-positive with odds ratios of 6.1 for hepatitis C virus and 5.9 for HIV infection [16].

## Metabolic Disease

The metabolic syndrome (clinically represented by dyslipidemia, central obesity, impaired glucose tolerance and hypertension) has been associated with an increased risk of intrahepatic CCA [17]. Several cohort and case-controlled studies have also demonstrated both type 2 diabetes mellitus and obesity as independent risk factors associated with increased incidence of iCCA, and this has been substantiated by meta-analyses of such studies [18, 19].

It remains unclear, however, whether diabetes and obesity are direct drivers of carcinogenesis or are merely surrogate markers for molecular derangement associated with the metabolic syndrome.

## Molecular Pathogenesis

Carcinogenesis involves specific cell genome derangements; the genetic pathways contributing to the selective growth advantage of cancer cells can be organised into those governing cell fate and differentiation, proliferation, cell survival, and maintenance of genome integrity [20]. The transition from normal biliary epithelium to malignant tissue occurs through a precursor lesion: intraductal papiliary neoplasia (IPMN) of the bile duct or biliary intraepithelial neoplasia (BilN). These lesions like pancreatic IPMN are classified due to the extent of cellular atypia [5].

A proposed model for carcinogenesis in cholangiocarcinoma showing interaction between environmental factors and host genetics is presented in Fig. 14.3. As with many cancers, there is a stepwise progression from normal cell biology to neoplasia, influenced by interplay between environmental and host factors.

Genetic polymorphisms in the cytochrome P450 enzymes or in the bile salt transporter proteins, for example, could lead to alterations in the efficiency with which environmental toxins (xenobiotics) are handled by the liver. The development of cholangiocarcinoma probably needs a 'second hit' to deconjugate such xenobiotics and to expose the bile duct epithelium to damage. Such secondary hits include chronic inflammation, viral hepatitis, worm infections, and recurrent cholangitis [21].

Recent molecular analysis has delineated the genomic landscape in CCA, and the diverse genetic targets identified have reinforced the evidence for heterogeneity. These concepts are explored in more depth in chapter "Oncotherapies for Cholangiocarcinoma".

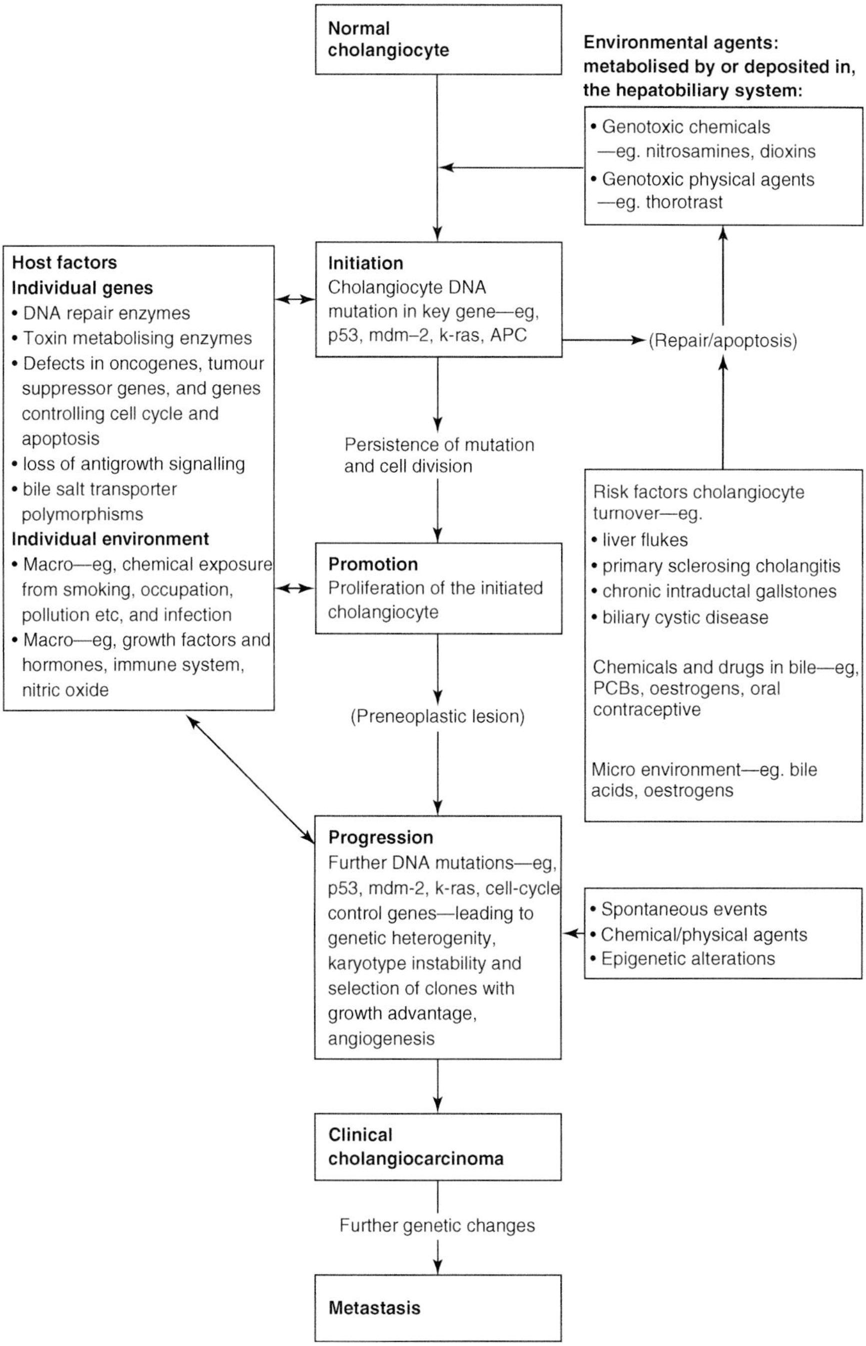


**Fig. 14.3** Proposed model for carcinogenesis in cholangiocarcinoma showing interaction between environmental factors and host genetics (Bridgewater et al. [2])

## References

1. Vauthey JN, Blumgart LH. Recent advances in the management of cholangiocarcinomas. Semin Liver Dis. 1994;14(2):109.
2. Bridgewater J, Galle PR, Khan SA, Llovet JM, Park J-W, Patel T, Pawlik TM, Gores GJ. Guidelines for the diagnosis and management of intrahepatic cholangiocarcinoma. J Hepatol. 2014;60(6):1268–89 pii: S0168-8278(14)00067-1. https://doi.org/10.1016/j.jhep.2014.01.021.
3. DeOliveira ML, Cunningham SC, Cameron JL, et al. Cholangiocarcinoma: thirty-one-year experience with 564 patients at a single institution. Ann Surg. 2007;245:755.
4. Kato T, Tsukamoto E, Kuge Y, et al. Clinical role of (18)F-FDG PET for initial staging of patients with extrahepatic bile duct cancer. Eur J Nucl Med Mol Imaging. 2002;29:1047–54.
5. Zen Y, Adsay NV, Bardadin K, et al. Biliary intraepithelial neoplasia: an international interobserver agreement study and proposal for diagnostic criteria. Mod Pathol. 2007;20:701.
6. Broome U, Olsson R, Loof L, et al. Natural history and prognostic factors in 305 Swedish patients with primary sclerosing cholangitis. Gut. 1996;38:610–5.
7. Watanapa P, Watanapa WB. Liver fluke-associated cholangiocarcinoma. Br J Surg. 2002;89:962–70.
8. Simeone DM. Gallbladder and biliary tree: anatomy and structural anomalies. In: Yamada T, editor. Textbook of gastroenterology. Philadelphia: Lippincott Willimas and Wilkins; 1999. p. 2244–57.
9. Ohtsuka T, Inoue K, Ohuchida J, et al. Carcinoma arising in choledochocele. Endoscopy. 2001;33:614–9.
10. Kubo S, Kinoshita H, Hirohashi K, Hamba H. Hepatolithiasis associated with cholangiocarcinoma. World J Surg. 1995;19:637–41.
11. Chen MF. Peripheral cholangiocarcinoma (cholangiocellular carcinoma): clinical features, diagnosis and treatment. J Gastroenterol Hepatol. 1999;14:1144–9.
12. Khan SA, Carmichael PL, Taylor-Robinson SD, Habib N, Thomas HC. DNA adducts, detected by 32P postlabelling, in human cholangiocarcinoma. Gut. 2003;52:586–91.
13. Sahani D, Prasad SR, Tannabe KK, Hahn PF, Mueller PR, Saini S. Thorotrast-induced cholangiocarcinoma: case report. Abdom Imaging. 2003;28:72–4.
14. Hardell L, Bengtsson NO, Jonsson U, Eriksson S, Larsson LG. Aetiological aspects on primary liver cancer with special regard to alcohol, organic solvents and acute intermittent porphyria: an epidemiological investigation. Br J Cancer. 1984;50:389–97.
15. Sorensen HT, Friis S, Olsen JH, et al. Risk of liver and other types of cancer in patients with cirrhosis: a nationwide cohort study in Denmark. Hepatology. 1998;28:921–5.
16. Donato F, Gelatti U, Tagger A, et al. Intrahepatic cholangiocarcinoma and hepatitis C and B virus infection, alcohol intake, and hepatolithiasis: a case-control study in Italy. Cancer Causes Control. 2001;12:959–64.
17. Welzel TM, Graubard BI, Zeuzem S, et al. Metabolic syndrome increases the risk of primary liver cancer in the United States: a study in the SEER-medicare database. Hepatology. 2011;54:463.
18. Palmer WC, Patel T. Are common factors involved in the pathogenesis of primary liver cancers? A meta-analysis of risk factors for intrahepatic cholangiocarcinoma. J Hepatol. 2012;57(1):69–76.
19. Jing W, Jin G, Zhou X, et al. Diabetes mellitus and increased risk of cholangiocarcinoma: a meta-analysis. Eur J Cancer Prev. 2012;21:24.
20. Razumilava N, Gores GJ. Cholangiocarcinoma. Lancet. 2014;383:2168–79.
21. Khan SA, Thomas HC, Davidson BR, Taylor-Robinson SD. Cholangiocarcinoma. Lancet. 2005;366:1303–14.

# Chapter 15
# Diagnosis and Staging of Cholangiocarcinoma

Jessica R. Hale and Olusola O. Faluyi

**Key Learning Points**

1. Cholangiocarcinoma (CCA), the most common biliary tract malignancy, is unfortunately often diagnosed late with resultant poor survival outcomes.
2. Accurate staging is of paramount importance both for identifying patients with potentially curable disease amenable to resection and for guiding treatment in patients with locally advanced or metastatic disease.
3. Radiological evaluation usually involves CT staging, with the option of MRI, PET, EUS, US and cholangiography for further clarification of disease status.
4. To guide treatment, CCA can be classified into early, locally advanced or metastatic stages. More detailed staging can also be achieved using the AJCC/UICC TNM system or other staging methods. Laparoscopic evaluation is capable of detecting sub-radiological disease.
5. Future considerations include the development of biomarkers to enhance early and specific diagnosis as well as to guide systemic treatment. Furthermore, improved imaging techniques to allow accurate identification of patients who may benefit from potentially curative surgical intervention.

J. R. Hale (✉) · O. O. Faluyi
Clatterbridge Cancer Centre, Wirral, UK
e-mail: jessica.hale3@nhs.net



T. Cross, D. H. Palmer (eds.), *Liver Cancers*,
https://doi.org/10.1007/978-3-319-92216-4_15

**Areas of Controversy and Uncertainty**

1. Due to the scirrhous nature of lesions as well as the histological and molecular features shared with other malignancies, the pathological diagnosis of Cholangiocarcinoma (CCA) can be challenging.
2. Currently there is no universal staging system in use for CCA; the AJCC/UICC system incorporates information on survival and is the most commonly used. Accurate staging is vital to guide treatment.
3. Radiological evaluation of CCA can be a challenge even with the most modern CT imaging techniques. Radiological distinction between CCA, HCC and metastases to the liver from non-hepatobiliary sites can be difficult; this often requires complex evaluation of arterial uptake of index lesions and the assessment of surrounding tissue as well as further imaging techniques such as MRI or possibly PET.
4. Meaningful improvement in outcomes for patients with CCA necessitates systematic evaluation, often requiring a multimodal approach to patient workup.

## Introduction

Cholangiocarcinoma (CCA) is the broad term for malignancies originating from biliary epithelial cells. CCA is the most common malignancy of the biliary tract. CCA can be classified based on anatomical location into intrahepatic (iCCA), perihilar (pCCA, Klatskin tumours), distal (dCCA, extrahepatic tumours) and gall bladder cancer. iCCA is located proximal to the second-degree bile ducts, pCCA is defined as tumour in the area between the second-degree bile ducts and the insertion of the cystic duct into the common bile duct, while dCCA is defined as tumour in the area between the insertion of the cystic duct to the bile duct and the ampulla of Vater [1].

The majority of CCAs occur in the perihilar region (60–70%) with the remainder occurring in the distal common bile duct (20–30%) or within the liver (5–15%) [2]. pCCA which accounts for the majority of tumours can be classified using the Bismuth-Corlette classification (Table 15.1; [3]).

**Table 15.1** Bismuth–Corlette classification of Perihilar (Klatskin) tumours (adapted from Bismuth and Corlette [3])

| Type | Description |
|---|---|
| Type I | Limited to the common hepatic duct, below the level of the confluence of the right and left hepatic ducts |
| Type II | Tumour extends into the bifurcation but not into intraphepatic bile ducts |
| Type IIIa | Tumour occlusion of the common hepatic duct and the right hepatic duct |
| Type IIIb | Tumour occlusion of the common hepatic duct and left hepatic duct |
| Type IV | Tumour involving the confluence and both right and left hepatic ducts |

# Diagnosis

## *Clinical Presentation*

The clinical presentation of CCA can be fairly unspecific. Extrahepatic tumours usually present with painless jaundice, steatorrhoea, dark urine and pruritus related to biliary obstruction. Conversely, iCCA can present with pain, most commonly localised to the right upper quadrant of the abdomen. Other clinical features include fatigue, weight loss and fever. Differential diagnosis is wide, including hepatocellular carcinoma (HCC), pancreatic carcinoma, cholangitis, cholelithiasis, parasitic infestations or metastases to the liver from non-hepatobiliary (non-HB) malignancies. While the definitive diagnosis of cholangiocarcinoma is histological, various less invasive tests are useful for the exclusion of differential diagnosis and staging of the disease.

## *Radiological Imaging Investigations*

### Ultrasonography (US)

Abdominal ultrasonography, although cheap, non-invasive and often the first line of investigation, is of limited value in the diagnosis of CCA. Large intrahepatic mass lesions may be identified on US. However, smaller intrahepatic, perihilar and gall bladder lesions can be more difficult to visualise. The sensitivity of US in detecting pCCA ductal masses or thickening is operator-dependent and reported to range from 87 to 96% [4]. Irregular thickening of the duct wall and polypoid intraluminal masses can also be seen in some cases of iCCA [5]. Despite its limitations, contrast-enhanced US can be utilised in the radiological exclusion of HCC for patients unable to tolerate contrast-enhanced CT or MRI [6].

### Endoscopic Ultrasound (EUS)

EUS allows clear visualisation of the distal biliary tree, gall bladder, local blood supply and regional lymph nodes. This modality can be utilised to facilitate fine needle aspiration of suspicious areas, allowing differentiation between malignant and benign lesions. However, the sensitivity and specificity of EUS are variable- and user-dependent. Meta-analysis has found a sensitivity of between 59 and 80% for EUS-FNA in the diagnosis of CCA [7].

### Computerised Axial Tomography (CT)

Triple-phase contrast-enhanced hepatobiliary CT is the routine initial test for assessment of HB tumours in many centres. Furthermore, thoraco-abdominal CT is a particularly useful tool in the perioperative evaluation and staging of early HB tumours (including CCA). Besides visualising masses and showing biliary duct stricturing or dilatation, CT allows clear delineation of macrovascular invasion which is imperative for estimating operative feasibility. In these respects, meta-analysis has suggested that CT has a sensitivity of over 80% and specificity of over 90% for staging CCA [8]. However, its sensitivity is lower for smaller lesions (<3 cm), excluding distant metastases (63%) and identifying regional lymph node metastases (54%) [9, 10].

As regards diagnosis, even with triple-phase (arterial, portal venous and delayed/washout phase) imaging on the most modern CT scanners, the radiological distinction between CCA, HCC and metastases to the liver from non-HB sites can be challenging. The best validated criteria are for distinguishing HCC where in a cirrhotic liver, HCC appears hypervascular compared with liver parenchyma on the hepatic arterial phase of scans. This hypervascularity diminishes during the washout phase. According to the American Association for the Study of Liver Diseases (AASLD) [11] and the European Association for the Study of the Liver (EASL) [12], in a cirrhotic liver, demonstration of intense arterial uptake followed by washout is diagnostic of HCC. However, these criteria are not diagnostic of HCC in non-cirrhotic livers. In comparison, CCA (more common in non-cirrhotic livers) appears as a hypo-dense lesion with rim enhancement, often accompanied by biliary duct dilatation and contrast enhancement on delayed images, similar to non-HB metastases. A previous study reported that iCCA in patients with cirrhosis had varied enhancement patterns on triple-phase contrast CT [13]. Additionally, the study suggested that even though most iCCA did not display the same radiological characteristics as HCC, the rate of misdiagnosis of iCCA for HCC was significant [13]. Consequently, histological confirmation of CT findings would be recommended when feasible. Nevertheless, typical radiological features of CCA and its common differential diagnoses are outlined in Table 15.2.

**Table 15.2** Summary of histological and molecular markers of the most common primary and secondary hepatobiliary malignancies

| Malignancy | Cholangiocarcinoma (CCA) | Hepatocellular carcinoma (HCC) | Metastatic adenocarcinoma |
|---|---|---|---|
| Expressed | *Common*: CK7, CK19, MOC31, Claudin 4, Ber-Ep4, mCEA, pCEA (non-canalicular), Mucin (Extra-hepatic): CK20 *Rare*: GPC3 | *Common*: Hep Par1, albumin (by in-situ hybridization), AFP, pCEA (canalicular), GPC3 *Rare*: CK7, CK19, MOC31, claudin 4, Ber-Ep4, mucin | *Common*: *Gastro-oesophaeal and pancreatic*: similar to CCA *Lower GI*: CK19, CK20, Ber-Ep4, pCEA (non-canalicular) |
| Radiology | Hypo-dense hepatic lesion with rim enhancement on portal venous or washout phase | In a cirrhotic liver, lesion with arterial phase enhancement and washout in portal venous or washout phase | Hypo-dense hepatic lesion with rim enhancement on portal venous or washout phase (primary tumour may be evident) |
| Serological marker | Ca19-9, CEA | AFP | Multiple markers including AFP, Ca19-9 and CEA |
| Not expressed | Hep Par1, AFP | mCEA | Hep Par1, AFP |

## Magnetic Resonance Imaging (MRI)

Triple-phase gadolinium-enhanced images of the liver can also be obtained during MRI evaluation. Better separation of the MRI phases can be achieved compared with CT, allowing hypervascular lesions and washout to be identified more clearly for radiological exclusion of HCC. During the arterial phase of gadolinium-enhanced MRI, iCCAs tend to appear hypointense compared with liver tissue on T1-weighted images. However, iCCAs tend to look hyperintense on T2-weighted images, due to fibrosis and the presence of mucin within tumours [14]. Given that the distinction between smaller iCCA and HCC on CT scans of cirrhotic livers remains a challenge [15], lesion intensity on T1-and T2-weighted MRI may help to further clarify the nature of such liver masses. In a study of the accuracy of MRI distinction between HCC and CCA (for lesions > 2 cm), MRI had a sensitivity of 85% and specificity of 89.7% [16]. However, MRI is less accurate for the differential diagnoses of smaller lesions or metastases from non-hepatobiliary primary sites. Furthermore, in livers with chronic biliary stricturing conditions such as primary sclerosing cholangitis, the specificity of typical MRI appearances for CCA can be as low as 37% [17]. As regards CCA staging, trials comparing the accuracy of contrast-enhanced CT with MRI (including MRCP) are yet to be conducted. However, from small studies, their overall accuracy is considered broadly equivalent [18]. Nevertheless, MRI may provide more detail on hepatic architecture and smaller iCCA particularly when radical surgery is feasible.

## Positron Emission Tomography (PET)

For lesions which remain indeterminate for malignancy after CT and MRI evaluation, PET may be useful, providing metabolic rather than anatomical information on tumours. The main limitations of PET imaging include poor resolution and anatomical localisation. The development of PET-CT fusion images has been of help in overcoming this issue to some degree. Studies evaluating the accuracy of PET-CT in staging CCA are fairly limited. However, they seem to suggest its utility for exclusion of distant metastatic disease. One small study found that only 25% of distant metastases detected on PET were evident on contrast-enhanced CT scan [19]. Another study has reported a sensitivity of 95% for detection of distant metastases by PET compared with 63% for CT [9]. Nevertheless, PET is less reliable for the detection of lymph node and peritoneal metastases. While PET may be a potential tool for preventing unnecessary radical surgery for cholangiocarcinoma, adequately powered studies are required to validate its role.

## Cholangiography

Magnetic resonance cholangiopancreatography (MRCP) is the most accurate non-invasive means of imaging of the entire biliary tree and is as sensitive as ERCP for detecting extrahepatic CCA [20]. This could be of value when selective bile duct dilatation is crucial to the differential diagnosis of periampullary lesions. Invasive cholangiography permits direct visualisation of the biliary tree utilising various techniques such as endoscopic retrograde cholangiopancreatography (ERCP), single-operator peroral cholangiopancreatography (SpyGlass endoscopy) or percutaneous transhepatic cholangiography (PTC). ERCP is useful in the diagnosis of pCCA and dCCA as well as obtaining brush samples of epithelium for cytological analysis. Specificity of cytology is high (60–100%); however, sensitivity is low (9–24%) [21]. In addition, ERCP and PTC both facilitate therapeutic stent deployment to relieve biliary obstruction. SpyGlass endoscopy is utilised as an option to overcome some of the limitations of standard ERCP. It provides a useful alternative technique of stent deployment and obtains a tissue diagnosis when ERCP is unsuccessful [22]. However, diagnostic radiological imaging is recommended to be obtained prior to any intervention, to prevent anatomical distortion precluding interpretation of imaging.

## Laboratory Investigations

### *Serology*

#### Liver Function Tests

Common biochemical abnormalities associated with CCA typically reflect biliary obstruction which include raised levels of bilirubin, alkaline phosphatase and gamma-glutamyltransferase. In more advanced cases, aspartate aminotransferase and alanine aminotransferase can also become deranged, along with impaired clotting and falling albumin levels indicative of failing synthetic liver function. However, these are non-specific for a cholangiocarcinoma diagnosis.

#### Tumour Markers

The value of tumour markers in the diagnosis of CCA is limited. Carbohydrate antigen (CA) 19-9 remains one of the best studied markers. Carcinoembryonic antigen (CEA) is another well-studied marker. Both markers are, however, rather non-specific and can be raised in a multitude of inflammatory conditions such as cholangitis and with other malignancies. On the other hand, patients who are Lewis antigen negative will not be able to produce CA 19-9. Thus the sensitivity and specificity of currently studied tumour markers are low for a cholangiocarcinoma diagnosis.

#### Histopathology

CCA is thought to develop through a series of stages from early biliary glandular hyperplasia, through metaplasia, to dysplasia and finally carcinoma. CCAs are adenocarcinomas comprising tubules, acini, solid nests or trabeculae, embedded in desmoplastic stroma [23]. As they can be surrounded by extensive fibrosis, it is often difficult to distinguish cholangiocarcinoma from chronically inflamed tissue morphologically. iCCA is usually found in non-cirrhotic livers. However, in the setting of an intrahepatic lesion on a background of cirrhosis, differentiation of CCA from HCC morphologically is sometimes problematic. Morphologically, iCCA can be classified into mass-forming, periductal-infiltrating, intraductal, superficial spreading and undefined subtypes [24]. Furthermore, pCCAs can be classified into exophytic mass-forming and intraductal subtypes. Periductal and mass-forming types harbour the poorest prognosis.

CCAs can range from being undifferentiated to well-differentiated. Papillary adenocarcinoma is by far the commonest variant. Subtypes of CCA other than papillary adenocarcinoma account for <10% of tumours and include mucinous, adenosquamous, squamous cell, signet-ring cell, mucoepidermoid, glycogen-rich clear-cell and spindle cell or undifferentiated carcinomas. Adenosquamous and spindle cell carcinomas are thought to have a worse prognosis than adenocarcinoma [23]. The difference between poorly differentiated CCA, HCC with a pseudoglandular pattern of differentiation and metastases to the liver from non-HB sites can be challenging. Immunohistochemical and molecular markers which could be of assistance in this respect are shown in Table 15.2.

## Staging

The staging of CCA guides management and helps with prognostication. The complexities of staging this tumour group are well documented due to the variation in anatomical location of the tumour as well as the limited sensitivity of even the most modern imaging modalities. To guide treatment, CCA can be simply classified into early, locally advanced (LA) or metastatic stages. Early CCA is potentially resectable, dependent upon patient suitability. LA CCA is deemed surgically unresectable due to macrovascular or lymph node involvement. However, there is ongoing interest in the role of locoregional ablative treatment approaches and the potential for conversion to resectable disease (particularly when LA by virtue of macrovascular invasion). Finally, metastatic CCA occurs with spread to adjacent or more distant organs, only amenable to palliative systemic treatment.

While no staging system has been universally adopted, at least three well-known comprehensive staging systems are currently available which incorporate prognostic factors to expand on the basic classification. Variations exist in each of these staging systems according to the anatomical location of tumour. These include the American Joint Committee on Cancer/Union for International Cancer Control (AJCC/UICC), the Liver Cancer Study Group of Japan (LCSGJ) and the National Comprehensive Cancer Network (NCCN) staging systems. The AJCC/UICC is the only system which has shown correlation between stage and survival, is the most often used and will be discussed in more detail. This staging system underwent recent revision with an 8th edition projected to come into effect globally in January 2018 [25].

## *Radiological Staging*

### Intrahepatic CCA

For iCCA, T classification (AJCC/UICC staging) is dependent upon the number of lesions present, the presence of macrovascular invasion and invasion of adjacent structures. Tumour size has been controversial as a prognostic factor; however, size has been shown to correlate with tumour grade which could confound such analysis [26]. The AJCC/UICC system for intrahepatic CCA (8th edition; [27]):

#### T Stage

*T1a*: solitary tumour, <5 cm without macrovascular involvement
*T1b*: solitary tumour >5 cm, also without macrovascular involvement
*T2*: solitary tumour with intrahepatic macrovascular invasion or multiple tumours, with or without macrovascular invasion
*T3*: tumours perforating visceral peritoneum
*T4*: tumours directly invading local extrahepatic structures

#### N Stage

*N0*: refers to no regional lymph node involvement
*N1*: refers to regional lymph node involvement

#### M Stage

*M0*: refers to no distant metastases or nodal involvement
*M1*: refers to distant metastatic spread or distant nodal involvement

The 8th edition (AJCC system) has been shown to be better able to stratify the risk of death for stage III and T3 patients [28]. A further study claimed the 8th edition provided more discrete stratification of patient prognostic groups in general [29].

### Perihilar CCA

For pCCA, the presence of lymph node metastases, differentiation, macrovascular invasion, perineural invasion and surgical resection margins has been shown to be of prognostic relevance [30, 31]. The Bismuth-Corlette system (Table 15.1) is not a staging system but can help guide surgical management. The two main staging systems in common use include AJCC/UICC and the Memorial Sloan Kettering Cancer Centre (MSKCC) staging system. The AJCC/UICC system for pCCA (8th Edition):

### T Stage

*T1*: tumour confined to the bile duct, with extension up to the muscle layer or fibrous tissue
*T2*: tumours which invade beyond the wall of the bile duct to surrounding adipose tissue or adjacent hepatic parenchyma
*T3*: tumours which invade unilateral branches of the portal vein or hepatic artery
*T4*: tumours which invade the main portal vein or its branches bilaterally, the common hepatic artery, the unilateral second-order biliary radicals with contralateral portal vein or hepatic artery involvement

### N Stage

*N0*: refers to no lymph node involvement
*N1*: refers to involvement of one to three lymph nodes within the hilar, cystic duct, common bile duct, hepatic artery, posterior pancreatoduodenal and/or portal vein lymph node groups
*N2*: refers to involvement of four or more lymph nodes from the sites mentioned for N1 (above)

### M Stage

*M0*: refers to no distant metastases or nodal involvement
*M1*: refers to distant metastases or distant nodal involvement

## Distal CCA

For distal CCA, factors such as depth of invasion, the presence of lymph node metastases, microscopic vascular invasion, direct invasion into the pancreas/adjacent structures, resection margins and perineural invasion have been suggested to be independent prognostic factors [31, 32]. The AJCC/UICC 8th edition is currently the only accepted staging system for distal CCA [33].

### T Stage

*T1*: tumours invading the bile duct wall with a depth less than 5 mm
*T2*: tumours invadeing the bile duct wall with a depth of 5–12 mm
*T3*: tumours invadeing the bile duct wall with a depth greater than 12 mm
*T4*: tumours are classed as involving the celiac axis, superior mesenteric artery and/or common hepatic artery

### N Stage

*N1*: disease encompasses metastasis in one to three regional lymph nodes
*N2*: disease is classed as four or more regional lymph nodes involved

### M Stage

*M0*: refers to no distant metastases or nodal involvement
*M1*: distant metastasis or distant nodal involvement

## *Laparoscopy and Surgical Staging*

Laparoscopy has been shown to be able to detect sub-radiological intra-abdominal metastases by facilitating closer evaluation of the liver surface, which may allow detection of occult hepatic metastases. Staging laparoscopy can also detect occult peritoneal metastases. A previous study [34] found that in patients with CCA that initially appeared resectable after combined imaging modalities, staging laparoscopy detected peritoneal and liver metastasis in one third of patients (accuracy was found to be 92% and 71%, respectively). It could not however detect lymph node or vascular involvement which was only observed during laparotomy [34]. Consequently preoperative laparoscopy has been said to prevent unnecessary laparotomy in up to 30% of patients. Expert consensus recommends preoperative laparoscopy in patient with high-risk localised CCA, such as defined by T stage and Ca 19-9 levels in secretors [35]. Nevertheless, a previous study suggested that the presence of metastases on laparoscopy was not contingent with radiological staging [36].

Furthermore, laparoscopy allows biopsy of lesions which appear indeterminate on imaging, providing histological confirmation in case of uncertainty. The addition of laparoscopic ultrasound also aids the diagnosis of hepatic metastases and should be combined with staging laparoscopy to determine local stage and rule out metastatic disease [37]. Nevertheless, surgical resectability cannot be guaranteed without complete abdominal exploration at the time of surgery.

## Future Considerations

With respect to the diagnosis of cholangiocarcinoma, further research into potential biomarkers to enhance early diagnosis with a high degree of sensitivity and specificity is ongoing [38]. Furthermore, improved resolution of imaging is crucial for accurate selection of cases which are potentially curable by surgery. Techniques such as PET-CT and PET-MR and the use of cholangiocyte-specific contrast media are currently undergoing evaluation [39]. Finally, in this era of genomic and precision medicine, molecular biomarkers to distinguish liver metastatic upper gastrointestinal malignancies from CCA and to identify clinically relevant subsets of cholangiocarcinoma may be crucial to optimising the benefit from systemic therapy for cancer [40].

## References

1. Razumilava N, Gores GJ. Combination of gemcitabine and cisplatin for biliary tract cancer: a platform to build on. J Hepatol. 2011;54:577–8.
2. Ahrendt SA, Pitt HA. Biliary tract. In: Townsend C, editor. Sabiston textbook of surgery. Philadelphia: W.B. Saunders Company; 2001. p. 1076–111.
3. Bismuth H, Corlette MB. Intrahepatic cholangioenteric anastomosis in carcinoma of the hilus of the liver. Surg Gynecol Obstet. 1975;140:170–8.

4. Hann LE, Greatrex KV, Bach AM, et al. Cholangiocarcinoma at the hepatic hilus: sonographic findings. AJR Am J Roentgenol. 1997;168(4):985–9.
5. Van Beers BE. Diagnosis of cholangiocarcinoma. HPB (Oxford). 2008;10(2):87–93.
6. Giorgio A, Montesarchio L, Gatti P, et al. Contrast-enhanced ultrasound: a simple and effective tool in defining a rapid diagnostic work-up for small nodules detected in cirrhotic patients during surveillance. J Gastrointestin Liver Dis. 2016;25(2):205–11.
7. Navaneethan U, Njei B, Venkatesh PG, Lourdusamy V, Sanaka MR. Endoscopic ultrasound in the diagnosis of cholangiocarcinoma as the etiology of biliary strictures: a systematic review and meta-analysis. Gastroenterol Rep (Oxf). 2015;3(3):209–15.
8. Ruys AT, van Beem BE, Engelbrecht MR, et al. Radiological staging in patients with hilar cholangiocarcinoma: a systematic review and meta-analysis. Br J Radiol. 2012;85(1017):1255–62.
9. Lee SW, Kim HJ, Park JH, et al. Clinical usefulness of 18F-FDG PET-CT for patients with gallbladder cancer and cholangiocarcinoma. J Gastroenterol. 2010;45(5):560–6.
10. Lee HY, Kim SH, Lee JM, et al. Preoperative assessment of resectability of hepatic hilar cholangiocarcinoma: combined CT and cholangiography with revised criteria. Radiology. 2006;239(1):113–21.
11. Tan CH, Low SC, Thng CH. APASL and AASLD consensus guidelines on imaging diagnosis of hepatocellular carcinoma: a review. Int J Hepatol. 2011;2011:519783.
12. Pugacheva O, Matsui O, Kozaka K, et al. Detection of small hypervascular hepatocellular carcinomas by EASL criteria: comparison with double-phase CT during hepatic arteriography. Eur J Radiol. 2011;80(3):e201–6.
13. Li R, Cai P, Ma KS, et al. Dynamic enhancement patterns of intrahepatic cholangiocarcinoma in cirrhosis on contrast-enhanced computed tomography: risk of misdiagnosis as hepatocellular carcinoma. Sci Rep. 2016;6:26772. https://doi.org/10.1038/srep26772.
14. Vilgrain V, Van Beers BE, Flejou JF, et al. Intrahepatic cholangiocarcinoma: MRI and pathologic correlation in 14 patients. Comput Assist Tomogr. 1997;21(1):59–65.
15. Huang B, Wu L, Lu XY, et al. Small intrahepatic cholangiocarcinoma and hepatocellular carcinoma in cirrhotic livers may share similar enhancement patterns at multiphase dynamic MR imaging. Radiology. 2016;281(1):150–7.
16. Forner A, Vilana R, Ayuso C, et al. Diagnosis of hepatic nodules 20 mm or smaller in cirrhosis: prospective validation of the noninvasive diagnostic criteria for hepatocellular carcinoma. Hepatology. 2008;47(1):97–104.
17. Charatcharoenwitthaya P, Enders FB, Halling KC, Lindor KD. Utility of serum tumor markers, imaging, and biliary cytology for detecting cholangiocarcinoma in primary sclerosing cholangitis. Hepatology. 2008;48(4):1106–17.
18. Ryoo I, Lee JM, Park HS, Han JK, Choi BI. Preoperative assessment of longitudinal extent of bile duct cancers using MDCT with multiplanar reconstruction and minimum intensity projections: comparison with MR cholangiography. Eur J Radiol. 2012;81(9):2020–6.
19. Petrowsky H, Wildbrett P, Husarik DB, et al. Impact of integrated positron emission tomography and computed tomography on staging and management of gallbladder cancer and cholangiocarcinoma. J Hepatol. 2006;45:43–50.
20. Park MS, Kim TK, Kim KW, et al. Differentiation of extrahepatic bile duct cholangiocarcinoma from benign stricture: findings at MRCP versus ERCP. Radiology. 2004;233(1):234–40.
21. Harewood GC, Baron TH, Stadheim LM, Kipp BR, Sebo TJ, Salomao DR. Prospective, blinded assessment of factors influencing the accuracy of biliary cytology interpretation. Am J Gastroenterol. 2004;99:1464–9.
22. Navaneethan U, Hasan MK, Lourdusamy V, Njei B, Varadarajulu S, Hawes RH. Single-operator cholangioscopy and targeted biopsies in the diagnosis of indeterminate biliary strictures: a systematic review. Gastrointest Endosc. 2015;82(4):608–14.
23. Esposito I. Schirmacher pathological aspects of cholangiocarcinoma. HPB (Oxford). 2008;10(2):83–6.
24. Nakanuma Y, Sato Y, Harada K, Sasaki M, Xu J, Ikeda H. Pathological classification of intrahepatic cholangiocarcinoma based on a new concept. World J Hepatol. 2010;2:419–27.

25. Blechacz B. Cholangiocarcinoma: current knowledge and new developments. Gut Liver. 2017;11(1):13–26.
26. Spolverato G, Ejaz A, Kim Y, Sotiropoulos GC, Pau A, Alexandrescu S, et al. Tumor size predicts vascular invasion and histologic grade among patients undergoing resection of intrahepatic cholangiocarcinoma. J Gastrointest Surg. 2014;18:1284–91.
27. Nagorney DM, Pawlik TM, Chun YS, et al. Perihilar bile ducts. In: Amin MB, editor. AJCC cancer staging manual. 8th ed. Chicago: AJCC; 2017. p. 311.
28. Spolverato G, Bagante F, Weiss M, et al. Comparative performances of the 7th and the 8th editions of the American Joint Committee on Cancer staging systems for intrahepatic cholangiocarcinoma. J Surg Oncol. 2017; https://doi.org/10.1002/jso.24569. [Epub ahead of print].
29. Aloia T, Pawlik TM, Taouli B, et al. Intrahepatic bile ducts. In: Amin MB, editor. AJCC cancer staging manual. 8th ed. Chicago: AJCC; 2017. p. 295.
30. Ercolani G, Zanello M, Grazi GL, et al. Changes in the surgical approach to hilar cholangiocarcinoma during an 18-year period in a Western single center. J Hepatobiliary Pancreat Sci. 2010;17(3):329–37.
31. Ghouri YA, Mian I, Boris Blechacz B. Cancer review: cholangiocarcinoma. J Carcinog. 2015;14:1. Published online 23 Feb 2015. https://doi.org/10.4103/1477-3163.151940.
32. Hong SM, Pawlik TM, Cho H, et al. Depth of tumor invasion better predicts prognosis than the current American Joint Committee on Cancer T classification for distal bile duct carcinoma. Surgery. 2009;146(2):250–7.
33. Krasinskas A, Pawlik TM, Mino-Kenudson M, Vauthey J-N. Distal bile duct. In: Amin MB, editor. AJCC cancer staging manual. 8th ed. Chicago: AJCC; 2017. p. 317.
34. Goere D, Wagholikar GD, Pessaux P, et al. Utility of staging laparoscopy in subsets of biliary cancers: laparoscopy is a powerful diagnostic tool in patients with intrahepatic and gallbladder carcinoma. Surg Endosc. 2006;20(5):721–5.
35. Weber SM, Ribero D, O'Reilly EM, Kokudo N, Miyazaki M, Pawlik TM. Intrahepatic cholangiocarcinoma: expert consensus statement. HPB (Oxford). 2015;17(8):669–80.
36. Bird N, Elmasry M, Jones R, et al. Role of staging laparoscopy in the stratification of patients with perihilar cholangiocarcinoma. Br J Surg. 2017;104(4):418–25.
37. Joseph S, Connor S, Garden OJ. Staging laparoscopy for cholangiocarcinoma. HPB (Oxford). 2008;10(2):116–9.
38. Macias RIR, Banales JM, Sangro B, et al. The search for novel diagnostic and prognostic biomarkers in cholangiocarcinoma. Biochim Biophys Acta. 2018;1864(4 Pt B):1468–77. pii: S0925-4439(17):30275-2.
39. Kirchner J, Sawicki LM, Deuschl C, et al. 18 F-FDG PET/MR imaging in patients with suspected liver lesions: value of liver-specific contrast agent Gadobenate dimeglumine. PLoS One. 2017;12(7):e0180349.
40. Sia D, Hoshida Y, Villanueva A, et al. Integrative molecular analysis of intrahepatic cholangiocarcinoma reveals 2 classes that have different outcomes. Gastroenterology. 2013;144(4):829–40.

# Chapter 16
# Cholangiocarcinoma: From Mechanisms to Management

**Leonard M. Quinn, Nicholas Bird, Robert Jones, David Vass, and Hassan Malik**

**Key Learning Points**
1. Symptomatically silent in the early stages, cholangiocarcinoma manifests a very poor prognosis with many patients having advanced disease at presentation.
2. None of the staging systems accurately predict survival. The most important staging and predictive issue is surgical resectability which represents the only treatment with curative intent.
3. Survival following resection is largely dependent on tumour-negative margin status, the absence of vascular invasion and lymph node metastasis and adequate functional liver remnant.
4. The UK BILCAP Phase III trial found improved median survival with adjuvant capecitabine following successful resection compared to observation alone.
5. Preoperative (neoadjuvant) chemotherapy and orthotopic liver transplantation are not standard treatment protocol at the current time.

L. M. Quinn · N. Bird · D. Vass
Hepatobiliary Surgery, Digestive Diseases Unit, Aintree University Hospital, Liverpool, UK
e-mail: L.M.Quinn@liverpool.ac.uk

R. Jones · H. Malik (✉)
Department of Liver Surgery, Aintree University Hospital NHS Foundation Trust, Liverpool, UK
e-mail: robjones@liv.ac.uk; Hassan.Malik@aintree.nhs.uk



T. Cross, D. H. Palmer (eds.), *Liver Cancers*,
https://doi.org/10.1007/978-3-319-92216-4_16

**Areas of Controversy and Uncertainty**
1. Disease staging and prediction of surgical resectability.
2. Preoperative biliary drainage and staging laparoscopy.
3. Neoadjuvant chemotherapy.
4. Neoadjuvant radiotherapy.
5. Adjuvant chemotherapy.
6. Orthotopic liver transplantation.

## Introduction

In this chapter we explore the following areas pertaining to cholangiocarcinoma (CCA):

- Anatomy, tumour classification and staging
- Epidemiology and risk factors
- Molecular spectrum of disease
- Clinical presentation
- Approach to investigation and staging
- Treatment for localized cholangiocarcinoma
- Treatment for advanced disease
- Future research perspectives
- References

## Anatomy

Intrahepatic cholangiocarcinoma (iCCA) originates in the small peripheral intrahepatic bile ducts or the large intrahepatic ducts proximal to the bifurcation of the left and right hepatic ducts.

In extrahepatic cholangiocarcinoma, the disease may arise in the large bile ducts of the perihilar region (pCCA), including the confluence itself, proximal to the insertion of the cystic duct into the common bile duct (CBD) or distal to the insertion of the cystic duct into the CBD down to but not including the ampulla of Vater (dCCA).

Tumours involving the common hepatic duct bifurcation are termed hilar cholangiocarcinoma or Klatskin tumours. These two terms do not account for whether or not the tumour originated from the intrahepatic or extrahepatic components [1].

In Western populations pCCA comprises 50%, dCCA 40% and iCCA 10% of cases, respectively [2].

Perihilar disease is subdivided according to the Bismuth-Corlette classification. Tumours located below the confluence of the left and right hepatic ducts are classified as Type I. Tumours reaching the confluence are Type II. Those tumours occluding the common hepatic duct and either the right or left hepatic duct are termed Type IIIa and IIIb, respectively. Multicentric tumours are Type IV [3].

## Staging of Disease

A number of staging systems are used to stage cholangiocarcinoma. The most commonly used is the Union for International Cancer Control/American Joint Committee on Cancer (UICC/AJCC) 2010 revision of the tumour, node and Metatasis (TNM) classification that separates cholangiocarcinoma into intrahepatic, hilar and distal disease, respectively [4]. A full description of TNM staging follows.

None of the staging systems accurately predict survival. The most important staging and predictive issue is surgical resectability. The AJCC system is based on pathological outcome following resection—this is therefore of use only for prognostication and not for predicting resectability.

Clinical staging systems for pCCA include the Bismuth-Corlette and Memorial Sloan Kettering Cancer Centre (MSKCC) systems.

The Bismuth-Corlette system (described previously) classifies patients on the extent of biliary involvement but does not incorporate important features such as vascular involvement or lobar atrophy. As such it cannot be used for predicting resectability.

MSKCC staging for pCCA, first proposed in 1998, builds on Bismuth-Corlette and includes longitudinal and radial extension of the tumour to more accurately predict resectability. Specifically the T staging compromises local tumour involvement, portal vein involvement and hepatic lobar atrophy (Table 16.3). This staging system has been externally validated and accurately predicted resectability, probability of metastatic disease and long-term survival in the preoperative setting [5].

## **iCCA Tumour Classification** (Table 16.1)

- Tis—Carcinoma in situ
- T1—Solitary tumour without vascular invasion
- T2a—Solitary tumour with vascular invasion
- T2b—Multiple tumours with or without vascular invasion
- T3—Tumour perforating visceral peritoneum or involving local extrahepatic structures through direct invasion
- T4—Tumour with periductal invasion (longitudinal)

**Table 16.1** UICC/AJCC TNM classification of intrahepatic cholangiocarcinoma

| Stage | T | N | M |
|---|---|---|---|
| 0 | Tis | N0 | M0 |
| I | T1 | N0 | M0 |
| II | T2 | N0 | M0 |
| III | T3 | N0 | M0 |
| IVa | T4 | N0 | M0 |
| | Any T | N1 | M0 |
| IVb | Any T | Any N | M1 |

## **pCCA Tumour Classification** (Table 16.2)

- Tis—Tumour in situ
- T1—Tumour confined to bile duct with extension to muscle or fibrous tissue
- T2a—Tumour invading beyond bile duct to surrounding adipose tissue
- T2b—Tumour invading adjacent hepatic parenchyma
- T3—Tumour invading unilateral branches of portal vein or hepatic artery
- T4—Tumour invading main portal vein or its branches bilaterally, the common hepatic artery and second biliary radicals bilaterally, or second-order biliary radicals unilaterally with contralateral portal vein or hepatic artery involvement

## **MSKCC T Staging Classification** (Table 16.3)

## **dCCA Tumour Classification** (Table 16.4)

- Tis—Tumour in situ
- T1—Tumour confined to bile duct
- T2—Tumour invades beyond wall of bile duct
- T3—Tumour invades adjacent structures but without involvement of superior mesenteric artery or coeliac axis
- T4—Tumour involves the coeliac axis or superior mesenteric artery.

**Table 16.2** UICC/AJCC TNM classification of peri-hilar cholangiocarcinoma

| Stage | T | N | M |
|---|---|---|---|
| 0 | Tis | N0 | M0 |
| I | T1 | N0 | M0 |
| II | T2a-b | N0 | M0 |
| IIIa | T3 | N0 | M0 |
| IIIb | T1–3 | N1 | M0 |
| IVa | T4 | N0–1 | M0 |
| IVb | Any T | N1 | M0 |
| | Any T | Any N | M1 |

**Table 16.3** MSKCC T Staging classification

| T-stage | Description |
|---|---|
| T1 | Tumour involving biliary confluence ± unilateral extension to 2nd-order biliary radicles |
| T2 | Tumour involving biliary confluence ± unilateral extension to 2nd-order biliary radicles and ipsilateral portal vein involvement ± ipsilateral hepatic lobar atrophy |
| T3 | Tumour involving biliary confluence and bilateral extension to 2nd-order biliary radicles or unilateral extension to 2nd-order biliary radicles with contralateral portal vein involvement, or unilateral extension to 2nd-order biliary radicles with contralateral hepatic lobar atrophy or main or bilateral portal venous involvement |

**Table 16.4** UICC/AJCC TNM classification of distal cholangiocarcinoma

| Stage | Tumour | Nodes | Metastasis |
|---|---|---|---|
| 0 | Tis | N0 | M0 |
| Ia | T1 | N0 | M0 |
| Ib | T2 | N0 | M0 |
| IIa | T3 | N0 | M0 |
| IIb | T1 | N1 | M0 |
| | T2 | N1 | M0 |
| | T3 | N1 | M0 |
| III | T4 | Any N | M0 |
| IV | Any T | Any N | M1 |

## Regional Lymph Nodes

- N0—No regional lymph node metastasis
- N1—Regional lymph node metastasis present

## Distant Metastasis

- M0—No evidence of distant metastasis
- M1—Distant metastasis present

## Histologic Grading

- G1—Well differentiated
- G2—Moderately differentiated
- G3—Poorly differentiated
- G4—Undifferentiated

## Epidemiology

Cholangiocarcinoma is a rare malignancy accounting for 3% of gastrointestinal cancers with an incidence of 1–2 per 100,000 population [6].

The incidence of iCCA is rising globally, whilst extra-hepatic is decreasing. This may be related to increases in cirrhosis, alcoholic liver disease and hepatitis C [7].

Cholangiocarcinoma occurs more frequently in males and increases with age [8].

## Risk Factors

There are well-recognized risk factors. However, in the vast majority of patients, no one specific risk factor is identified [9].

Risk factors in Western cohorts include primary sclerosing cholangitis [10], congenital fibropolycystic liver disease, e.g. choledochal cysts [11]; chronic intrahepatic ductal stones [12], and hepatitis C infection [13].

Asian cohorts demonstrate strong associations with parasitic liver fluke infection (genera Clonorchis and Opisthorcis) [14].

## Mechanisms of Disease

The molecular understanding of CCA is far less understood and described compared to other gastrointestinal cancers and exhibits marked heterogeneity on the basis of location. iCCA has been more fully examined at the present time.

Currently, there are no molecular markers for early diagnosis, prognostication or therapy selection. With the advent of next-generation sequencing and multi-omics approaches, it is hoped that advances in understanding CCA biology will lead to biomarker development and personalized medicine.

Diverse candidates for cellular origin include hepatic stem cells, immature neural cell adhesion molecule-positive cholangiocytes, mature interlobular cholangiocytes and peri-biliary glands [15].

CCA expresses cancer stem cells (with capacity for self-renewal) in >30% of tumour mass [16].

Precursor biliary epithelial lesions harbour mutations in p53 [17].

The most prevalent tumour genetic alterations affect key networks such as DNA repair (TP53) and tyrosine kinase signalling (KRAS, BRAF, SMAD4, FGFR) and chromatin remodelling (ARID1A, BAP1) and lead to more aggressive phenotypes.

One third of tumours overexpress TP53 suggesting mutation in this suppressor. Abnormal K-ras expression is found in 45–54% of iCCA and 10–15% of extrahepatic [18].

Fusion gene products involving the kinase receptor FGFR2 gene drive cell proliferation and are well described in iCCA and are suppressed with FGFR kinase inhibitors [19].

Epigenetic profiles differ. iCCA demonstrates mutated isocitrate dehydrogenase-1 (associated with CpG shore hypermethylation) in 25% of cases. It is not present in extrahepatic [20].

Immunohistochemistry demonstrated epidermal growth factor receptor is overexpressed. EGFR activation triggers the MAPK-ERK pathway in cholangiocytes and is targetable [21]. CCAs are oestrogen sensitive with increased expression of alpha- and beta-oestrogen receptors [22].

CCA arises in biliary inflammation with overexpression of interleukin-6, crucial in activating MAPK [23]. TGF-B receptors promote invasion and migration [24].

CCA is characterized by a prominent desmoplastic stroma with high densities of tumour-associated macrophages suggesting a role in CCA progression through the Wnt pathway. Wnt inhibition in animal CCA models increases apoptosis [25].

## Clinical Presentation

Both iCCA and extrahepatic cholangiocarcinomas present late with subtle early symptoms [26].

iCCA is often detected during surveillance in cirrhosis and hepatitis B and C infection. Jaundice is unlikely without significant metastatic burden. The symptoms include:

- Dull right upper quadrant pain
- Weight loss

Extrahepatic cholangiocarcinoma presents when the bile ducts are occluded. Cholangitis is a rare presentation. The symptoms and signs include:

- Jaundice
- Pale stools
- Dark urine
- Pruritus
- Night sweats/malaise
- Right upper quadrant pain/tenderness/mass.
- Hepatomegaly
- Weight loss

## Investigation and Workup

### *Laboratory Analyses*

Extrahepatic CCA reflects biliary obstruction with elevation of bilirubin and alkaline phosphatase. Transaminases are normal in early stages but may elevate as biliary obstruction progresses. The prothrombin time and international normalized ratio similarly elevate.

iCCA will demonstrate elevated alkaline phosphatase levels but normal bilirubin.

The tumour marker CA 19-9 is suggestive of CCA but not specific [27]. CA 19-9 has significant overlap with pancreatic cancer and may also rise in the presence of biliary obstruction alone [28]. CA 19-9 levels greater than 1000 units/ml are suggestive of advanced disease [29].

CEA is associated with colorectal cancer and liver metastases [30]. AFP suggests hepatocellular carcinoma [31].

## Investigation and Staging

Most jaundiced patients will undergo transabdominal ultrasound initially. This confirms the presence or absence of ductal dilatation, helps localize site of biliary obstruction and determines the presence of gallstones [32]. When US cannot confirm benign causation, cross-sectional imaging is required.

Multiphase contrast CT can detect intrahepatic tumours, clarify the level of biliary obstruction and assist in differentiating benign and malignant strictures [33].

Ductal dilatation in both liver lobes, with a contracted gall bladder or non-union of left and right ducts, with or without a thickened wall, suggests perihilar. A distended gall bladder with both dilated intrahepatic and extrahepatic ducts is typical of tumours involving CBD, ampulla of Vater or head of the pancreas.

For intra-hepatic lesions in the non-cirrhotic liver, iCCA (hypodense) must be differentiated from distant metastasis. In the cirrhotic liver, HCC hyperenhances [34].

CT visualizes lymph node basins but with low sensitivity. Preoperative lymph node enlargement is not evidence of non-curability [35]. CT has limited sensitivity for extra-regional metastases, particularly peritoneal [36].

MRI and MRCP provide non-invasive assessment with CCA appearing hypodense on T1 and heterogeneously hyperintense on T2 imaging [37].

In extra-hepatic, if CT and MRI fail to confirm diagnosis, endoscopic ultrasound (EUS) or ERCP (endoscopic retrograde cholangiopancreatography) permits direct visualization and enables biopsy or brush cytology for tissue diagnosis. ERCP enables therapeutic stenting.

Tissue diagnosis is not absolutely necessary prior to curative or palliative intervention, provided characteristic radiology is present [38].

Positron emission tomography (with fluorodeoxyglucose) scanning offers greater sensitivity for detection of occult metastases [39].

Where staging radiology is satisfactory, patients proceed to staging laparoscopy. This identifies many patients with unresectable disease and peritoneal metastases not found on radiology [40]. Unfortunately, true resectability can often only be determined at laparotomy [41].

Biliary drainage is indicated in cholangitis or jaundice in conjunction with malnutrition, hepatic/renal insufficiency and portal vein embolization [42]. In the palliative setting, biliary drainage may prolong survival. Self expanding metal stents offer higher patency duration [43].

## Surgical Resection of Localized Cholangiocarcinoma

Complete surgical resection of CCA represents the only treatment with curative intent.

In iCCA, resection of affected liver segments or of the affected lobe is undertaken. pCCA resection is dependent on the extent of disease but may mandate resection of involved intra- and extrahepatic bile ducts, ipsilateral liver, gallbladder and regional lymph nodes. Pancreatoduodenectomy is performed for dCCA with pylorus-preserving procedures preferable.

Unfortunately, a minority of patients have disease considered to be resectable at time of diagnosis due to local tumour infiltration, peritoneal or distant metastases, lack of biliary reconstructive options or inadequate future liver remnant. dCCA has a higher resectability rate than more proximal pCCA and iCCA [26].

Traditional guidance on the resectability of CCA is as follows [44]:

- Absence of retropancreatic and paracoeliac nodal metastases or distant liver metastases
- Absence of invasion of portal vein and main hepatic artery (some centres do support en bloc resection with vascular reconstruction)
- Absence of adjacent extrahepatic organ invasion
- Absence of disseminated disease

Resectability is ultimately determined at the time of surgery particularly in pCCA, as these tumours often extend into the liver and major vascular structures and accurate preoperative evaluation of these areas is difficult. Therefore, surgical exploration with or without trial resection is appropriate for potentially resectable disease [41].

Survival following resection is largely dependent on tumour-negative margin status, the absence of vascular invasion and lymph node metastasis and adequate functional liver remnant [45].

The majority of cases still recur despite complete resection. Relapse patterns are local and distant, forming the basis for adjuvant chemotherapy.

Overall 5-year survival following resection is reported as 22–44% for iCCA, 11–41% for pCCA and 27–37% for dCCA.

## Orthotopic Liver Transplantation

Liver transplantation is not considered a standard treatment approach due to issues surrounding donor allocation and the poor sensitivity of invasive staging for CCA [46]. Transplantation for iCCA is associated with rapid metastatic formation and has thus been abandoned [47].

The US Mayo Clinic considers liver transplantation in highly selected cases of early stage local unresectable perihilar CCA, in patients who have completed thorough staging, assessment and neoadjuvant chemoradiotherapy [48]. Vascular encasement of the hilar vessels is not a contraindication to transplantation. The upper limit of tumour size is 3 cm and with the absence of intra- or extrahepatic metastases and excludes iCCA or GB cancer. Prior to resection patients undergo exploratory laparotomy. Regional lymph node metastases and peritoneal and locally extensive disease preclude surgery.

The published Mayo experience found a statistically significant improved survival following their transplantation protocol with 92% 1 year, 82% 3 year and 82% 5 year survival. This compared to 82%, 48% and 21%, respectively, following resection only [49]. The ongoing French Phase III Transphil trial compares this strategy with standard surgical resection.

## Adjuvant Therapy

The role of adjuvant therapy remains ill defined. The European Society for Medical Oncology and the National Comprehensive Cancer Network suggest chemotherapy for both margin-negative and margin-positive resected patients [50].

On the basis of improved survival in periampullary cancer in the ESPAC-3 trial, gemcitabine or flurouracil is considered acceptable adjuvant chemotherapy for CCA [51].

The U.K. BilCap Phase III trial found improved median survival with Capecitabine compared to observation which was not statistically significant. This included large numbers of R1 resections but was deemed clinically relevant. Per protocol analysis demonstrated a statistically significant survival benefit. The authors recommend adjuvant capecitabine as standard of care [52].

No prospective clinical trials have identified if benefit is achieved with adjuvant radiotherapy.

## Systemic Therapy for Advanced Disease

In advanced disease, for first-line treatment, the UK ABC-01 and ABC-02 trial found the gemcitabine in combination with cisplatin was superior to gemcitabine alone with improved tumour control rate, time to progression and progression free survival [53]. If cisplatin is not well tolerated, oxaliplatin is an excellent alternative (GEMOX) [54]. Gemcitabine and capecitabine combinations are also beneficial [55]. In patients with borderline performance status, monotherapy is reasonable.

The second line treatment can be offered and include FOLFOX (Folinic acid, flurouracil, oxaliplatin) [56], capecitabine and oxaliplatin [57] or GEMOX plus bevacizumab/rituximab [58], or FOLFIRI (folinic acid, flurouracil and irinotecan) and Bevacizumab [59].

In selected cases, improved outcomes were found using erlotinib (targets epidermal growth factor receptor), an oral tyrosine kinase inhibitor [60]. The monoclonal antibody bevacizumab can be added as salvage (targeting vascular endothelial growth factor) [61].

# Future Perspectives

## *Neoadjuvant Therapy*

Preoperative chemotherapy or radiotherapy is not considered a routine treatment. Many patients are jaundiced and malnourished.

However, the potential benefit cannot be ignored in selected patients. A small study identified complete pathological response and margin-negative resection in extrahepatic CCA [62]. Further work identified survival benefit despite the neoadjuvant cohort having more advanced disease [63].

These promising early findings warrant further investigation with appropriately powered clinical trials.

# References

1. Nagorney DM, Pawlik TM, Chun YS, et al. Perihilar bile ducts. In: Amin MB, editor. AJCC cancer staging manual. 8th ed. Chicago: AJCC; 2017. p. 312.
2. DeOliveira ML, Cunningham SC, Cameron JL, et al. Cholangiocarcinoma: thirty-one-year experience with 564 patients at a single institution. Ann Surg. 2007;245(5):755.
3. Bismuth H, Nakache R, Diamond T. Management strategies in resection for hilar cholangiocarcinoma. Ann Surg. 1992;215(1):31.
4. Edge SB, Byrd DR, Compton CC, et al., editors. American Joint Committee on Cancer staging manual. 7th ed. New York: Springer; 2010. p. 201.
5. Janargin WR, Fong Y, DeMatteo RP, et al. Staging, resectability and outcome in 225 patients with hilar cholangiocarcinoma. Ann Surg. 2001;234(4):507–17.
6. Vauthey JN, Blumgart LH. Recent advances in the management of cholangiocarcinomas. Semin Liver Dis. 1994;14(2):109.
7. Shaib YH, El-Serag HB, Davila JA, Morgan R, McGlynn KA. Risk factors of intrahepatic cholangiocarcinoma in the United States: a case-control study. Gastroenterology. 2005;128(3):620.
8. Henson DE, Albores-Saavedra J, Corle D. Carcinoma of the extrahepatic bile ducts. Histologic types, stage of disease, grade, and survival rates. Cancer. 1992;70(6):1498.
9. Chapman RW. Risk factors for biliary tract carcinogenesis. Ann Oncol. 1999;10(Suppl 4):308.
10. Bergquist A, Ekbom A, Olsson R, et al. Hepatic and extrahepatic malignancies in primary sclerosing cholangitis. J Hepatol. 2002;36(3):321.
11. Lipsett PA, Pitt HA, Colombani PM, Boitnott JK, Cameron JL. Choledochal cyst disease. A changing pattern of presentation. Ann Surg. 1994;220(5):644.
12. Hsing AW, Gao YT, Han TQ, et al. Gallstones and the risk of biliary tract cancer: a population-based study in China. Br J Cancer. 2007;97(11):1577.
13. Mahale P, Torres HA, Kramer JR, Hwang LY, Li R, Brown EL, Engels EA. Hepatitis C virus infection and the risk of cancer among elderly US adults: a registry-based case-control study. Cancer. 2017;123(7):1202. Epub 2017 Jan 24.
14. Watanapa P, Watanapa WB. Liver fluke-associated cholangiocarcinoma. Br J Surg. 2002;89(8):962.

15. Cardinale V, Carpino G, Reid L, Gaudio E, Alvaro D. Multiple cells of origin in cholangiocarcinoma underlie biological, epidemiological and clinical heterogeneity. World J Gastrointest Oncol. 2012;4:94–102.
16. Cardinale V, et al. Profiles of cancer stem cell subpopulations in cholangiocarcinomas. Am J Pathol. 2015;185:1724–39.
17. Nakanishi Y, Zen Y, Kondo S, Itoh T, Itatsu K, Nakanuma Y. Expression of cell cycle-related molecules in biliary premalignant lesions: biliary intraepithelial neoplasia and biliary intraductal papillary neoplasm. Hum Pathol. 2008;39(8):1153.
18. Isa T, Tomita S, Nakachi A, Miyazato H, Shimoji H, Kusano T, Muto Y, Furukawa M. Analysis of microsatellite instability, K-ras gene mutation and p53 protein overexpression in intrahepatic cholangiocarcinoma. Hepatogastroenterology. 2002;49(45):604.
19. Arai Y, et al. Fibroblast growth factor receptor 2 tyrosine kinase fusions define a unique molecular subtype of cholangiocarcinoma. Hepatology. 2014;59:1427–34.
20. Borger DR, Tanabe KK, Fan KC, et al. Frequent mutation of isocitrate dehydrogenase (IDH)1 and IDH2 in cholangiocarcinoma identified through broad-based tumor genotyping. Oncologist. 2012;17(1):72–9. Epub 2011 Dec 16.
21. Yoshikawa D, et al. Clinicopathological and prognostic significance of EGFR, VEGF and HER2 expression in cholangiocarcinoma. Br J Cancer. 2008;98:418–25.
22. Alvaro D, et al. Estrogens and insulin-like growth factor 1 modulate neoplastic cell growth in human cholangiocarcinoma. Am J Pathol. 2006;169:877–88.
23. Webhe H, Henson R, Meng F, Mize-Berge J, Patel T. Interleukin-6 contributes to growth in cholangiocarcinoma cells by aberrant promoter methylation and gene expression. Cancer Res. 2006;66:10517–24.
24. Sato Y, et al. Epithelial-mesenchymal transition induced by transforming growth factor B-1/Snail activation aggravates invasive growth of cholangiocarcinoma. Am J Pathol. 2010;177:141–52.
25. Boulter L, et al. WNT signaling drives cholangiocarcinoma growth and can be pharmacologically inhibited. J Clin Invest. 2015;125:1269–85.
26. Nakeeb A, Pitt HA, Sohn TA, et al. Cholangiocarcinoma. A spectrum of intrahepatic, perihilar, and distal tumors. Ann Surg. 1996;224(4):463.
27. Malaguarnera G, Paladina I, Giordano M, Malaguarnera M, Bertino G, Berretta M. Serum markers of intrahepatic cholangiocarcinoma. Dis Markers. 2013;34(4):219.
28. Kim HJ, Kim MH, Myung SJ, et al. A new strategy for the application of CA19-9 in the differentiation of pancreaticobiliary cancer: analysis using a receiver operating characteristic curve. Am J Gastroenterol. 1999;94(7):1941.
29. Patel AH, Harnois DM, Klee GG, LaRusso NF, Gores GJ. The utility of CA 19-9 in the diagnoses of cholangiocarcinoma in patients without primary sclerosing cholangitis. Am J Gastroenterol. 2000;95(1):204.
30. Siqueira E, Schoen RE, Silverman W, et al. Detecting cholangiocarcinoma in patients with primary sclerosing cholangitis. Gastrointest Endosc. 2002;56(1):40.
31. Maeda T, Adachi E, Kajiyama K, Sugimachi K, Tsuneyoshi M. Combined hepatocellular and cholangiocarcinoma: proposed criteria according to cytokeratin expression and analysis of clinicopathologic features. Hum Pathol. 1995 Sep;26(9):956–64.
32. Saini S. Imaging of the hepatobiliary tract. N Engl J Med. 1997;336(26):1889.
33. Choi SH, Han JK, Lee JM, et al. Differentiating malignant from benign common bile duct stricture with multiphasic helical CT. Radiology. 2005;236(1):178. Epub 2005 Jun 13.
34. Iavarone M, Piscaglia F, Vavassori S, et al. Contrast enhanced CT-scan to diagnose intrahepatic cholangiocarcinoma in patients with cirrhosis. J Hepatol. 2013;58(6):1188–93. Epub 2013 Feb 26.
35. Adachi T, Eguchi S, Beppu T, et al. Prognostic impact of preoperative lymph node enlargement in intrahepatic cholangiocarcinoma: a multi-institutional study by the Kyushu Study Group of Liver Surgery. Ann Surg Oncol. 2015;22(7):2269–78. Epub 2015 Jan 13.
36. Tillich M, Mischinger HJ, Preisegger KH, Rabl H, Szolar DH. Multiphasic helical CT in diagnosis and staging of hilar cholangiocarcinoma. AJR Am J Roentgenol. 1998;171(3):651.

37. Manfredi R, Barbaro B, Masselli G, Vecchioli A, Marano P. Magnetic resonance imaging of cholangiocarcinoma. Semin Liver Dis. 2004;24(2):155.
38. Pelsang RE, Johlin FC. A percutaneous biopsy technique for patients with suspected biliary or pancreatic cancer without a radiographic mass. Abdom Imaging. 1997;22(3):307.
39. Corvera CU, Blumgart LH, Akhurst T, et al. 18F-fluorodeoxyglucose positron emission tomography influences management decisions in patients with biliary cancer. J Am Coll Surg. 2008;206(1):57. Epub 2007 Oct 1.
40. Weber SM, RP DM, Fong Y, Blumgart LH, Jarnagin WR. Staging laparoscopy in patients with extrahepatic biliary carcinoma. Analysis of 100 patients. Ann Surg. 2002;235(3):392.
41. Su CH, Tsay SH, Wu CC, et al. Factors influencing postoperative morbidity, mortality, and survival after resection for hilar cholangiocarcinoma. Ann Surg. 1996;223(4):384.
42. Khan SA, et al. Guidelines for the diagnosis and treatment of cholangiocarcinoma: an update. Gut. 2012;61:1657–69.
43. Liberato MJ, Canena JM. Endoscopic stenting for hilar cholangiocarcinoma: efficacy of unilateral and bilateral placement of plastic and metal stents in a retrospective review of 480 patients. BMC Gastroenterol. 2012;12:103.
44. Tsao JI, Nimura Y, Kamiya J, et al. Management of hilar cholangiocarcinoma: comparison of an American and a Japanese experience. Ann Surg. 2000;232(2):166.
45. Edge SB, Byrd DR, Compton CC, et al., editors. American Joint Committee on Cancer staging manual. 7th ed. New York: Springer; 2010. p. 219.
46. Panjala C, Nguyen JH, Al-Hajjaj AN, et al. Impact of neoadjuvant chemoradiation on the tumor burden before liver transplantation for unresectable cholangiocarcinoma. Liver Transpl. 2012;18(5):594.
47. Meyer CG, Penn I, James L. Liver transplantation for cholangiocarcinoma: results in 207 patients. Transplantation. 2000;69:1633–7.
48. Croome KP, Rosen CB, Heimbach JK, Nagorney DM. Is liver transplantation appropriate for patients with potentially resectable De Novo hilar cholangiocarcinoma? J Am Coll Surg. 2015;221(1):130–9. Epub 2015 Mar 11.
49. Rea DJ, Heimback JK, Rosen CB, et al. Ann Surg. 2005;242(3):451–8.
50. Eckel F, Brunner T, Jelic S, ESMO Guidelines Working Group. Biliary cancer: ESMO clinical practice guidelines for diagnosis, treatment and follow-up. Ann Oncol. 2011;22(Suppl 6):vi40–4.
51. Neoptolemos JP, Moore MJ, Cox TF, et al. European Study Group for Pancreatic Cancer. Effect of adjuvant chemotherapy with fluorouracil plus folinic acid or gemcitabine vs observation on survival in patients with resected periampullary adenocarcinoma: the ESPAC-3 periampullary cancer randomized trial. JAMA. 2012;308(2):147.
52. Primrose JN, Fox R, Palmer DH, et al. Adjuvant capecitabine for biliary tract cancer: the BILCAP randomized study (abstract). J Clin Oncol. 2017; 35 (suppl; abstr 4006).
53. Valle J, Wasan H, Palmer DH, et al. Cisplatin plus gemcitabine versus gemcitabine for biliary tract cancer. N Engl J Med. 2010;362(14):1273.
54. André T, Tournigand C, Rosmorduc O, et al. Gemcitabine combined with oxaliplatin (GEMOX) in advanced biliary tract adenocarcinoma: a GERCOR study. Ann Oncol. 2004;15(9):1339.
55. Knox JJ, Hedley D, Oza A, et al. Combining gemcitabine and capecitabine in patients with advanced biliary cancer: a phase II trial. J Clin Oncol. 2005;23(10):2332.
56. Novarino AM, Satolli MA, Chiappino I, et al. FOLFOX-4 regimen or single-agent gemcitabine as first-line chemotherapy in advanced biliary tract cancer. Am J Clin Oncol. 2013;36(5):466–71.
57. Nehls O, Oettle H, Hartmann JT, et al. Capecitabine plus oxaliplatin as first-line treatment in patients with advanced biliary system adenocarcinoma: a prospective multicentre phase II trial. Br J Cancer. 2008;98(2):309. Epub 2008 Jan 8.
58. Zhu AX, Meyerhardt JA, Blaszkowsky LS, et al. Efficacy and safety of gemcitabine, oxaliplatin, and bevacizumab in advanced biliary-tract cancers and correlation of changes

in 18-fluorodeoxyglucose PET with clinical outcome: a phase 2 study. Lancet Oncol. 2010;11(1):48–54. Epub 2009 Nov 20.
59. Guion-Dusserre JF, Lorgis V, Vincent J, Bengrine L, Ghiringhelli F. FOLFIRI plus bevacizumab as a second-line therapy for metastatic intrahepatic cholangiocarcinoma. World J Gastroenterol. 2015;21(7):2096–101.
60. Philip PA, Mahoney MR, Allmer C, et al. Phase II study of erlotinib in patients with advanced biliary cancer. J Clin Oncol. 2006;24(19):3069.
61. Lubner SJ, Mahoney MR, Kolesar JL, et al. Report of a multicenter phase II trial testing a combination of biweekly bevacizumab and daily erlotinib in patients with unresectable biliary cancer: a phase II Consortium study. J Clin Oncol. 2010;28(21):3491. Epub 2010 Jun 7.
62. McMasters KM, Tuttle TM, Leach SD, et al. Neoadjuvant chemoradiation for extrahepatic cholangiocarcinoma. Am J Surg. 1997;174(6):605.
63. Nelson JW, Ghafoori AP, Willett CG, et al. Concurrent chemoradiotherapy in resected extrahepatic cholangiocarcinoma. Int J Radiat Oncol Biol Phys. 2009;73(1):148. Epub 2008 Sep 19.

# Chapter 17
# Oncotherapies for Cholangiocarcinoma

**Oliver Pickles and Yuk Ting Ma**

**Key Learning Points**

1. Although biliary tract cancers are relatively rare tumours, large-scale randomised clinical trials are feasible with multicentre collaboration and have helped to inform the evidence base.
2. First-line chemotherapy for patients with advanced disease should be with gemcitabine and cisplatin.
3. There is no proven second-line chemotherapy and patients should be enrolled into clinical trials where possible.
4. Adjuvant capecitabine chemotherapy should be considered in all patients following surgical resection.
5. The role of adjuvant radiotherapy and adjuvant chemoradiotherapy remains uncertain, and further randomised trials in this setting are indicated.

**Areas of Controversy and Uncertainty**

1. Conflicting data exists for the role of radiotherapy and chemoradiotherapy in the management of biliary tract cancers and randomised trials in this setting are indicated.

O. Pickles · Y. T. Ma (✉)
Department of Medical Oncology, Queen Elizabeth Hospital, Birmingham, UK



T. Cross, D. H. Palmer (eds.), *Liver Cancers*,
https://doi.org/10.1007/978-3-319-92216-4_17

## Chemotherapy for Advanced Disease

Cholangiocarcinoma is frequently diagnosed at a late and therefore inoperable stage and the aims of treatment in this setting are to palliate symptoms and to control disease. Management of patients with advanced disease is often complicated by the presence of biliary obstruction and sepsis as well as age-related comorbidities. For patients with a good performance status, chemotherapy has been shown to improve cancer-related symptoms and median survival, although the overall median survival still remains poor (less than 1 year).

Due to the rarity of these tumours, nearly all of the clinical trials performed have broadened their eligibility to include all biliary tract cancers. Two randomised phase III trials have demonstrated a survival benefit of chemotherapy over best supportive care (BSC) in patients with advanced disease [1, 2]. The first study by Glimelius et al., compared 5-fluorouracil (5FU), leucovorin and etoposide with BSC in patients with pancreatic and biliary tract cancers. Chemotherapy significantly improved median survival (6 vs 2.5 months, $p < 0.01$) and quality of life [1]. The second study by Sharma et al., randomised patients with unresectable gallbladder cancer to gemcitabine and oxaliplatin (GEMOX), 5FU and folinic acid or BSC. Chemotherapy with GEMOX significantly improved survival compared with 5-fluorouracil and folinic chemotherapy or BSC (9.5 vs 4.6 vs 4.5 months, $p = 0.39$) and was associated with a much higher response rate [2].

Many chemotherapeutic agents have been investigated in biliary tract cancers, although the majority have been small single-arm phase II studies. A pooled analysis comprising 104 trials and 2810 patients revealed fluoropyrimidines, gemcitabine and platinum analogues to be the most active agents, with the highest response and disease-control rates observed with gemcitabine in combination with cisplatin or oxaliplatin [3].

The UK phase III Advanced Biliary tract Cancer (ABC)-02 study finally established combination chemotherapy with gemcitabine and cisplatin as the first-line standard-of-care chemotherapy for advanced biliary tract cancers in 2010 [4]. This study was initiated as a randomised phase II study (ABC-01), which was then extended to a phase III study [5]. Four hundred and ten patients with locally advanced or metastatic cholangiocarcinoma, gallbladder cancer or ampullary cancer were randomised to either cisplatin (25 mg/m$^2$) followed by gemcitabine (1000 mg/m$^2$) each given on days 1 and 8 every 21 days for eight cycles, or gemcitabine alone (1000 mg/m$^2$) given on days 1, 8 and 15 every 28 days for six cycles. This study demonstrated a statistically improved median overall survival in patients treated with the gemcitabine-cisplatin doublet compared to gemcitabine alone (11.7 vs 8.1 months, HR 0.64, 95% CI 0.52–0.80; $p < 0.001$), without the addition of significant toxicity [4]. A similar magnitude of benefit was seen in the parallel randomised phase II Biliary Tract (BT)-22 study performed in Japan using the same treatment regimen (median overall survival 11.2 vs 7.7 months, HR 0.69, 95% CI 0.42–1.13) [6]. The BT-22 trial was developed to evaluate the same dose and regimens used in the ABC-02 trial in Japanese patients with advanced biliary tract cancer. In a subsequent pre-planned meta-analysis of both studies, representing the largest prospectively evaluated patient pool with nearly 500 patients, gemcitabine and cisplatin chemotherapy was confirmed to significantly improve progression-free survival (8.8 vs 6.7 months, HR 0.64, $p < 0.001$) and overall survival (11.6 vs 8.0 months, HR 0.65, $p < 0.001$) [7]. Exploratory subgroup analyses demonstrated that all subgroups benefit from treatment but patients with ampullary tumours and poor performance status [2] were least likely to benefit [7]. The ABC-02 and BT22 studies have shown that even though biliary tract cancers are relatively rare tumours, large-scale prospective studies can be successfully undertaken with multicentre and multinational collaboration.

## *Second Line Chemotherapy*

There is no phase III data to support any chemotherapy regimen over best supportive care after failure of first-line chemotherapy in advanced disease. A number of regimes have been used, most notably fluoropyrimidine-based where patients have been treated with gemcitabine in the first line. In the ABC-02 study, 15% of patients received second-line chemotherapy, whereas in the BT-22 study, 75% of patients received second-line chemotherapy. Despite this difference, the median overall survival observed in both studies was very similar, suggesting that subsequent lines of treatment may be of limited benefit. Prospective randomised trials are clearly needed to answer this question definitively [8].

In the absence of randomised phase III studies, a systematic review was undertaken to evaluate the level of evidence supporting the use of second-line chemotherapy in patients with advanced biliary tract cancers [8]. Twenty-five studies comprising 761 patients were included in the final analysis: 14 phase II clinical trials, 9 retrospective analyses and 2 case reports. There was marked heterogeneity with respect to both first- and second-line chemotherapies used in these studies, and it was concluded that there is a poor level of evidence (level C) to recommend a second-line chemotherapy schedule in patients with advanced biliary tract cancer. Of note, the weighted mean overall survival in the 20 studies with survival data available was 7.2 months (95% CI 6.2–8.2), which is much higher than the 4-month expected median overall survival following progression observed in the ABC-02 study. This clearly reflects a highly selected population as patients eligible for second-line chemotherapy usually have a better performance status and thus better prognosis, and combined with the observation that 15–25% of patients may be fit enough for second-line treatment, it is evident that a cohort of patients exist who may benefit from second-line treatment. This issue will hopefully be addressed in the ongoing UK ABC-06 (NCT 01926236) study, a randomised phase III clinical trial that is comparing combination chemotherapy with oxaliplatin and 5FU against active symptom control alone in patients with advanced biliary tract cancers, following progression on first-line gemcitabine and cisplatin chemotherapy. With recruitment likely to complete in late 2017, the results of this study are eagerly awaited.

## *Summary*

- First-line systemic treatment for unresectable biliary tract cancer should be with gemcitabine and cisplatin chemotherapy.
- The role of target therapy will be discussed in the next chapter.
- At present, in the second line, no treatment can be recommended with a robust evidence base over best supportive care. Where possible these patients should be enrolled into clinical trials.

## Chemotherapy in the Adjuvant Setting

The outcome following surgery for biliary tract cancer remains poor, with the majority of patients succumbing to local recurrent or metastatic disease. Until recently, there was sparse data supporting the routine use of adjuvant therapy. Due to the relative rarity of these tumours and the even fewer patients who are eligible for surgical resection, one of the challenges is the difficulty in completing a large randomised controlled trial that is adequately powered to show a survival advantage. Consequently the majority of the publications consist of uncontrolled institutional series and registry analyses.

The first prospective study was published in 2002. Takada et al. randomised 508 patients with resected pancreatic ($n = 173$), bile duct ($n = 139$), gallbladder ($n = 140$) or ampullary carcinoma ($n = 56$) to chemotherapy with mitomycin C and 5FU (MF) or to surgery alone [9]. In a per-protocol analysis, the 5-year survival in patients with gallbladder cancer was significantly better in the MF group compared to surgery alone (26% vs 14.4%, $p = 0.0367$), but this was no longer statistically significant in the intention-to-treat analysis. There were no significant differences found in the 5-year survival in patients with pancreatic, bile duct or ampullary carcinomas. Major limitations of this study include the inclusion of patients who underwent both curative and non-curative resections, as well as a large number of ineligible patients who were imbalanced between the two gallbladder carcinoma groups.

The ESPAC-3 periampullary trial was a randomised phase III trial designed to compare the survival benefit of adjuvant chemotherapy versus observation following resection for patients with periampullary cancers and to compare 5FU plus folinic acid chemotherapy to that of gemcitabine alone [10]. Four hundred and twenty-eight patients with resected ampullary ($n = 297$), bile duct ($n = 96$) or other periampullary ($n = 35$) cancers were randomised in a 1:1:1 ratio to 5FU and folinic acid, gemcitabine or to observation alone. In the primary analysis, no difference in median overall survival was observed between the three groups, but after correcting for independent prognostic variables (age, bile duct cancer, poor differentiation, positive lymph nodes), a statistically significant survival benefit was observed for chemotherapy (HR 0.75, 95% CI 0.57–0.98, $p = 0.03$) and specifically for gemcitabine (HR 0.70, 95% CI 0.51–0.97, $p = 0.03$) compared to observation. This study also revealed significant differences in survival based on tumour type with a median survival of 53.1 months for ampullary cancers, 20.9 months for bile duct cancers and 32.6 months for patients with other cancers. This study was not powered to reveal a survival advantage for each specific tumour type due to the relatively low incidence of each tumour type, but it is notable that amongst the patients with bile duct cancers, the median survival was 27.2 months in those randomised to observation alone, 18.3 months in the 5FU and folinic acid group and 19.5 months in the gemcitabine group; thus, the value of adjuvant chemotherapy specifically in bile duct cancers remains uncertain from this trial, and the authors recommend investigating bile duct cancers as a separate entity in future studies.

Horgan et al. performed a systematic review of all the published, mainly nonrandomised, studies evaluating adjuvant therapy for biliary tract cancers up to 2010 to try and inform the design of subsequent prospective randomised controlled trials [11]. Twenty studies involving 6712 patients were included, and the pooled analysis revealed a non-significant improvement in overall survival with any adjuvant therapy compared with surgery alone (pooled OR 0.74, $p = 0.06$), with the greatest benefit observed in those with lymph node-positive disease (OR 0.49, $p = 0.004$) and R1 disease (OR 0.36, $p = 0.002$). There was no difference observed between gallbladder and bile duct cancers [11].

Recently, two randomised phase III trials of adjuvant chemotherapy, designed specifically for patients with biliary tract cancers, have been presented. The French PRODIGE 12-ACCORD 18 study was presented at the 2016 ASCO GI meeting [12]. This study randomised 196 patients to GEMOX chemotherapy or to surveillance alone following an R0 or R1 resection of a localised biliary tract cancer (intrahepatic, perihilar, extrahepatic cholangiocarcinoma or gallbladder cancer). Tolerability of treatment was satisfactory, and although there was a trend towards an improvement in relapse-free survival with GEMOX chemotherapy (30.4 vs 22 months, HR 0.83, 95% CI 0.58–1.19, $p = 0.31$), this was not statistically significant. This study was also underpowered to detect an overall survival difference. The second, the UK BILCAP study, is the first adequately powered randomised trial of adjuvant chemotherapy in patients with resected biliary tract cancer, and was presented at the 2017 ASCO meeting [13]. This study randomised 447 patients with a completely resected cholangiocarcinoma or gallbladder cancer to oral capecitabine (1250 mg/m$^2$ twice daily on days 1–14 of a 21 day cycle for 24 weeks) or to surveillance alone. The primary analysis was not statistically significant (51.1 vs 36.4 months, HR 0.80, 95% CI 0.63–1.04, $p = 0.097$) but in the pre-planned sensitivity analysis adjusting for prognostic factors (nodal status, grade of disease and gender), a statistically significant improvement in median overall survival was observed (HR 0.70, 95% CI 0.55–0.91, $p = 0.007$). The full publication of both datasets is awaited but it is likely that oral capecitabine will now become the standard-of-care adjuvant therapy.

The ongoing ACTICCA-1 (NCT02170090) trial is a European randomised phase III trial comparing chemotherapy with gemcitabine and cisplatin (as per the ABC-02 study) with surveillance alone, in patients with curatively resected cholangiocarcinoma or gallbladder cancer. Following the publication of the results of the BILCAP study, a substantial amendment has been submitted to replace the surveillance arm with oral capecitabine, providing an opportunity to compare the two regimens head-to-head. The primary end point is disease-free survival, and the study plans to enrol 280 patients with cholangiocarcinoma and 80 patients with gallbladder cancer. The UK-wide BILCAP study took 10 years to complete, and it is hoped that with more collaborative working, future adjuvant studies will be completed more quickly.

### *Summary*

- There is a high risk of recurrence following surgery in biliary tract cancer and poor 5-year survival.
- Given the results of the BILCAP trial, patients with resected biliary tract cancer should be offered adjuvant capecitabine. Full results from this study will likely be published shortly.

## Radiotherapy in Cholangiocarcinoma

The role of radiotherapy remains poorly defined in biliary tract cancers, and efforts to study the effectiveness of treatment have been hampered by small patient numbers and heterogeneous patients and trial designs. Currently no randomised phase III data exists. Besides the usual palliative role of radiotherapy, e.g. treating painful bone metastases, groups have sought to establish the effectiveness in the palliative, adjuvant and neoadjuvant setting, with conflicting data frequently seen in the literature.

### *Adjuvant Radiotherapy*

There is limited evidence to support the use of radiotherapy alone following surgical resection. There has been no prospective clinical trial investigating its role as a sole adjuvant modality, and given the results from adjuvant chemotherapy, it is unlikely that such a study will be performed in the future. The available data comes from retrospective series and population-based registries only.

In the systematic review of nonrandomised studies undertaken by Horgan et al., pooled analysis suggested a significant benefit of adjuvant therapy in patients with R1 disease (OR 0.36, 95% CI 0.19–0.68, $p = 0.004$). Sixty-three percent of these R1 patients received radiotherapy alone, compared to mostly chemoradiotherapy in the R0 studies. A significant benefit was observed with adjuvant radiotherapy in patients with R1 disease, irrespective of disease site (OR 0.33, 95% CI 0.014–0.81, $p = 0.01$), whereas treatment with radiotherapy was associated with a nonsignificant odds of harm (OR 1.26, 95% CI 0.88–1.79, $p = 0.20$) in those with R0 status. This difference in effect size was statistically significant suggesting that adjuvant radiotherapy may be of benefit only in patients with R1 disease [11].

Population-based analyses using data from the US Surveillance, Epidemiology and End Results (SEER) database have formed the largest datasets to examine the role of adjuvant radiotherapy. Hyder et al. reported on the outcomes of 5011 patients with gallbladder cancer who underwent surgical resection between 1988 and 2009. Eight hundred ninety-nine (18%) patients received external beam radiotherapy; these patients were more likely to be younger, have more extensive disease, poorly differentiated tumours and lymph node involvement. On a propensity-matched multivariate model, radiotherapy was associated with a better long-term survival at 1 year (HR 0.45; $p < 0.001$) but not at 5 years (HR 1.06; $p = 0.50$) [14]. The lack of information regarding chemotherapy administration and the inclusion of patients with metastatic disease in these datasets means that it is difficult to draw any conclusions regarding the role of adjuvant radiotherapy.

### *Summary*

- Given the limited available evidence, adjuvant radiotherapy is not routinely recommended.

## Adjuvant Chemoradiotherapy

Adjuvant chemoradiotherapy (CRT) has been investigated by some groups in an attempt to combine the local control effect of radiotherapy with the systemic effects of adjuvant chemotherapy. There is a lack of randomised data in this area, and conflicting results have been reported from pooled analyses of retrospective series and population registries.

Wang et al. performed an analysis of patients treated in the SEER-Medicare database with adjuvant chemoradiotherapy for gallbladder cancer between 1995 and 2005. Of the 1137 patients included in this analysis, 126 patients (11%) had received adjuvant chemoradiotherapy. The authors developed a nomogram to help make individualised survival estimates and found that in their model, adjuvant chemoradiotherapy outperformed adjuvant chemotherapy for virtually all patient subsets [15].

Conversely, in the systematic review by Horgan et al., subgroup analysis of the different adjuvant modalities showed the greatest benefit with adjuvant chemotherapy (OR 0.39, 95% CI 0.23–0.66, $p < 0.01$) followed by chemoradiotherapy (OR 0.61, 95% CI 0.38–0.99, $p = 0.049$) with no benefit observed with adjuvant radiotherapy alone (OR 0.98, 95% CI 0.67–1.43, $p = 0.90$) [11].

Recently, the results from the SWOG S0809 study have been published [16]. This was a prospective, multicentre (intergroup) nonrandomised phase II study that assessed the efficacy of adjuvant chemoradiotherapy with four cycles of adjuvant gemcitabine (1000 mg/m$^2$ on days 1 and 8) in combination with capecitabine (1500 mg/m$^2$ on days 1–14) every 21 days, followed by concurrent capecitabine

(1330 mg/m$^2$ per day) with radiotherapy (45Gy to regional lymphatics, 54–59.4 Gy to tumour bed). High-quality radiotherapy with either three-dimensional planning or intensity-modulated radiotherapy (IMRT) was used in this study. Per protocol radiotherapy was given in 85% of patients. A total of 79 patients were enrolled and encouraging 2 year survival of 65% (95% CI 53–74%) for all patients was observed. Treatment was also well tolerated; the most common grade 3 or 4 toxicity was neutropenia in 44%, and other grade 3 toxicities were rare. One patient died from GI haemorrhage [16]. The main limitation of this study is the absence of a control arm, but this study demonstrates the feasibility of conducting a national clinical trial for a relatively rare tumour, and future randomised phase III clinical trials in this setting are indicated.

## Neoadjuvant Chemoradiotherapy

At present the role of neoadjuvant, as well as downstaging techniques, remains poorly defined in biliary tract cancer and is generally only performed in an experimental setting. Chemotherapy, CRT and other techniques, e.g. photodynamic therapy, have all been considered. Given the lack of clear guidance on this topic, it is not uncommon for patients with unresectable disease at presentation to be commenced on standard palliative therapy. During routine response assessment, it is important to consider those with significant response for surgical exploration following MDT discussion. One systemic review of neoadjuvant therapy in hilar cholangiocarcinoma prior to standard resection was limited by study quality and heterogeneity but was unable to favourably recommend neoadjuvant therapy in this group [17].

A notable exception to this is with hilar cholangiocarcinoma where an approach with neoadjuvant CRT followed by liver transplantation has been compared to liver transplantation alone. This approach developed by the Mayo Clinic involved patients initially receiving external beam irradiation with bolus 5FU, followed by brachytherapy with iridium and concomitant 5FU infusion, and then continuous 5FU until laparoscopy. The early results from this pilot study revealed a prolonged disease-free survival (DFS) in those undergoing liver transplantation after neoadjuvant treatment (92% after a median follow-up of 37 months). However, these patients were highly selected with 40% of patients being excluded following exploratory laparotomy due to progressive disease [18]. A retrospective multicentre analysis of this approach from 12 large-volume transplant centres in the United States confirmed these initial findings. Of the 287 patients included who received neoadjuvant CRT followed by liver transplantation, 65% remained recurrence free at 5 years. In total 25% of patients starting CRT dropped out prior to transplantation [19]. The French phase III TRANSPHIL study (NCT02232932) is ongoing and looks to formally assess the effectiveness of this approach in this highly selected group of patients (using CRT with capecitabine followed by liver transplantation vs surgical resection alone).

### *Summary*

- Adjuvant chemoradiotherapy is not routinely recommended in biliary tract cancers.
- Promising results have been observed in a prospective phase II trial but there is a need for randomised controlled studies in this area.
- A role for neoadjuvant CRT in hilar cholangiocarcinoma prior to liver transplantation may exist for highly selected patients, though remains specialised, and further trial data is awaited.

## Chemoradiotherapy for Locally Advanced Disease

The role of chemoradiotherapy in a palliative setting for locally advanced disease is poorly defined. As with many treatment modalities in the biliary tract, there is a lack of randomised prospective evidence. One French randomised phase II study has been performed comparing CRT (EBRT 50Gy in 25 fractions with cisplatin and 5FU) with GEMOX chemotherapy. Unfortunately the study closed early due to slow recruitment, with only 34 patients included [20]. Further retrospective analyses have been performed including a single-centre retrospective analysis of CRT (with either 5FU or gemcitabine) against best supportive care alone. One hundred six patients were treated with CRT versus 70 with BSC, and the CRT patients were on average 5 years younger with lower T stage (T2) compared to the BSC group. Median overall survival was better in the CRT group (OS 42.6 weeks vs 13.3 weeks, $p < 0.001$) [21].

At present there is insufficient evidence to recommend the routine use of CRT in locally advanced biliary tract disease. Emerging techniques including stereotactic body radiotherapy (SBRT) will need to be assessed in the coming years. In the UK, a feasibility study which hopes to extend to a randomised phase II is currently recruiting (ABC-07). This looks at randomising to SBRT versus two further cycles of chemotherapy in patients who have disease control following six cycles of gemcitabine and cisplatin chemotherapy.

### *Summary*

- It is not possible to recommend CRT for locally advanced biliary tract cancer at present.
- Data in existing retrospective series is unlikely to be comparable with modern radiotherapy techniques and emerging technologies (e.g. SBRT), and direct comparison with standard-of-care gemcitabine and cisplatin chemotherapy is required.

## References


1. Glimelius B, Hoffman K, Sjoden PO, Jacobsson G, Sellstrom H, Enander LK, et al. Chemotherapy improves survival and quality of life in advanced pancreatic and biliary cancer. Ann Oncol. 1996;7(6):593–600.
2. Sharma A, Dwary AD, Mohanti BK, Deo SV, Pal S, Sreenivas V, et al. Best supportive care compared with chemotherapy for unresectable gall bladder cancer: a randomized controlled study. J Clin Oncol. 2010;28(30):4581–6.
3. Eckel F, Schmid RM. Chemotherapy in advanced biliary tract carcinoma: a pooled analysis of clinical trials. Br J Cancer. 2007;96:896–902.
4. Valle J, Wasan H, Palmer DH, Cunningham D, Anthoney A, Maraveyas A, et al. Cisplatin plus gemcitabine versus gemcitabine for biliary tract cancer. N Engl J Med. 2010;362(14):1273–81.
5. Valle JW, Wasan H, Johnson P, Jones E, Dixon L, Swindell R, et al. Gemcitabine alone or in combination with cisplatin in patients with advanced or metastatic cholangiocarcinomas or other biliary tract tumours: a multicentre randomised phase II study—The UK ABC-01 study. Br J Cancer. 2009;101(4):621–7.
6. Okusaka T, Nakachi K, Fukutomi A, Mizuno N, Ohkawa S, Funakoshi A, et al. Gemcitabine alone or in combination with cisplatin in patients with biliary tract cancer: a comparative multicentre study in Japan. Br J Cancer. 2010;103(4):469–74.
7. Valle JW, Furuse J, Jitlal M, Beare S, Mizuno N, Wasan H, et al. Cisplatin and gemcitabine for advanced biliary tract cancer: a meta-analysis of two randomised trials. Ann Oncol. 2014;25(2):391–8.
8. Lamarca A, Hubner RA, David Ryder W, Valle JW. Second-line chemotherapy in advanced biliary cancer: a systematic review. Ann Oncol. 2014;25(12):2328–38.
9. Takada T, Amano H, Yasuda H, Nimura Y, Matsushiro T, Kato H, et al. Is postoperative adjuvant chemotherapy useful for gallbladder carcinoma? A phase III multicenter prospective randomized controlled trial in patients with resected pancreaticobiliary carcinoma. Cancer. 2002;95(8):1685–95.
10. Neoptolemos JP, Moore MJ, Cox TF, Valle JW, Palmer DH, McDonald AC, et al. Effect of adjuvant chemotherapy with fluorouracil plus folinic acid or gemcitabine vs observation on survival in patients with resected periampullary adenocarcinoma: the ESPAC-3 periampullary cancer randomized trial. JAMA. 2012;308(2):147–56.
11. Horgan AM, Amir E, Walter T, Knox JJ. Adjuvant therapy in the treatment of biliary tract cancer: a systematic review and meta-analysis. J Clin Oncol. 2012;30(16):1934–40.
12. Edeline J, Bonnetain F, Philip JM, Watelet J, Hammel P, Joly JP, et al. GEMOX versus surveillance following surgery of localized biliary tract cacner: results of the PRODIGE 12-ACCORD 18 (UNICANCER GI) phase III trial. J Clin Oncol. 2017;35(4 suppl):225.
13. Primrose JN, Fox R, Palmer DH, Prasad R, Mirza D, Anthoney DA, et al. Adjuvant capecitabine for biliary tract cancer: the BILCAP randomized study. J Clin Oncol. 2017;35(15 suppl):4006.
14. Hyder O, Dodson RM, Sachs T, Weiss M, Mayo SC, Choti MA. Impact of adjuvant external beam radiotherapy on survival in surgically resected gallbladder adenocarcinoma: a propensity score-matched Surveillance, Epidemiology, and End Results analysis. Surgery. 2014;155(1):85–93.
15. Wang SJ, Lemieux A, Kalpathy-Cramer J, Ord CB, Walker GV, Fuller CD, et al. Nomogram for predicting the benefit of adjuvant chemoradiotherapy for resected gallbladder cancer. J Clin Oncol. 2011;29(35):4627–32.
16. Ben-Josef E, Guthrie KA, El-Khoueiry AB, Corless CL, Zalupski MM, Lowy AM, et al. SWOG S0809: a phase II intergroup trial of adjuvant capecitabine and gemcitabine followed by radiotherapy and concurrent capecitabine in extrahepatic cholangiocarcinoma and gallbladder carcinoma. J Clin Oncol. 2015;33(24):2617–22.
17. Grendar J, Grendarova P, Sinha R, Dixon E. Neoadjuvant therapy for downstaging of locally advanced hilar cholangiocarcinoma: a systematic review. HPB. 2014;16(4):297–303.

18. De Vreede I, Steers JL, Burch PA, Rosen CB, Gunderson LL, Haddock MG, et al. Prolonged disease-free survival after orthotopic liver transplantation plus adjuvant chemoirradiation for cholangiocarcinoma. Liver Transpl. 2000;6(3):309–16.
19. Darwish Murad S, Kim WR, Harnois DM, Douglas DD, Burton J, Kulik LM, et al. Efficacy of neoadjuvant chemoradiation, followed by liver transplantation, for perihilar cholangiocarcinoma at 12 US centers. Gastroenterology. 2012;143(1):88–98.
20. Phelip JM, Vendrely V, Rostain F, Subtil F, Jouve JL, Gasmi M, et al. Gemcitabine plus cisplatin versus chemoradiotherapy in locally advanced biliary tract cancer: Federation Francophone de Cancerologie Digestive 9902 phase II randomised study. Eur J Cancer. 2014;50(17):2975–82.
21. Yi SW, Kang DR, Kim KS, Park MS, Seong J, Park JY, et al. Efficacy of concurrent chemoradiotherapy with 5-fluorouracil or gemcitabine in locally advanced biliary tract cancer. Cancer Chemother Pharmacol. 2014;73(1):191–8.

# Part III
# Neueoendocrine Tumours

# Chapter 18
# Novel Treatments for Advanced Cholangiocarcinoma

**Jenny Cotton, Angela Lamarca, Mairéad G. McNamara, and Juan W. Valle**

**Key Learning Points**

1. A modest gain in survival in advanced cholangiocarcinoma using systemic chemotherapy highlights the need for improved therapies at all stages of treatment.
2. Locoregional therapies show promising results in locally advanced and palliative settings; however liver toxicity can occur in up to 40% of patients.
3. The use of targeted therapies remains investigational; to date none have demonstrated an improvement in patient outcomes.
4. The use of antiangiogenic agents has not yet resulted in a significant improvement in survival.
5. As the field of molecular medicine advances, systemic therapies may now focus on targeted therapies and immunotherapies.
6. Further research into novel treatments is warranted and further targeted molecular profiling developments may result in improved survival in advanced cholangiocarcinoma in the future.
7. Palliative care needs to be introduced earlier in the disease for better overall outcomes and quality of life.

J. Cotton
Department of Medical Oncology, The Christie NHS Foundation Trust, Manchester, UK

Department of Medical Oncology, The Clatterbridge Cancer Centre, Wirral, UK

A. Lamarca
Department of Medical Oncology, The Christie NHS Foundation Trust, Manchester, UK
e-mail: Angela.Lamarca@christie.nhs.uk

M. G. McNamara · J. W. Valle (✉)
Department of Medical Oncology, The Christie NHS Foundation Trust, Manchester, UK

Division of Cancer Sciences, University of Manchester, Manchester, UK
e-mail: Mairead.McNamara@christie.nhs.uk; Juan.Valle@christie.nhs.uk



T. Cross, D. H. Palmer (eds.), *Liver Cancers*,
https://doi.org/10.1007/978-3-319-92216-4_18

**Areas of Controversy and Uncertainty**

1. High-level evidence for the efficacy of locoregional therapy in cholangiocarcinoma is lacking.
2. Where locoregional therapies will be included in a patient's disease management plan is uncertain.
3. To date, the addition of targeted therapy to the treatment algorithm for cholangiocarcinoma has not resulted in increases in overall survival, and novel agents are needed.
4. The use of immunotherapy has demonstrated encouraging response rates in numerous cancers, and final results of prospective clinical trials in patients with a diagnosis of cholangiocarcinoma are awaited.

## Introduction

Cholangiocarcinoma, which may be intrahepatic, hilar or extrahepatic (distal bile duct), according to primary location, is an aggressive malignancy with unmet treatment needs in advanced stages. The incidence and mortality rates for intrahepatic cholangiocarcinoma (ICC), in particular, have risen steeply over recent decades [1]. Radical surgery with lymphadenectomy (tailored for the site of primary) is the only option which provides the possibility of cure, but most patients have advanced disease at presentation, and disease relapse is common, with 5-year survival rates of only 38.8% [2, 3].

With the rise in cholangiocarcinoma incidence, and the anticipation that novel agents will improve overall survival (OS), symptom palliation will become an ever-increasing challenge. Stenting to relieve biliary obstruction provides essential palliation of cholangiocarcinoma involving the main bile ducts and is associated with improved quality of life, particularly for patients with unresectable disease [4]. Patient education and encouragement of self-reporting of symptoms may help with early detection of obstructive and/or infective disease-related complications and lead to improved outcomes such as OS and quality of life, as has been shown in other cancer types [5]. Early palliative care should be considered for all patients with advanced cholangiocarcinoma, so that optimal benefit with systemic treatment, where appropriate, is achieved.

The current standard treatment for patients with locally advanced or metastatic biliary tract cancer is cisplatin plus gemcitabine (CisGem) chemotherapy [6]. The median survival in patients with advanced biliary tract cancers who receive CisGem is 11.7 months with a median progression-free survival (PFS) of 8 months [6]. There is no second-line therapy with established benefit for patients with advanced cholangiocarcinoma [7].

Whilst there is evidence to support the use of standard-of-care treatments, a number of novel treatments remain in early phases of clinical trial development [8, 9]. These trials are required to establish the efficacy of novel treatments and identify associated toxicity, the role of biomarkers and their place in the patient therapeutic pathway. This chapter will highlight novel treatments and some ongoing clinical trials in locally advanced and metastatic cholangiocarcinoma and identify where they might be used in the disease trajectory. Locoregional approaches are discussed first, followed by systemic therapy options.

## Locoregional Approaches in Cholangiocarcinoma

Locoregional therapies are used for the treatment of ICC, although high-level evidence for their efficacy is lacking [3]. Transcatheter arterial chemoembolisation (TACE) and radioembolisation have been used for some years to treat cancer in the liver (primary or secondary). Technical advances over the last decade have allowed more precise tumour treatment with focused delivery of chemotherapy and radiotherapy, whilst sparing adjacent normal tissues as much as possible.

Novel approaches such as hepatic arterial-based therapies (HAT) now focus on minimising toxicity and improving quality of life. A meta-analysis of 20 studies of the use of HAT in ICC suggested that hepatic arterial infusion offered the best outcomes in terms of tumour response and survival, compared to other locoregional therapies. However, its use is limited by hepatic toxicity, including raised liver enzymes, hepatic abscess formation and hepatic failure [10].

## Chemotherapy-Based Therapies

### *Chemosaturation*

Most recently, chemosaturation allows delivery of potentially lethal doses of melphalan to the liver via an indwelling hepatic artery catheter, followed by external filtering of the drug before blood is returned to the systemic circulation. By this mechanism, the liver can be exposed to doses of chemotherapy that are not feasible by conventional infusion. It is associated with a degree of bone marrow suppression due to the limited systemic escape of melphalan (approx. 3% of the total delivered dose) [11]. It is resource-intensive, requiring an expert team including interventional radiology, perfusionist and anaesthetist, with oncological and surgical backup, if necessary.

Chemosaturation has resulted in improved PFS in liver metastases in patients with cutaneous or ocular melanoma. A phase III trial comparing the use of chemosaturation with best standard of care reported that patients had an improved median hepatic PFS of 7.0 months compared to 1.6 months with standard-of-care treatment, with an overall PFS of 5.4 months compared to 1.6 months. Median OS, however, was not significantly different [12]. It has been investigated in patients with cholangiocarcinoma [13], as well as primary liver tumours [14] and unresectable hepatic metastases [12]. There has been one documented case of a complete response when used in metastatic cholangiocarcinoma [14]. In order to clarify the potential role of this treatment in cholangiocarcinoma, randomised-controlled trials are needed.

### *Drug-Eluting Bead Transcatheter Arterial Chemoembolisation (DEB-TACE) in Unresectable Cholangiocarcinoma*

Drug-eluting bead transcatheter arterial chemoembolisation is a procedure where drug-eluting microspheres can be delivered directly to the tumour via an arterial catheter. This process allows sustained delivery of chemotherapy into the liver, therefore avoiding peak concentrations which may be associated with toxicity, as well as arterial embolisation. In a small study of 11 patients with ICC using doxorubicin drug-eluting beads (loaded with 100–150 mg), there was a 100% response rate according to response evaluation criteria in solid tumours (RECIST), with a median OS of 13 months [15]. In a further study where 26 patients were given irinotecan DEB-TACE and ten patients were given mitomycin-C DEB-TACE, irinotecan produced a better PFS of 3.9 months and OS of 11.7 months versus a PFS of 1.8 months and OS of 5.7 months in the mitomycin-C group. Doxorubicin appears to be the most effective agent in DEB-TACE. A recognised risk of such therapy is "post-embolisation syndrome" which is characterised by a low-grade fever, nausea and abdominal pain [16].

## Ablative Therapies

### *Irreversible Electroporation in Unresectable Cholangiocarcinoma*

Irreversible electroporation (IRE) is a novel image-guided ablation technique that has been used in the treatment of metastatic or primary tumours in the liver, kidney, lung and prostate [17, 18]. It uses a pulsed electric current to create irreversible pores in the cell membrane causing cell death through non-thermal ablation. Patients who have undergone palliative metal stenting are required to have the metal stent changed for a plastic one before the procedure can be performed, as power conduction tissue heating may lead to thermal complications. Currently, a single-arm pilot clinical trial focussing on the effectiveness of IRE for the treatment of metastatic cholangiocarcinoma or liver cancer is evaluating the response of IRE-treated lesions according to modified RECIST evaluation (clinicaltrials.gov identifier, NCT02807181). Case reports on the use of this technique in cholangiocarcinoma exist, but no randomised trial data is available yet.

### *Radiofrequency Ablation in Unresectable or Advanced Cholangiocarcinoma*

Several small studies in recent years have suggested that percutaneous ultrasound-guided thermal ablation for unresectable ICC is safe and potentially effective, particularly for primary and relatively small tumours (see Table 18.1). The evidence demonstrates that smaller tumours, particularly those <5 cm [19] and a small

**Table 18.1** Retrospective studies including patients with intrahepatic cholangiocarcinoma treated with radiofrequency ablation

| Treatment intent | *N* | Median f/u (months) | No. of nodules | Successful ablation | Largest nodule | OS at 6 months | Median OS (months) |
|---|---|---|---|---|---|---|---|
| Curative /palliative (Giorgio et al.) [19] | 10 | 19.5 | 12 | 8 (75%) | 7 cm | 83.3% | – |
| Curative (Xu et al.) [20] | 18 | 8.7 | 25 | 23 (92%) | 4.3 cm | 30% | – |
| Curative /palliative (Fu et al.) [21] | 17 | 29 | 26 | – | 4.4 cm | – | 33 |
| Curative (Kim et al.) [22] | 13 | 19.5 | 17 | 15 (88%) | 8 cm | 15%. | 38.5 |

*N* number of participants; *f/u* follow-up; *OS* overall survival

number of nodules [20], have a better recurrence-free survival but not OS. Identification of prognostic factors might allow better patient selection and outcomes with this technique [19]. This suggests that radiofrequency ablation may be an option for the treatment of small lesions.

## Radiation-Based Therapies

### *Stereotactic Body Radiation Therapy (SBRT) in Locally Advanced Cholangiocarcinoma*

Stereotactic body radiation therapy allows safe delivery of one to five fractions of high-dose radiotherapy compared with small fractions of daily radiotherapy over many weeks. It has been used in the treatment of unresectable, locally advanced ICC, though experience is limited. There are, to date, no randomised trials comparing this technique with conventional radiotherapy in biliary tract cancer.

Toxicity may limit use, but case reports and retrospective case series have shown that SBRT can give good local control [23, 24]. One report of ten patients with hilar cholangiocarcinoma, where 30 Gy in three fractions was delivered with gemcitabine, resulted in 80% local control and 80% 2-year survival [25]. A phase I study of 41 patients receiving individualised SBRT for unresectable hepatocellular carcinoma and ICC, who were not suitable for standard therapies, received 6 fractions of SBRT over a 2-week period. Seventeen of the 41 patients had received no prior therapy, and patients who had received previous radiotherapy to the right upper abdomen were excluded. This study reported a median survival of 15.0 months in the ICC group. No radiotherapy-induced liver disease or treatment-related grade 4/5 toxicity was seen within 3 months of SBRT [26].

The ongoing multicentre UK randomised phase II, ABC-07, clinical trial randomises patients in a 2:1 ratio between CisGem chemotherapy + SBRT and CisGem chemotherapy alone. If feasibility of recruitment is demonstrated (feasibility phase), the study will then continue to full accrual. It will evaluate the efficacy of six cycles of CisGem chemotherapy followed by SBRT (experimental arm) compared to eight cycles of CisGem chemotherapy (control arm). The primary endpoint is improvement in PFS at 12 months (EudraCT number 2014-003656-31).

### *Selective Internal Radiation Therapy (SIRT) in Unresectable Cholangiocarcinoma*

Selective internal radiation therapy consists of the injection of millions of tiny beads or microspheres into the hepatic artery feeding the tumour or region of the liver containing malignancy. They embed and irradiate surrounding tissue with yttrium-90, via radioembolisation. A meta-analysis of 12 relevant studies demonstrated a partial radiological-based tumour response in 28% of patients, and stable disease in 54%, at three months, in the setting of unresectable disease. The complication profile of radioembolisation is similar to that of other intra-arterial treatment modalities with elevated liver enzymes, radiotherapy-induced hepatitis and ascites [27]. The SIRCCA trial (clinicaltrials.gov identifier, NCT02807181) is a first-line randomised phase II trial for patients with inoperable ICC, investigating standard of treatment CisGem in one arm versus SIRT preceding CisGem in the other arm; this study is currently recruiting.

### *Proton Beam Irradiation in Locally Advanced Cholangiocarcinoma*

Proton beam therapy, a method of delivering high-dose radiotherapy, minimising normal tissue dose because of the unique physical properties of heavy particles, has been used as a successful method of gaining local control in cholangiocarcinoma. A phase II multi-institutional study of 83 evaluable patients has been conducted to determine the efficacy and safety of proton beam therapy in patients with hepatocellular carcinoma and unresectable ICC. Thirty-seven of these patients had ICC, and OS at 2 years was 46.5% for this patient population [28]. As expected, the larger tumour sizes and worse performance status were associated with inferior survival. The most common associated toxicities were gastrointestinal symptoms and cholangitis (seen in 40% of patients).

## Conclusion on Use of Locoregional Therapies in Cholangiocarcinoma

Locoregional therapies can be used in the locally advanced or palliative settings in cholangiocarcinoma, and Fig. 18.1 demonstrates where they can potentially be included in a patient's disease trajectory. These treatments have only been assessed

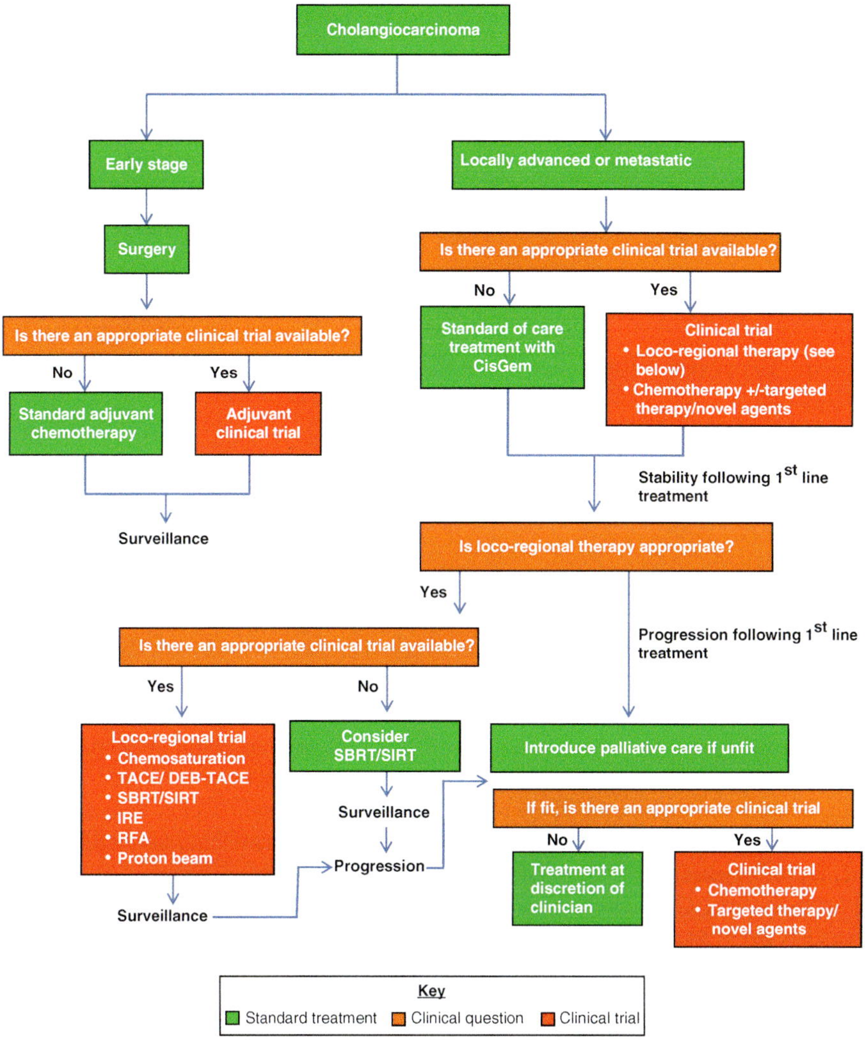


**Fig. 18.1** Algorithm for the potential future management of patients with cholangiocarcinoma (modified from ESMO guidelines, Ann Oncol (2016) 27 (suppl 5): v28-v3, Valle et al.). *TACE* transcatheter arterial chemoembolisation, *DEB-TACE* drug-eluting bead transcatheter arterial chemoembolisation, *SBRT* Stereotactic body radiation therapy, *SIRT* selective internal radiation therapy, *IRE* irreversible electroporation, *RFA* radiofrequency ablation

in small, early phase trials and retrospective series, but have shown some promise in local control and OS. Toxicity to the liver and other abdominal organs is prevalent (occurring in up to 40% of patients). Clinical trials and good patient selection, considering performance status and tumour size, are imperative prior to offering these novel treatments. Results of prospective randomised trials will evaluate the magnitude of benefit compared to currently available options.

## Systemic Therapies in the Treatment of Cholangiocarcinoma

Advances in technology for drug delivery and an improved understanding of advanced cholangiocarcinoma and its microenvironment are aiding researchers in identification of potential future treatment options, including targeted agents and immunotherapies. This section will review the current evidence supporting these potential treatment options. For standard systemic therapy options, please refer to the previous Chap. 16 in this book.

## Some Targeted Therapies Investigated in Biliary Tract Cancers

### *Targeting Epidermal Growth Factor Receptor (EGFR) Mutations in Biliary Tract Cancer*

Common carcinoma-associated gene mutations are found in the epidermal growth factor receptor (*EGFR*), providing a rationale for targeting EGFR-tyrosine kinase (*EGFR-TK*) with novel treatment approaches. The *EGFR-TK* is strictly controlled in normal cells and activated in many tumour cells, and it provides signals that drive dysregulated proliferation, invasion and metastasis, angiogenesis and enhanced cell survival [29]. The use of agents to inhibit this pathway has been investigated as a therapeutic strategy in cholangiocarcinoma [30, 31]. Erlotinib is an oral tyrosine kinase inhibitor which acts on the intracellular kinase domain. Cetuximab and panitumumab are intravenously administered anti-EGFR monoclonal antibodies; they act on the extracellular receptors of the same pathway.

The use of EGFR-TK inhibitors and anti-EGFR antibodies in biliary tract cancers has led to mixed results. Some of the randomised phase II and III studies utilising these agents are summarised in Table 18.2.

Although the data reported in Table 18.2 include all biliary tract cancers, there have been further subgroup analyses of the use of EGFR-TK inhibitors within some of these studies.

An early phase II trial suggested that there could be therapeutic benefit for EGFR blockade with erlotinib as a monotherapy in biliary tract cancer [36]. However, erlotinib compared with standard chemotherapy in a phase III trial [32] showed no OS advantage and no significant difference in PFS. A subgroup analysis of the 180 patients with cholangiocarcinoma reported that those who received erlotinib with gemcitabine and oxaliplatin (GEMOX), versus GEMOX alone, had a significantly better PFS of 5.9 months versus 3 months ($p = 0.049$). Although grade 3 and 4 toxicities were not significantly more frequent in the erlotinib group, toxicity-related dose reductions were more common in the combination therapy arm (64% versus 43%) [32]. In a randomised phase II trial subgroup analysis [34] of the use of panitumumab in cholangiocarcinoma, patients with ICC treated with panitumumab plus

**Table 18.2** Trials using EGFR inhibitors in patients with advanced biliary tract cancers

| Name of study | Drug (dose) | Phase of trial | *N* | Median f/u (months) | EGFR expression | Most common toxicity | PFS (months) | OS (months) | ORR |
|---|---|---|---|---|---|---|---|---|---|
| NCT01149122 | Erlotinib (100 mg) and GEMOX versus GEMOX alone [32] | III | 268 | 15 | Not reported | Febrile neutropenia | 5.8 vs. 4.2 | 9.5 in both groups | 40 (30%) vs. 21 (16%) |
| BINGO | Cetuximab and GEMOX versus GEMOX alone [33] | II | 150 | 31.1 | 23% | Peripheral neuropathy, neutropenia and aminotransferase elevation | 6.1 vs. 5.5 | 11.0 vs. 12.4 | 24% vs. 23% |
| TCOG T1210 | Cetuximab (500 mg/m$^2$) and GEMOX versus GEMOX alone [31] | II | 122 | – | (KRAS)-36.1% | – | 6.7 vs. 4.1 | 10.6 vs. 9.8 | 27% vs. 17% |
| Vecti-BIL | Panitumumab (6 mg/kg) and GEMOX versus GEMOX alone [34] | II | 89 | 10.1 | Not reported | Skin toxicity | 5.3 vs. 4.4 | 9.9 vs. 10.2 | 26.6% vs. 18.1% |
| PICCA | Panitumumab (6 mg/kg) and Cis/Gem versus Cis/Gem alone [35] | II | 93 | – | (p53 34%) | Skin toxicity | 6.7 vs. 8.2 | 12.4 vs. 21.4 | 45% vs. 39% |

Abbreviations: *N* number of participants; *f/u* follow-up; *PFS* progression-free survival; *OS* overall survival; *ORR* objective response rate; *EGFR* epidermal growth factor receptor; *GEMOX* gemcitabine plus oxaliplatin; *Cis/Gem* cisplatin and gemcitabine chemotherapy had a non-significant survival benefit in comparison with chemotherapy alone (15.1 vs. 11.8 months, $p = 0.13$).

Cetuximab has been associated with improved outcomes in various malignancies including colorectal, lung and head and neck cancer [37]. Cetuximab and panitumumab have shown antitumour activity in *RAS* wild-type colorectal cancer [35, 37]. The *KRAS* or *EGFR* mutation status is not related to outcome in advanced ICC [33, 34].

The use of EGFR-targeted agents in combination with chemotherapy in this disease group has shown no benefit in OS compared to standard chemotherapy, and only one study showed a significant difference in PFS [31]. With no effective targeted therapy for cholangiocarcinoma identified in the face of several negative trials, further investigation of chemotherapy in combination with EGFR-targeted agents is not yet warranted.

## Targeting Angiogenesis in Biliary Tract Cancer

Vascular endothelial growth factor (VEGF) is overexpressed in biliary tract cancers and has been proposed as a therapeutic target [38]. It is one of the main growth factors regulating angiogenesis. Receptors for this ligand are also expressed in the adjacent endothelial cells and are named VEGF receptor-1 (VEGFR1) and VEGFR2.

Bevacizumab is a recombinant humanised monoclonal antibody that blocks angiogenesis by inhibiting vascular endothelial growth factor-A (VEGF-A). It has demonstrated efficacy in a number of other solid tumours, including colorectal cancer, renal cell cancer, non-small cell lung cancer and metastatic breast cancer [39]. In phase I and II trials, bevacizumab in combination with erlotinib demonstrated no pharmacokinetic interaction [40, 41]; but there are no randomised trials to establish whether bevacizumab can improve standard-of-care outcomes in biliary tract cancer. A phase II trial exploring its use in patients diagnosed with advanced cholangiocarcinoma in combination with erlotinib reported a small response rate of just 12%, with a median OS of 9.9 months and median time to disease progression of 4.4 months [39].

Cediranib is an oral tyrosine kinase inhibitor acting on VEGFR1, VEGFR2 and VEGFR3, with additional activity against platelet-derived growth factor (PDGF) receptors and the proto-oncogene c-KIT. A multicentred, placebo-controlled, randomised phase II trial [38] of 124 patients (ABC-03) reported that PFS did not improve with the addition of cediranib to CisGem chemotherapy (median PFS 7.4 months vs. 8.0 months in the standard CisGem and placebo group). The study did not meet its primary endpoint (to detect an improvement in PFS), maybe due to lack of efficacy, but also perhaps due to the fact that patients on cediranib discontinued treatment at a median of 4.6 months, mainly due to toxic effects. The most common grade 3 toxicity was hypertension (37%). The partial response rate of 41% in the cediranib group and improved 6-month PFS of 70.5% in the cediranib group versus 61.3% in the placebo group suggest that cediranib may have had some beneficial effect. However, its toxicity profile, and therefore limited exposure to treatment, prevents longer-term benefit.

The role of VEGF inhibition in addition to chemotherapy for patients with advanced biliary tract cancer remains investigational. Whether a better-tolerated anti-VEGF treatment can improve overall survival in combination with chemotherapy remains to be seen.

## *The Use of Isocitrate Dehydrogenase 1 (IDH-1) Mutation Inhibitors in Cholangiocarcinoma.*

Somatic mutations in *IDH-1* produce the oncometabolite D-2-hydroxyglutarate (2-HG) which promotes oncogenesis. Mutant IDH-1 *(mIDH-1)* was first detected in an integrated genomic analysis of human glioblastoma. Mutations in *IDH-1* occur in up to 25% of ICC [9]. The ongoing ClarIDHy trial is a phase III multicentred, randomised, placebo-controlled trial of AG-120, an inhibitor of the *mIDH-1* enzyme; it plans to enrol 186 patients with an *IDH-1* mutation [9]. In the small phase I trial (500 mg daily versus placebo) in advanced cholangiocarcinoma, AG-120 demonstrated a favourable safety profile and some clinical activity (with 40% PFS rate at 6 months) (clinicaltrials.gov identifier, NCT02073994).

## *The Role of Fibroblast Growth Factor Receptor 2 (FGFR2) Fusion Mutations in Cholangiocarcinoma*

Fibroblast growth factor receptor *(FGFR)* alterations are implicated in the development and progression of ICC. There are four subtypes of *FGFR* identified in multiple cancers, including breast, bladder, lung, gastric, endometrial and multiple myeloma [42]. Using fluorescent in situ hybridisation (FISH) or next-generation sequencing (NGS), mutations are seen in up 20% of ICC [43], with *FGFR2* translocations occurring in approximately 13% of patients [44]. The presence of *FGFR* fusions is therefore a potential therapeutic target and is currently being investigated in clinical trials.

The highly potent and selective irreversible *FGFR* inhibitor, TAS-120, inhibits all four *FGFR* subtypes. It has been shown in vitro to inhibit growth of human cancer cell lines with *FGFR* gene abnormalities selectively, cellular phosphorylation of *FGFR*, intercellular signalling pathways downstream of *FGFR* and tumour growth in human tumour xenograft mouse models [42].

Other *FGFR* inhibitors, such as ARQ 087 and INCB054828 are currently being investigated in clinical trials in this patient group [8, 43]. The pan-*FGFR* inhibitor, ARQ 087, is undergoing a phase I/phase II open-label clinical trial for patients with identified *FGFR2* status positivity in ICC. An interim analysis following post-treatment radiographic assessment has reported partial response, stable disease and progressive disease in 20%, 57% and 23% of patients, respectively. This indicates encouraging antitumour activity with a manageable safety profile.

A selective *FGFR* inhibitor to *FGFR1, FGFR2* and *FGFR3,* INCB054828 [8] is being investigated in a phase II open-label study recruiting patients with unresectable cholangiocarcinoma.

A phase I study by Nogova et al. has recently reported that oral BGJ398, a selective FGFR1-3 tyrosine kinase inhibitor, demonstrated antitumour activity in several advanced solid tumour types. Common adverse effects at the maximum tolerated dose were hyperphosphataemia (82.5%), constipation (50.9%), decreased appetite (45.6%) and stomatitis (45.6%) [45]. A phase II study has evaluated BGJ398 antitumor activity in patients with advanced or metastatic cholangiocarcinoma containing FGFR2 fusions or other FGFR alterations whose disease had progressed whilst receiving prior therapy, and promising antitumor activity was demonstrated, with an overall response rate of 14.8% (18.8% FGFR2 fusions only), disease control rate of 75.4% (83.3% FGFR2 fusions only) and estimated median PFS of 5.8 months (95% CI, 4.3 to 7.6 months) [46].

## *Mitogen-Activated Protein/Extracellular Signal-Regulated Kinase Kinase (MEK) Inhibitors in Biliary Tract Cancer*

Trametinib is a MEK inhibitor which acts downstream in the mitogen-activated protein kinase (MAPK) pathway. Mitogen-activated protein kinase pathway alterations have been identified in biliary cancers [47]. A randomised phase II trial of 80 patients with cholangiocarcinoma or gallbladder cancer who failed platinum/gemcitabine therapy, and then received oral trametinib versus chemotherapy with oral capecitabine or infusional 5-fluorouracil, reported that survival was not improved in a planned interim analysis of objective response of 14 patients registered to the trametinib arm. Consequently, the study was interrupted early [47]. Further research is required to ascertain if there is a strong enough scientific rationale for pursuing MEK inhibition with or without chemotherapy in this disease group.

## Immunotherapies in Biliary Tract Cancer

Immune checkpoint inhibitors have demonstrated encouraging response rates in numerous cancer groups including melanoma, renal cell cancer, colorectal, bladder and urothelial carcinoma and non-small cell lung cancer [48]. This negative feedback pathway supresses the T-cell immune response and is upregulated in many tumours and their surrounding microenvironment. Expression of programmed death-ligand-1 (PD-L1) and programmed death-ligand-2 (PD-L2) on the surface of tumour cells is important. However, it is not an entirely reliable predictive marker of response to treatment with immune checkpoint inhibitors [49]. Another factor which may be used as a predictive marker of response is mismatch repair (MMR) deficiency in cholangiocarcinoma, which is strongly associated with therapeutic response to PD-1 blockade in colorectal cancer [50]. The presence of MMR deficiency leads to a high mutational load and microsatellite instability (MSI) (accumulation of numerous insertion/deletion mutations affecting microsatellites). This, in turn, leads to T-cell neoantigen production with a pronounced antitumour immune response resulting in successful immune checkpoint blockade [50]. The MSI phenotype is most frequently found in colorectal and endometrial cancers, but also occurs in a variety of other malignancies [51]. The availability of MSI analysis may open new therapeutic options for biliary tract cancer after (or even prior to) standard treatment.

## *Targeting Programmed Death-1 and Programmed Death-Ligand 1*

Even tumours without PD-L1 expression or dense infiltration with cytotoxic cells can show a good response to immunotherapies. A case series characterising PD-L1 and PD-1 expression and density of tumour-infiltrating lymphocytes (TILs) in 99 cholangiocarcinoma specimens reported that PD-L1 expression by neoplastic cells was observed in only nine patients, but PD-L1 positive inflammatory cell aggregates were identified in 46. Expression of PD-L1 by either neoplastic or inflammatory cells was associated with a high density of CD3-positive TILs. The results highlight that cholangiocarcinomas with dense intra-tumoral lymphocytic infiltration might represent good candidates for PD-L1/PD-1 blocking agents [48].

There is a case report of a patient with extrahepatic cholangiocarcinoma who had a strong and durable response to the immune checkpoint inhibitor pembrolizumab (a highly selective humanised monoclonal antibody against PD-1 and its ligands, PD-L1 and PD-L2) [50]. The patient's tumour displayed deoxyribonucleic acid (DNA) MMR deficiency and MSI, but lacked other features commonly discussed as predictors of response to checkpoint blockade, such as PD-L1 expression or dense infiltration with cytotoxic T cells. Notably, high levels of human leukocyte antigen (HLA) class I and II expression were detected in the tumour, suggesting a potential causal relationship between functionality of the tumour's antigen presentation machinery and the success of immune checkpoint blockade. This suggests that it is worthwhile to determine MSI status in combination with HLA class I and II antigen expression in tumours potentially eligible for immune checkpoint blockade, even in the absence of conventional markers predictive for anti-PD-1/PD-L1 therapy or in entities not commonly linked to MSI phenotype [50]. Defects in HLA class I expression may allow tumour cells to escape immune recognition [52]. A phase II trial to evaluate the clinical activity of pembrolizumab (anti-PD-1 immune checkpoint inhibitor), in patients with progressive metastatic disease, identified MMR deficiency in one case of cholangiocarcinoma; however the response to pembrolizumab was not discussed [53].

No large phase II/III clinical trials have been conducted to ascertain if PD-L1/PD-1 blockade results in improved survival in cholangiocarcinoma. KEYNOTE-028 is a phase Ib multicohort trial designed to assess the safety and antitumour activity of pembrolizumab in patients with PD-L1-positive advanced biliary tract cancer. Preliminary results report that 17% had a partial response, 17% had stable disease, and 52% had progressive disease. The treatment was generally well tolerated, but these data again demonstrate that targeting the PD-L1 ligand does not guarantee response to treatment, even in the presence of PD-L1 expression [54].

## Mesothelin in Cholangiocarcinoma

Mesothelin is a tumour differentiation antigen present at low levels in a restricted set of normal adult tissues and is expressed at high levels in mesothelioma and also in ovarian, pancreatic and lung cancers [55]. Its use as a therapeutic target in cholangiocarcinoma has yet to be fully investigated. An anti-mesothelin recombinant immunotoxin, SS1P, has been found to be active in cholangiocarcinoma in vitro and may be a relevant antigenic target for future immunotherapies [55].

## Conclusion on the Use of Systemic Therapy Options in Cholangiocarcinoma

Understanding of cholangiocarcinoma biology, the oncogenic landscape of this disease and its complex interaction with the tumour microenvironment and immune response could lead to optimum therapies with improvement in patient survival. Studies to characterise the mutational landscape of cholangiocarcinoma further may help to identify appropriate future lines of treatment following standard of care. However, there have been instances where genetic alterations do not stratify risk of disease recurrence or death. More research is required to understand the tumour microenvironment and relevant antigenic targets better. The use of immunotherapy and targeted therapy in cholangiocarcinoma in the UK remains investigational, and therefore these agents remain available only to those patients eligible for clinical trials.

## References

1. Khan SA, et al. Guidelines for the diagnosis and treatment of cholangiocarcinoma: an update. Gut. 2012;61(12):1657–69.
2. Tabata M, et al. Surgical treatment for hilar cholangiocarcinoma. J Hepato-Biliary-Pancreat Surg. 2000;7(2):148–54.
3. Razumilava N, Gores GJ. Cholangiocarcinoma. Lancet. 2014;383(9935):2168–79.

4. Salgado SM, Gaidhane M, Kahaleh M. Endoscopic palliation of malignant biliary strictures. World J Gastrointest Oncol. 2016;8(3):240–7.
5. Basch E, et al. Overall survival results of a trial assessing patient-reported outcomes for symptom monitoring during routine cancer treatment. JAMA. 2017;318(2):197–8.
6. Valle J, et al. Cisplatin plus gemcitabine versus gemcitabine for biliary tract cancer. N Engl J Med. 2010;362(14):1273–81.
7. Lamarca A, et al. Second-line chemotherapy in advanced biliary cancer: a systematic review. Ann Oncol. 2014;25(12):2328–38.
8. Borad MJ, et al. Phase 2, open-label, multicenter study of the efficacy and safety of INCB054828 in patients (pts) with advanced, metastatic, or surgically unresectable cholangiocarcinoma (CCA) with inadequate response to prior therapy. J Clin Oncol. 2017;35(15_suppl):TPS4145.
9. Lowery MA, et al. ClarIDHy: a phase 3, multicenter, randomized, double-blind study of AG-120 vs placebo in patients with an advanced cholangiocarcinoma with an IDH1 mutation. J Clin Oncol. 2017;35(15_suppl):TPS4142.
10. Boehm LM, et al. Comparative effectiveness of hepatic artery based therapies for unresectable intrahepatic cholangiocarcinoma. J Surg Oncol. 2015;111(2):213–20.
11. Vogel A, et al. Chemosaturation percutaneous hepatic perfusion: a systematic review. Adv Ther. 2017;33(12):2122–38.
12. Hughes MS, et al. Results of a randomized controlled multicenter phase III trial of percutaneous hepatic perfusion compared with best available care for patients with melanoma liver metastases. Ann Surg Oncol. 2016;23(4):1309–19.
13. Vogl TJ, et al. Chemosaturation with percutaneous hepatic perfusions of melphalan for hepatic metastases: experience from two European centers. Rofo. 2014;186(10):937–44.
14. Pingpank JF, et al. Phase I study of hepatic arterial melphalan infusion and hepatic venous hemofiltration using percutaneously placed catheters in patients with unresectable hepatic malignancies. J Clin Oncol. 2005;23(15):3465–74.
15. Aliberti C, et al. Chemoembolization (TACE) of unresectable intrahepatic cholangiocarcinoma with slow-release doxorubicin-eluting beads: preliminary results. Cardiovasc Intervent Radiol. 2008;31(5):883–8.
16. Kuhlmann JB, et al. Treatment of unresectable cholangiocarcinoma: conventional transarterial chemoembolization compared with drug eluting bead-transarterial chemoembolization and systemic chemotherapy. Eur J Gastroenterol Hepatol. 2012;24(4):437–43.
17. Ball C, Thomson KR, Kavnoudias H. Irreversible electroporation: a new challenge in "out of operating theater" anesthesia. Anesth Analg. 2010;110(5):1305–9.
18. Onik G, Mikus P, Rubinsky B. Irreversible electroporation: implications for prostate ablation. Technol Cancer Res Treat. 2007;6(4):295–300.
19. Giorgio A, et al. Radiofrequency ablation for intrahepatic cholangiocarcinoma: retrospective analysis of a single centre experience. Anticancer Res. 2011;31(12):4575–80.
20. Xu HX, et al. Percutaneous ultrasound-guided thermal ablation for intrahepatic cholangiocarcinoma. Br J Radiol. 2012;85(1016):1078–84.
21. Fu Y, et al. Radiofrequency ablation in the management of unresectable intrahepatic cholangiocarcinoma. J Vasc Interv Radiol. 2012;23(5):642–9.
22. Kim JH, et al. Radiofrequency ablation for the treatment of primary intrahepatic cholangiocarcinoma. AJR Am J Roentgenol. 2011;196(2):W205–9.
23. Jung DH, et al. Outcomes of stereotactic body radiotherapy for unresectable primary or recurrent cholangiocarcinoma. Radiat Oncol J. 2014;32(3):163–9.
24. Mahadevan A, et al. Stereotactic body radiotherapy (SBRT) for intrahepatic and hilar cholangiocarcinoma. J Cancer. 2015;6(11):1099–104.
25. Polistina FA, et al. Chemoradiation treatment with gemcitabine plus stereotactic body radiotherapy for unresectable, non-metastatic, locally advanced hilar cholangiocarcinoma. Results of a five year experience. Radiother Oncol. 2011;99(2):120–3.
26. Tse RV, et al. Phase I study of individualized stereotactic body radiotherapy for hepatocellular carcinoma and intrahepatic cholangiocarcinoma. J Clin Oncol. 2008;26(4):657–64.

27. Al-Adra DP, et al. Treatment of unresectable intrahepatic cholangiocarcinoma with yttrium-90 radioembolization: a systematic review and pooled analysis. Eur J Surg Oncol. 2015;41(1):120–7.
28. Hong TS, et al. Multi-institutional phase II study of high-dose hypofractionated proton beam therapy in patients with localized, unresectable hepatocellular carcinoma and intrahepatic cholangiocarcinoma. J Clin Oncol. 2016;34(5):460–8.
29. Ritter CA, Arteaga CL. The epidermal growth factor receptor-tyrosine kinase: a promising therapeutic target in solid tumors. Semin Oncol. 2003;30(1 Suppl 1):3–11.
30. Paule B, et al. Cetuximab plus gemcitabine-oxaliplatin (GEMOX) in patients with refractory advanced intrahepatic cholangiocarcinomas. Oncology. 2007;72(1–2):105–10.
31. Chen L-T, et al. KRAS mutation status-stratified randomized phase II trial of GEMOX with and without cetuximab in advanced biliary tract cancer (ABTC): The TCOG T1210 trial. J Clin Oncol. 2013;31(15_suppl):4018.
32. Lee J, et al. Gemcitabine and oxaliplatin with or without erlotinib in advanced biliary-tract cancer: a multicentre, open-label, randomised, phase 3 study. Lancet Oncol. 2012;13(2):181–8.
33. Malka D, et al. Gemcitabine and oxaliplatin with or without cetuximab in advanced biliary-tract cancer (BINGO): a randomised, open-label, non-comparative phase 2 trial. Lancet Oncol. 2014;15(8):819–28.
34. Leone F, et al. Panitumumab in combination with gemcitabine and oxaliplatin does not prolong survival in wild-type KRAS advanced biliary tract cancer: a randomized phase 2 trial (Vecti-BIL study). Cancer. 2016;122(4):574–81.
35. Vogel A, et al. Panitumumab in combination with gemcitabine/cisplatin (GemCis) for patients with advanced kRAS WT biliary tract cancer: a randomized phase II trial of the Arbeitsgemeinschaft Internistische Onkologie (AIO). J Clin Oncol. 2015;33(15_suppl):4082.
36. Philip PA, et al. Phase II study of erlotinib in patients with advanced biliary cancer. J Clin Oncol. 2006;24(19):3069–74.
37. Gruenberger B, et al. Cetuximab, gemcitabine, and oxaliplatin in patients with unresectable advanced or metastatic biliary tract cancer: a phase 2 study. Lancet Oncol. 2010;11(12):1142–8.
38. Valle JW, et al. Cediranib or placebo in combination with cisplatin and gemcitabine chemotherapy for patients with advanced biliary tract cancer (ABC-03): a randomised phase 2 trial. Lancet Oncol. 2015;16(8):967–78.
39. Lubner SJ, et al. Report of a multicenter phase II trial testing a combination of biweekly bevacizumab and daily erlotinib in patients with unresectable biliary cancer: a phase II Consortium study. J Clin Oncol. 2010;28(21):3491–7.
40. Herbst RS, et al. Phase I/II trial evaluating the anti-vascular endothelial growth factor monoclonal antibody bevacizumab in combination with the HER-1/epidermal growth factor receptor tyrosine kinase inhibitor erlotinib for patients with recurrent non-small-cell lung cancer. J Clin Oncol. 2005;23(11):2544–55.
41. Thomas MB, et al. Phase II trial of the combination of bevacizumab and erlotinib in patients who have advanced hepatocellular carcinoma. J Clin Oncol. 2009;27(6):843–50.
42. Ochiiwa H, et al. Abstract A270: TAS-120, a highly potent and selective irreversible FGFR inhibitor, is effective in tumors harboring various FGFR gene abnormalities. Mol Cancer Ther. 2013;12(11 Supplement):A270.
43. Mazzaferro V, et al. ARQ 087, an oral pan-fibroblast growth factor receptor (FGFR) inhibitor, in patients (pts) with advanced intrahepatic cholangiocarcinoma (iCCA) with FGFR2 genetic aberrations. J Clin Oncol. 2017;35(15_suppl):4017.
44. Arai Y, et al. Fibroblast growth factor receptor 2 tyrosine kinase fusions define a unique molecular subtype of cholangiocarcinoma. Hepatology. 2014;59(4):1427–34.
45. Nogova L, et al. Evaluation of BGJ398, a fibroblast growth factor receptor 1-3 kinase inhibitor, in patients with advanced solid tumors harboring genetic alterations in fibroblast growth factor receptors: results of a global phase I, dose-escalation and dose-expansion study. J Clin Oncol. 2017;35(2):157–65.

46. Javle M, et al. Phase II study of BGJ398 in patients with FGFR-altered advanced cholangiocarcinoma. J Clin Oncol. 2018;36(3):276–82.
47. Kim RD, et al. SWOG S1310: randomized phase II trial of single agent MEK inhibitor trametinib vs. 5-fluorouracil or capecitabine in refractory advanced biliary cancer. J Clin Oncol. 2017;35(15_suppl):4016.
48. Fontugne J, et al. PD-L1 expression in perihilar and intrahepatic cholangiocarcinoma. Oncotarget. 2017;8(15):24644–51.
49. Topalian SL, et al. Safety, activity, and immune correlates of anti-PD-1 antibody in cancer. N Engl J Med. 2012;366(26):2443–54.
50. Czink E, et al. Successful immune checkpoint blockade in a patient with advanced stage microsatellite unstable biliary tract cancer. Cold Spring Harb Mol Case Stud. 2017;3(5)
51. Hause RJ, et al. Classification and characterization of microsatellite instability across 18 cancer types. Nat Med. 2016;22(11):1342–50.
52. Sabbatino F, et al. PD-L1 and HLA Class I antigen expression and clinical course of the disease in intrahepatic cholangiocarcinoma. Clin Cancer Res. 2016;22(2):470–8.
53. Le DT, et al. PD-1 blockade in tumors with mismatch-repair deficiency. N Engl J Med. 2015;372(26):2509–20.
54. Bang YJ, et al. 525 Safety and efficacy of pembrolizumab (MK-3475) in patients (pts) with advanced biliary tract cancer: interim results of KEYNOTE-028. Eur J Cancer. 2015;51:S112.
55. Yu L, et al. Mesothelin as a potential therapeutic target in human cholangiocarcinoma. J Cancer. 2010;1:141–9.

# Chapter 19
# Making the Diagnosis of Neuroendocrine Tumour Disease

**Vandana M. Sagar, Mona Elshafie, and Tahir Shah**

**Key Learning Points**

1. The incidence of neuroendocrine tumours (NETs) is rising in the United Kingdom.
2. NETs are slow-growing tumours that are often discovered incidentally on imaging or histology. Their presentation is dependent on location of disease and hormone-related symptoms.
3. Majority of pancreatic NETs (panNETs) are 'non-functioning'. Functioning panNETs present with symptoms related to the hormone they may secrete—such as insulin or gastrin.
4. Bronchial carcinoids usually present early with usual chest symptoms—cough, infection and haemoptysis.
5. Expert histopathological assessment is essential. Cross-sectional and functional imaging modalities are used for staging and planning treatments.
6. NET management can be complex and should always be arranged in conjunction with a centre with comprehensive expertise.
7. All cases should be discussed in a multidisciplinary neuroendocrine tumour multidisciplinary meeting (NET MDM) in order to deliver optimal care.

V. M. Sagar (✉) · M. Elshafie · T. Shah
Birmingham Neuroendocrine Tumour Centre, Queen Elizabeth Hospital, Birmingham, UK
e-mail: Mona.Elshafie@uhb.nhs.uk; Tahir.Shah@uhb.nhs.uk



T. Cross, D. H. Palmer (eds.), *Liver Cancers*,
https://doi.org/10.1007/978-3-319-92216-4_19

**Areas of Controversy and Uncertainty**

1. Strategies for earlier diagnosis: most patients continue to be diagnosed with metastatic disease such that cure is not possible. However there is no agreement on ways to improve this situation through the use of available diagnostic modalities as screening tools.

**Areas of Likely Future Progress**

1. Somatostatin receptor-targeted imaging modalities such as DOTA PET are improving resolution and accuracy. There will likely be further improvement through the use of somatostatin receptor antagonists as tracers.
2. Telotristat may be licenced in the near future as a new therapy for carcinoid syndrome.
3. There is a need for highly effective systemic treatments that can either cure or effectively control the disease for very long periods, hence providing a normal or near normal life expectancy.

## Introduction

### *Epidemiology*

Neuroendocrine tumours (NETs) are rare, but their incidence is on the rise in the United Kingdom. Public Health England identified 8726 neuroendocrine neoplasms (3978 NETs) diagnosed between 2013 and 2014 in England yielding an overall incidence rate of 8 per 100,000 persons [1]. According to the World Health Organisation (WHO) 2010 classification, NETs are graded from 1 to 3 (G1–G3) which is based on the cellular proliferation rate (i.e. Ki-67 index) and the mitotic count [2, 3]. G1 and G2 tumours are generally well-differentiated NETs, and G3 can either be well-differentiated NETs or poorly differentiated neuroendocrine carcinomas (NECs) [2]. It is important to identify the G3 NETs from poorly differentiated NECs as treatments used will differ markedly. There are as many NECs diagnosed as NETs. There is a growing body of evidence to aid the management of NETs, whereas very little evidence exists to help manage NECs. The NECs are often referred to the neuroendocrine tumour multidisciplinary meeting (NET MDM) for treatment decision. Much smaller groups consist of the mixed adenoneuroendocrine carcinomas, Merkel cell carcinomas and a few rarer morphologies [1].

The majority of well-differentiated NETs arise in the gastrointestinal (GI) tract and pancreas. The lung is the second commonest site of origin. Other, albeit rarer, primary sites for NETs include the breast, ovaries, head and neck, renal tract and skin. The primary site is unknown in approximately 8.7% [1]. There is equal distribution between males and females. Even at an advanced stage of disease at diagnosis, NETs have a better overall 1-year survival (at least 90%) compared to NECs and other subtypes (as low as 40%) [1]. Unsurprisingly, survival for patients with NECs and other subtypes is dependent on the stage of the tumour at diagnosis [1].

## *Aetiology*

NETs are slow-growing tumours originating from cells containing neuroendocrine properties (known as enterochromaffin or Kulchitsky cells) [4, 5]. These cells express particular proteins including neuron-specific enolase and synaptophysin, which are classically identified in neural cells. In addition, they produce certain amines and peptide hormones including serotonin, somatostatin, substance P and vasoactive intestinal peptide (VIP) [5].

NETs originating in the GI tract were traditionally classified into tumours of the foregut, midgut and hindgut according to their embryological origin but now commonly follow the WHO 2010 classification system as described above [4]. There is currently emerging data on the molecular biology of NETs suggesting the presence of a role for molecular profiling and common genetic characteristics that may play a pivotal role in the classification of these tumours, in addition to identifying possible molecular targets involved in tumour progression [4].

## *Genetics*

The majority of NETs occur sporadically, but a small group of patients will have an inheritable condition [4]. NETs may be associated with familial endocrine cancer syndromes such as multiple endocrine neoplasia 1 (MEN1), multiple endocrine neoplasia 2 (MEN2), Von Hippel-Lindau (VHL) and tuberous sclerosis (TS) [2, 4]. In gastroenteropancreatic (GEP) NETs, the incidence of MEN1 varies from nearly nil in GI NETs to 5% in insulinomas and 25–30% in gastrinomas [6]. Some patients with midgut NETs have shown mutations in the succinate-ubiquinone oxidoreductase subunit D (SDHD) gene which is usually associated with phaeochromocytomas and paragangliomas [7]. It is therefore imperative to take a detailed family history and perform a thorough examination in patients with NETs and attempt to identify patients at risk for inherited conditions. Appropriate patients should then be referred for genetic testing to confirm the diagnosis [4]. A diagnosis of MEN1, MEN2, TS, neurofibromatosis type 1 (NF1) or a paraganglioma syndrome should necessitate screening for other associated tumours and genetic testing of patients' relatives [4].

Another significant risk factor for developing any type of NET is a family history of cancer, with the risk found to be greater in females than in males [8]. It has also been shown that pre-existing diabetes mellitus, particularly in women, has a strong association with gastric NETs, with one study showing the development of synchronous cancer (mostly colon adenocarcinoma) occurring in 25% of patients with a GI NET [8, 9].

## Clinical Features

In this chapter, the clinical features of the two commonest sites for NETs to occur (GEP NETs and pulmonary NETs) will be explained.

### *GEP NETs*

GI NETs can present with symptoms related to local mass effect or desmoplasia. Symptoms from distant metastases, commonly to the liver, can also occur. Around 60% of pancreatic NETs are non-functioning, which may present with symptoms from the pancreatic mass and/or liver metastases. Functioning pancreatic NETs have clinical features resulting from peptide and hormone release, and these are discussed below [4].

#### Gastric NETs

Gastric NETs (g-NETs) are the most frequently diagnosed digestive NETs, with an increasing recognition related to growing performance of upper GI endoscopies for various diagnostic purposes [10]. They are usually benign in nature but can occasionally be malignant. They are classified into three types: type 1, type 2 and type 3.

Type 1 is the commonest g-NET representing around 70–80% of all g-NETs and is related to atrophic gastritis that leads to chronic hypergastrinaemia. Type 2 is due to raised gastrin from a gastrinoma and is associated with Zollinger-Ellison syndrome (ZES) and MEN1. Type 1 and 2 are diagnosed relatively early due to symptoms related to underlying conditions, such as abdominal discomfort, reflux, diarrhoea and GI haemorrhage. Type 1 g-NET is usually asymptomatic, diagnosed on histology taken endoscopically. Type 1 and 2 g-NETs are well-differentiated tumours. Type 3 are sporadic and do not cause symptoms until the tumour has metastasised. They can be more aggressive with some expressing features of G3 NEC histologically. Around 50–100% of type 3 have evidence of metastases, compared to 2–5% of type 1 and 10–30% of type 2 [10, 11].

#### Proximal Small Bowel NETs

These include the duodenal NETs (d-NETs), whereas distal small bowel NETs include the jejunal and ileal NETs which will later be explained.

The d-NETs are usually sporadic but can be associated with MEN1. They are usually non-functioning but may also present with a functional syndrome: ZES occurring in duodenal gastrinomas [10, 12].

## Distal Small Bowel NETs

These represent at least the third largest cohort within the GEP NETs. The most frequent clinical symptom encountered is abdominal pain, which may be as a result of small bowel obstruction (SBO), small bowel wall dysmotility or secondary to transient mesenteric ischaemia from mesenteric fibrosis due to a desmoplastic reaction. Other non-specific symptoms that can occur including nausea and vomiting in SBO, weight loss, fatigue and occasionally GI bleeding [13]. Approximately 20% of cases may present with carcinoid syndrome: diarrhoea, flushing, palpitations, intermittent abdominal pain and occasionally lacrimation and rhinorrhoea [4] (Fig. 19.1).

## Colorectal NETs

Colorectal NETs are usually diagnosed incidentally on histology from tissue taken at the time of colonoscopy or sigmoidoscopy. Common indications for performing these endoscopic investigations include diarrhoea, abdominal pain, GI bleeding, change in bowel habit, anorectal symptoms or weight loss. Some patients (more so in colon NETs) may present with bowel obstruction. Colonic NETs usually present late with extensive metastatic disease, whereas 75–80% of rectal carcinoids are localised at diagnosis [14].

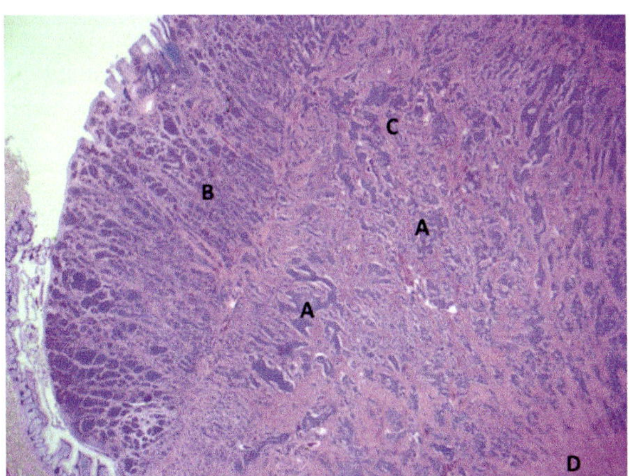


**Fig. 19.1** Haematoxylin and eosin (H&E) staining. Histology specimen demonstrating a polypoid ileal neuroendocrine tumour. Nests and trabecular growth pattern of neuroendocrine tumour cells (**A**) infiltrating the mucosa (**B**), submucosa (**C**) and muscularis propria (**D**)

**Functioning Pancreatic NETs**

Table 19.1 summarises the symptoms associated with functioning pancreatic NETs (F-P-NETs).

## *Pulmonary NETs*

Pulmonary NETs encompass the typical carcinoids that are low-grade NETs and atypical carcinoids that are intermediate-grade NETs. We will not be considering the large cell neuroendocrine carcinomas and small cell lung carcinomas which are the most aggressive and are high-grade malignant tumours with neuroendocrine differentiation. Typical and atypical carcinoids may be detected incidentally on imaging, or patients may present with symptoms of haemoptysis, recurrent chest infections, shortness of breath and wheezing [15]. These tumours may also be rarely associated with Cushing's syndrome or ectopic adrenocorticotropic hormone secretion [4, 15]. The majority of bronchial carcinoids are diagnosed at an early stage where surgical cure is possible (Fig. 19.2).

## *Carcinoid Syndrome*

Carcinoid syndrome is commonest in GI NET patients with sizeable metastases in the liver. It also occurs with advanced bronchial carcinoids. Carcinoid syndrome is rare in NETs of pancreatic origin. It usually results from the release of vasoactive compounds, such as serotonin and tachykinins, into the systemic circulation, via the hepatic vein, from liver metastases. However, in bronchial carcinoids, retroperitoneal or ovarian metastases, carcinoid syndrome may occur due to direct hormone release into the systemic venous system, bypassing the degradation capacity of the liver [4, 16]. Another presenting feature may be of right upper quadrant pain

**Table 19.1** F-P-NETs

| Type of F-P-NET | Symptoms |
|---|---|
| Insulinoma | Hypoglycaemic symptoms including sweating, confusion, loss of consciousness and dizziness. Improvement with eating |
| Gastrinoma | Profound peptic ulceration and diarrhoea in ZES or diarrhoea alone |
| Glucagonoma | Diabetes mellitus, rash (necrolytic migratory erythema), weight loss |
| Vasoactive intestinal peptide-secreting tumour: VIPoma | Verner-Morrison syndrome with marked watery diarrhoea and hypokalaemia |
| Somatostatinoma | Cholelithiasis, diabetes mellitus and diarrhoea/steatorrhoea |

Adapted from Ramage JK et al. [4]

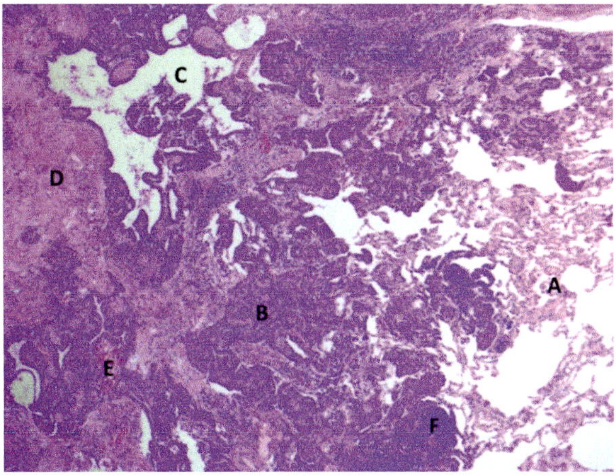


**Fig. 19.2** Haematoxylin and eosin (H&E) staining. Histology specimen demonstrating background lung tissue (**A**) with an ill-defined bronchial carcinoid lesion with trabecular (**B**) and microcystic (**C**) growth pattern of neuroendocrine tumour cells. Background fibrosis (**D**) and fresh haemorrhage (**E**) with chronic inflammation (**F**)

secondary to hepatic enlargement, haemorrhage into the tumour or necrosis of hepatic secondaries. Around 20% of patients with carcinoid syndrome present with features of carcinoid heart disease (CHD) at diagnosis [4].

### *Carcinoid Heart Disease*

CHD results from high levels of serotonin, in addition to other vasoactive substances, secreted by the metastatic tumour cells in the liver, reaching the right side of the heart and causing deposition of carcinoid plaques. The resulting fibrosis and thickening of the endocardial surface of the heart and valves lead to incompetence of tricuspid and pulmonary valves [17]. Left-sided lesions occur in around 15% of patients with carcinoid heart disease [4]. Foramen ovale patency is commonly involved in those with a left-sided lesion [4].

## Diagnosis

### *Biochemical Assessment*

Measuring secretory biomarkers can assist clinicians in various ways: firstly, to aid in making the diagnosis in functional duodenal or pancreatic NETs, by measuring the secretory peptides or hormones, secondly to monitor the efficacy of treatments, and thirdly to help determine the prognosis [2, 4]. Biochemical levels of calcium, phosphate, parathyroid hormone and prolactin, in addition to taking a thorough family history, may help in diagnosing MEN1. If Cushing's syndrome is suspected in pulmonary NETs, biochemical analysis of serum cortisol, 24-h urinary-free cortisol and ACTH should be performed. Chromogranin A (CgA), a secretory protein found in neuroendocrine cells, is currently the sole generic marker for all NETs, with levels related to tumour bulk rather than neuroendocrine tumour type or symptoms [2]. Chromogranin B (CgB) has also been raised but is perhaps less clinically relevant [4]. Pancreatic polypeptide (PP), normally secreted by cells in the endocrine pancreas, is found to be secreted in high concentrations from GEP NETs: 50–80% of pancreatic NETs and >30% of GI NETs. PP can therefore be a useful biomarker in certain cases, especially when CgA and CgB are within normal values [4].

Serotonin is secreted by the majority of NETs (>70%) found in the distal small bowel (jejunum and ileum), proximal colon and appendix, as well as 10–35% of gastric and pulmonary NETs. 5-Hydroxyindoleacetic acid (5-HIAA) is the breakdown product of serotonin which can be measured in the urine usually over a 24-hour collection. However, there are specific dietary restrictions and drug interaction problems associated with serotonin and the detection of 5-HIAA, and therefore careful instructions need to be provided to the patient to exclude certain foods and drugs prior to urine collection [4]. Rising tumour markers after surgery, particularly CgA, can be early indicators of tumour recurrence. Many NETs in the ileum and colon are diagnosed histopathologically after presentation with bowel obstruction. Biochemical samples are therefore taken post-operatively when the serum markers and 24-hour urinary 5-HIAA levels may have normalised. CgA together with neurokinin A and 24-hour urinary 5-HIAA will point towards residual disease in >90% of patients [4]. Excluding small appendiceal NETs, surgical cure is rare, and therefore patients should be followed up long term with serial laboratory and radiological investigations [4].

24-hour urinary 5-HIAA has a high sensitivity but low specificity in diagnosing CHD and is therefore not an appropriate marker for this indication. Neurohormones (called natriuretic peptides) released by the atria and ventricles secondary to wall stress are a useful screening tool for CHD [4]. Levels of NTproBNP that are above the normal range are an indication for an echocardiogram followed by a specialist cardiology review if appropriate.

## *Histopathology*

Histopathology is essential in the diagnosis and classification of NETs. A large proportion of NETs are diagnosed histologically after presentation with non-specific signs and symptoms. NETs should be classified in accordance with the WHO 2010 classification, which takes into consideration the malignant potential of all NETs. The WHO 2010 classification has a grading system: grade 1 (G1), grade 2 (G2) or grade 3 (G3), depending on their differentiation and proliferative activity as measured by Ki-67 immunostaining and mitotic count. Whilst tumours are graded according to the WHO 2010 classification, they should also follow the

**Table 19.2** WHO 2010 classification

| Type | Grade | Ki-67 index (%) | Mitotic count (per 10HPF) |
|---|---|---|---|
| NET | G1 | ≤2 | <2 |
| NET | G2 | 3–20 | 2–20 |
| NET or NEC | G3 | >20 | >20 |

*NET* neuroendocrine tumour; *NEC* neuroendocrine carcinoma; *HPF* high-power field. Adapted from Niederle B et al. [13]

Union for International Cancer Control (UICC) TNM staging system. For appendiceal, stomach and pancreas NETs, the ENETS TNM staging system should be used where the T-staging criteria differs from the UICC TNM staging system [4] (Table 19.2).

## *Radiological Assessment*

The radiological assessment of NETs can be divided into ‘anatomic imaging’ and ‘functional imaging’. Computed tomography (CT), ultrasound (US) and magnetic resonance imaging (MRI) are examples of anatomic imaging modalities that can provide information on the extent and staging of disease. Functional imaging, including somatostatin receptor scintigraphy (SRS), positron emission tomography (PET)/CT scan and tracers that mark NET metabolism, such as 3,4-dihydroxy-6-$^{18}$F-fluoro-l-phenylalanine (18F-FDOPA) and $^{18}$F-fluoro-2-deoxyglucose (18F-FDG), gives evidence of biologic behaviour and targets for specific medical treatment in managing the disease [4, 18].

Patients at risk of genetic conditions, such as those with a family history of MEN1, should be considered for screening according to MEN syndrome guidelines. Generally, asymptomatic individuals should be screened with investigations that avoid exposure to radiation, and therefore MRI is often most appropriate in this group [4].

A number of imaging modalities may be required to diagnose and detect lesions (in particular small lesions), stage the disease and assess response to treatment.

### Anatomic Imaging

CT is the most widely used anatomic imaging modality for NETs. It shows evidence of avid early enhancement on biphasic and triphasic contrast-enhanced CT (CECT), in particular with pancreatic NETs. In around 20% of pancreatic NETs, an isodense lesion with calcification can be seen on unenhanced scans in contrast to pancreatic adenocarcinomas that lack calcification [18].

More than 40% of pulmonary NETs can be detected incidentally on a chest x-ray. A CECT is the gold standard showing common features of a round or ovoid shape peripheral lung nodule with lobular or smooth margins. Pulmonary NETs are very vascular and typically show enhancement following administration of intravenous contrast [15]. If the tumour is located centrally, features of obstruction including obstructive pneumonitis, atelectasis or air trapping may be seen. High-resolution CT (HRCT) with an expiration study is the modality of choice for diffuse interstitial pulmonary neuroendocrine cell hyperplasia (DIPNECH) which shows air trapping and nodules [15].

Small bowel NETs are often associated with mesenteric nodules and mesenteric fibrosis due to desmoplastic reaction resulting in stranding, tethering and fat changes seen on CT. Radiological signs of bowel ischaemia can also be identified occurring as a result of nodal metastases encasing key vessels such as the superior mesenteric vein and superior mesenteric artery. Liver metastases enhance in a similar way to the primary NET, and the hepatic arterial phase of the scan will help identify these lesions [18].

Given the regular imaging surveillance required for patients with NETs, MRI may be preferred to reduce the risk of ionising radiation exposure. MRI has a 94% sensitivity in diagnosing pancreatic lesions. Pancreatic NETs show hyperintensity in T2-weighted images and hypointensity in T1-weighted images [4, 18]. Two-thirds of small bowel NETs can be detected on MRI and are better identified on postgadolinium contrast T1-weighted fat-suppressed images [18]. MRI is significantly better than CT for imaging NET liver metastases, including assessing response to liver targeted therapy [18].

## Functional Imaging

Functional imaging was used to corroborate the findings of anatomic imaging in terms of the visible lesions being likely NET and complement the findings in terms of lesions such as small bowel primaries that are not normally well seen on anatomic imaging. However, the advent of DOTA PET imaging has made functional imaging pre-eminent in terms of sensitivity and specificity for highlighting various cancer lesions. DOTA PET is particularly useful as part of staging imaging prior to surgery.

NETs overexpress somatostatin receptors (SSTRs) of subtypes 1–5. Most somatostatin receptor scintigraphy (SSRS) agents target the SSTR2 and SSTR5 subtypes. The sensitivity and specificity of SSRS are improved with the use of single-photon emission computed tomography (SPECT) or with SPECT-CT imaging. The diagnostic performance for pancreatic NETs using SSRS varies between specific tumour types, gastrinomas, VIPomas and glucagonomas, and non-functioning tumours have a sensitivity of around 75–100% compared to 50–60% sensitivity for primary insulinomas [19]. This is mainly because insulinomas can present with symptoms when too small for resolution by any of these imaging modalities. There are a few limitations associated with SSRS: firstly, the scan is performed over 2 days; secondly there is a reduced sensitivity in detecting <1 cm lesions; thirdly concurrent use of somatostatin analogues (SSAs) can interfere with SSTR imaging; and lastly the tumours may not express SSTRs [4].

Imaging using $^{111}$Indium ($^{111}$I)-octreotide, or $^{123}$I or $^{131}$I-meta-iodobenzylguanidine (mIBG), is used to identify patients with inoperable or metastatic disease who may benefit from targeted radiotherapy with radiolabelled mIBG [4, 18]. The main indication for performing mIBG imaging is to identify patients where $^{131}$I-mIBG-targeted radionuclide therapy would be an option. Pancreatic NETs rarely take up mIBG, and small bowel NETs have a better sensitivity for $^{111}$In scintigraphy than $^{123}$I-mIBG scintigraphy [4]. Lutetium and yttrium peptide receptor radionuclide therapy (PRRT) has superseded the use of mIBG treatment, and mIBG imaging is mostly used in locating phaeochromocytomas.

PET/CT imaging with $^{68}$Gallium-labelled somatostatin analogues, such as DOTA-octreotide (DOTATOC) and DOTA-octreotate (DOTATATE), bind avidly to SSTR2 and SSTR5. In addition to these SSTR subtypes, DOTA-Nal-octreotide (DOTANOC) also binds to SSTR3 [4]. One study showed an improved diagnostic efficacy of using $^{68}$Ga-DOTATOC as a radiotracer with PET imaging compared with SPECT and diagnostic CT imaging in detecting the primary lesion, the staging of disease and follow-up [20]. $^{68}$Ga-DOTATATE PET has been found to have a greater sensitivity and specificity compared to $^{111}$In-octreotide scintigraphy [18]. The major disadvantage of $^{68}$Ga-peptide PET/CT is the limited availability in the United Kingdom and elsewhere [4].

$^{18}$F-FDG PET/CT imaging is commonly used in bronchial NETs as part of standard workup for bronchial lesions. It is often not positive in well-differentiated bronchial NETs; however, if the scan is positive, then this indicates a poorer prognosis, as the tumour will usually then be of a less well-differentiated phenotype (Figs. 19.3 and 19.4).

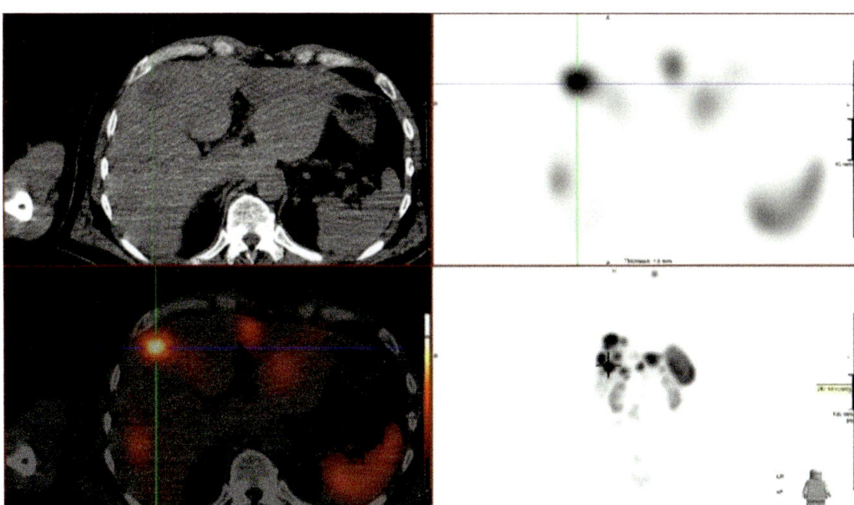

**Fig. 19.3** Multiplanar reconstructions of an octreotide SPECT-CT scan demonstrating strong radiotracer uptake in a focal liver neuroendocrine metastatic deposit (crosshairs). Less avid uptake in other neuroendocrine metastatic deposits seen around this lesion

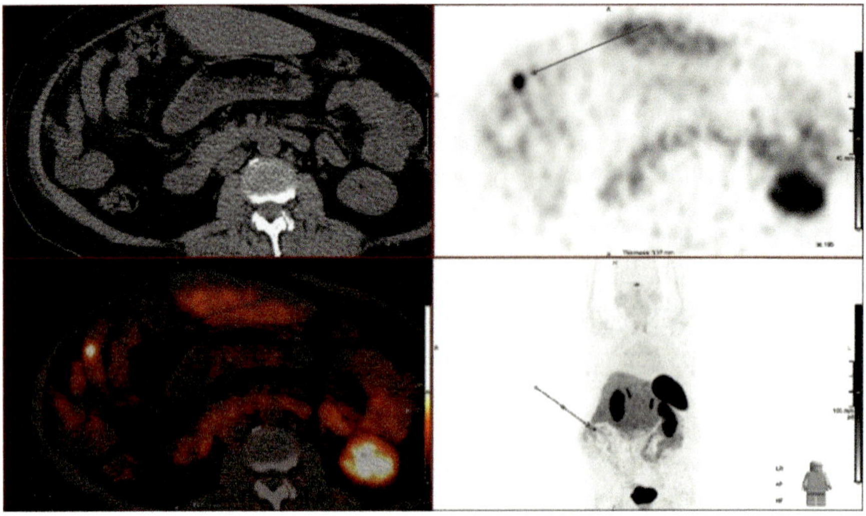

**Fig. 19.4** Multiplanar reconstructions of $^{68}$Ga-DOTA-PET/CT scan demonstrating focal radiotracer uptake (arrow) in a loop of small bowel representing a neuroendocrine lesion

**Table 19.3** Summary of diagnostic modalities for primary NET detection

| Type of diagnostic technique | Type of NET diagnosed |
|---|---|
| Upper GI endoscopy and biopsy | Gastric and duodenal |
| Lower GI endoscopy and biopsy | Colonic and rectal |
| Bronchoscopy and biopsy | Pulmonary |
| Endoscopic ultrasound (EUS) and biopsy | Pancreatic |
| Capsule endoscopy | Small bowel |
| DSA with intra-arterial calcium stimulation | Gastrinomas |

*GI* Gastrointestinal, Lower GI endoscopy includes colonoscopy and flexible sigmoidoscopy. *DSA* digital subtraction angiography. Information from Ramage JK et al. [4]

## Other Diagnostic Assessments

In addition to the diagnostic tools listed above, various other diagnostic modalities may be used when clinically indicated. The table below summarises some of these investigations (Table 19.3).

## Strategies for Earlier Diagnosis

Unless associated with hormonal symptoms, such as due to insulin or gastrin, NETs present late with non-specific GI symptoms or are discovered incidevntally. The majority of patients have metastatic disease at diagnosis. Unfortunately, we do not have accurate and easy-to-administer screening tools for diagnosing neuroendocrine tumours. Nevertheless, there has been a steady increase in diagnosis and a perceived improvement in earlier discovery of cancer, i.e. before the onset of carcinoid or other tumour-related symptoms. This is very likely due to the increased general use of imaging in the general population and a lowering of threshold for using US or CT imaging for abdominal symptoms after negative endoscopic tests. Whether earlier diagnosis could be achieved without causing severe harm to population under review remains debatable. At present there is lack of consensus on possible strategies for earlier diagnosis.

**Acknowledgements** We would like to thank Dr. Salil Karkhanis for his contribution in writing this chapter.

## References

1. Incidence and survival in neuroendocrine tumours and neuroendocrine carcinomas (NETs/NECs) in England, 2013–2014. Public Health England. 2016.
2. Oberg K, Castellano D. Current knowledge on diagnosis and staging of neuroendocrine tumors. Cancer Metastasis Rev. 2011;30(Suppl 1):3–7.
3. Jernman J, Välimäki MJ, Louhimo J, Haglund C, Arola J. The Novel WHO 2010 classification for gastrointestinal neuroendocrine tumour correlates well with the metastatic potential of rectal neuroendocrine tumours. Neuroendocrinology. 2012;95(4):317–24.
4. Ramage JK, Ahmed A, Ardill J, Bax N, Breen DJ, Caplin ME, et al. Guidelines for the management of gastroenteropancreatic neuroendocrine (including carcinoid) tumours (NETs). Gut. 2012;61(1):6–32.
5. Xavier S, Rosa B, Cotter J. Small bowel neuroendocrine tumors: from pathophysiology to clinical approach. World J Gastrointest Pathophysiol. 2016;7(1):117–24.
6. Debas HT, Mulvihill SJ. Neuroendocrine gut neoplasms. Important lessons from uncommon tumors. Arch Surg. 1994;129(9):965–71.
7. Kytölä S, Nord B, Elder EE, Carling T, Kjellman M, Cedermark B, et al. Alterations of the SDHD gene locus in midgut carcinoids, Merkel cell carcinomas, pheochromocytomas, and abdominal paragangliomas. Genes Chromosomes Cancer. 2002 Jul;34(3):325–32.
8. Hassan MM, Phan A, Li D, Dagohoy CG, Leary C, Yao JC. Risk factors associated with neuroendocrine tumors: A U.S.-based case-control study. Int J Cancer. 2008;123(4): 867–73.
9. Saha S, Hoda S, Godfrey R, Sutherland C, Raybon K. Carcinoid tumors of the gastrointestinal tract: a 44-year experience. South Med J. 1989;82(12):1501–5.
10. Delle Fave G, O'Toole D, Sundin A, Taal B, Ferolla P, Ramage JK, et al. ENETS consensus guidelines update for gastroduodenal neuroendocrine neoplasms. Neuroendocrinology. 2016;103(2):119–24.
11. Li TT, Qiu F, Qian ZR, Wan J, Qi XK, Wu BY. Classification, clinicopathologic features and treatment of gastric neuroendocrine tumors. World J Gastroenterol. 2014;20(1):118–25.
12. Hoffmann KM, Furukawa M, Jensen RT. Duodenal neuroendocrine tumors: Classification, functional syndromes, diagnosis and medical treatment. Best Pract Res Clin Gastroenterol. 2005;19(5):675–97.
13. Niederle B, Pape UF, Costa F, Gross D, Kelestimur F, Knigge U, et al. ENETS consensus guidelines update for neuroendocrine neoplasms of the jejunum and ileum. Neuroendocrinology. 2016;103(2):125–38.
14. Ramage JK, Goretzki PE, Manfredi R, Komminoth P, Ferone D, Hydrel R, et al. Consensus guidelines for the management of patients with digestive neuroendocrine tumours: well-differentiated colon and rectum tumour/carcinoma. Neuroendocrinology. 2008;87(1):31–9.

15. Caplin ME, Baudin E, Ferolla P, Filosso P, Garcia-Yuste M, Lim E, et al. Pulmonary neuroendocrine (carcinoid) tumors: European Neuroendocrine Tumor Society expert consensus and recommendations for best practice for typical and atypical pulmonary carcinoids. Ann Oncol. 2015;26(8):1604–20.
16. Bhattacharyya S, Davar J, Dreyfus G, Caplin ME. Carcinoid heart disease. Circulation. 2007;116(24):2860–5.
17. Bhattacharyya S, Burke M, Caplin ME, Davar J. Utility of 3D transoesophageal echocardiography for the assessment of tricuspid and pulmonary valves in carcinoid heart disease. Eur J Echocardiogr. 2011;12(1):E4.
18. Basuroy R, Srirajskanthan R, Ramage JK. Neuroendocrine tumors. Gastroenterol Clin N Am. 2016;45(3):487–507.
19. Dde Herder WW, Kwekkeboom DJ, Valkema R, Feelders RA, van Aken MO, Lamberts SW, et al. Neuroendocrine tumors and somatostatin: imaging techniques. J Endocrinol Invest. 2005;28(11 Suppl International):132–6.
20. Gabriel M, Decristoforo C, Kendler D, Dobrozemsky G, Heute D, Uprimny C, et al. 68Ga-DOTA-Tyr3-octreotide PET in neuroendocrine tumors: comparison with somatostatin receptor scintigraphy and CT. J Nucl Med. 2007;48(4):508–18.

# Chapter 20
# Treatment of Neuroendocrine Tumour Disease

**Andrew R. Moore and Vincent S. Yip**

**Key Learning Points**
1. NENs are increasing in incidence and, taken as a group, are more common than either oesophagogastric or pancreatic/hepatobiliary cancers.
2. The management of neuroendocrine tumours should be coordinated by specialist multidisciplinary teams.
3. Treatment is based on careful multimodal assessment to characterise and accurately stage NEN disease.
4. Tumours should be graded using the WHO 2010 classification and staged using a validated TNM classification such as that proposed by ENETS.
5. Resection of primary lesions and—in selected cases—of metastases potentiates the effectiveness of medical treatment.
6. Somatostatin receptor-positive NENs should be treated with somatostatin analogues as first line.

A. R. Moore
Liverpool Regional Neuroendocrine Tumour Service, Royal Liverpool University Hospital, Liverpool, UK
e-mail: Andrew.Moore@rlbuht.nhs.uk

V. S. Yip (✉)
Department of Hepatobiliary and Pancreatic Surgery, Royal Liverpool University Hospital, Liverpool, UK

Department of Hepatobiliary and Pancreatic Surgery, Royal London Hospital, London, UK
e-mail: vincent.yip@bartshealth.nhs.uk



T. Cross, D. H. Palmer (eds.), *Liver Cancers*,
https://doi.org/10.1007/978-3-319-92216-4_20

**Areas of Controversy and Uncertainty**

1. The timing of initiation of somatostatin analogues in metastatic grade 1 and 2 NEN disease
2. The tumour size above which colorectal NENs should be resected surgically
3. The follow-up protocol for patients following resection of duodenal, appendix and colorectal NENs
4. The role of novel targeted molecular therapies in combination with other agents

**Areas of Likely Future Progress**

1. Use of telotristat for carcinoid syndrome in functional NENs
2. Use of pasireotide for refractory carcinoid syndrome
3. Use of gastrin antagonist agents for types 1 and 2 gastric NENs and in Zollinger-Ellison syndrome

## Introduction

Neuroendocrine neoplasms (NENs) are a diverse group of uncommon tumours with widely divergent behaviour dependent on their site of origin, degree of cellular differentiation and proliferative activity. Their heterogeneity and relative scarcity have made their management challenging and have historically limited opportunities for large-scale research. In the past decade, however, the publication of several phase 3 trials has altered the landscape of treatment for NENs.

The treatment for NENs is dependent on various patient and disease characteristics. In this chapter, we outline the treatments commonly used for NEN disease of the gastrointestinal (GI) tract and pancreas and the means by which specialist multidisciplinary teams classify disease to determine the appropriate treatment.

## Gastroduodenal Neuroendocrine Neoplasms

### *Characteristics*

Gastric neuroendocrine neoplasms (g-NENs), though said to be rare, are the most prevalent of the GI NENs, and their incidence is increasing as a result of increased usage of upper GI fibre-optic endoscopy [1, 2]. They are most commonly found incidentally and can be classified according to their endoscopic, histopathological and clinical features (Table 20.1).

Types 1 and 2 g-NENs are both derived from the enterochromaffin-like (ECL) cells native to the proximal gastric mucosa and arise as the result of chronic hypergastrinaemia due to chronic autoimmune gastritis and Zollinger-Ellison

**Table 20.1** Characteristics of the types of gastric NET

| | Type 1 | Type 2 | Type 3 |
|---|---|---|---|
| Associated pathology | AIG and PA | ZES and MEN-1 | Sporadic |
| Proportion of gastric NETs (from La Rosa et al. [3]) | 46% | 6% | 15% |
| Site | Corpus/ fundus | Corpus/fundus | Any |
| Typical number | Multiple | Multiple | Single |
| Typical size of tumours | <10 mm | <10 mm | 20–50 mm |
| Serum gastrin concentration | Increased | Increased | Normal |
| Gastric acid production | Decreased | Increased | Normal |
| Prognosis | Very good | Good | Poor |
| Typical WHO grade | Grade 1 | Grade 1 | Grade 2 > grade1 > NEC |

*AIG* autoimmune atrophic gastritis, *PA* pernicious anaemia, *ZES* Zollinger Ellison syndrome, *MEN-1* multiple endocrine neoplasia type 1. Adapted from Burkitt et al. [4]

syndrome, respectively. They typically appear as multiple, small nodules or polyps in the proximal stomach and are generally found to have a low proliferative index (WHO grade 1).

In contrast, type 3 g-NENs are typically sporadic, large and solitary lesions of higher WHO grade and with a polypoidal appearance.

## *Disease Classification and Staging*

The initial assessment of g-NENs is accomplished by means of upper GI endoscopy. Careful inspection of visible gastric lesions and the background mucosa is made with representative biopsies taken. Endoscopic ultrasonography (EUS) is of value when assessing larger lesions prior to resection. Cross-sectional and functional imaging are not routinely recommended for small type 1 g-NENs but are employed for the staging of types 2 and 3 tumours to facilitate treatment selection [5, 6].

Haematological and biochemical analyses should be performed including full blood count, serum B12 concentration, fasting serum gastrin concentration and anti-gastric parietal cell/intrinsic factor antibody serology.

## *Treatment*

In type 1 tumours, the overall risk of metastases is low though the risk increases with tumour size. Lesions ≥10 mm have a significantly greater potential for malignant behaviour, and so endoscopic resection is recommended for these [7].

Other strategies for treatment of type 1 g-NENs include surgical antrectomy (to obviate endogenous gastrin secretion), the use of somatostatin analogues (SSAs) and administration of gastrin-receptor antagonists. All have been shown to bring about regression of type 1 tumours in small series, but there are no randomised controlled trials (RCTs) to support their use in what is generally considered to be a relatively benign, indolent disease, and so these are not recommended for use in routine clinical practice [8–10].

The treatment of type 2 g-NENs is generally directed towards the treatment of the associated gastrin-secreting NENs arising in the setting of multiple endocrine neoplasia type-1 (MEN-1) though larger gastric tumours are managed endoscopically as described for type 1 lesions [11].

Type 3 g-NENs are staged and managed along the same lines as more common gastric malignancies such as adenocarcinoma. Staging by means of computed tomography (CT) and diagnostic laparoscopy are employed prior to surgical resection with formal lymph node dissection in suitable cases [7].

Duodenal NENs (d-NENs) are generally treated by resection after staging using EUS and CT (and functional imaging where indicated). Small tumours can be safely resected endoscopically, whilst larger lesions or those involving the submucosa are resected surgically. The treatment of functional d-NENs associated with Zollinger-Ellison syndrome (ZES) is discussed along with pancreatic gastrinomas later [12, 13].

### *Follow-Up*

There are limited data to support any given surveillance regime for g-NENs and d-NENs, but the pragmatic approach adopted in international guidelines is to recommend biennial upper GI endoscopy [13, 14].

## Small Intestinal Neuroendocrine Neoplasms

### *Overview*

NENs of the jejunum and ileum (small intestinal NENs, si-NENs) arise from native enterochromaffin cells and are typically of low grade (WHO grades 1–2). Despite their innate indolence, the majority present following the development of locally advanced or metastatic disease [1].

### *Disease Classification and Staging*

Staging is achieved using cross-sectional (CT or MR) and functional ($^{68}$Ga-labelled somatostatin analogue PET-CT) imaging, whilst prognostic (and monitoring) information can be gleaned from the measurement of serum chromogranin A (CgA) concentration. In the majority of cases, tissue is obtained for diagnostic and grading purposes.

### *Treatment*

In patients with disease limited to the primary site, with or without involved regional lymph nodes, curative surgery with primary tumour resection and lymph node dissection should be considered. This surgical approach has been shown to confer 5-year survival rates of 100% for T1–T3 disease and >95% for T4 or regional nodal disease [15]. International guidelines advocate opportunistic cholecystectomy at the time of surgery, particularly for patients likely to be treated with somatostatin analogues (SSAs) to mitigate the risk of the complications of treatment-related cholelithiasis [16].

In patients with distant metastases, surgical resection may be employed as a palliative measure when the primary tumour or associate mesenteric fibrosis threatens small bowel obstruction.

## Appendix Neuroendocrine Neoplasms

Appendiceal NENs are most commonly identified incidentally following appendicectomy and are generally asymptomatic except in rare cases of locally advanced or widely metastatic disease. Treatment selection therefore is largely dependent on postoperative staging and disease characterisation. The most important features appear to be anatomical location, tumour size and local stage. Small (<10 mm) tumours at the tip of the appendix (hence more likely to be completely resected) without infiltration beyond the muscularis propria (ENETS stage T1) are thought to confer a very small risk of disease recurrence or metastases and do not usually require additional surgery [17]. CT/MRI can be used to complete staging and exclude metastatic disease in such cases. Large (<20 mm) tumours or those with significant (>3 mm) subserosal/mesoappendix invasion are uncommon but carry a substantial risk of metastases. For these, CT and functional imaging are used to complete staging and to exclude metastatic disease prior to formal oncological resection by means of right hemicolectomy with lymph node dissection. The appropriate treatment for intermediate disease (tumour size 1–2 cm, minimal subserosal/mesoappendix invasion) is less clear. In this group, the presence of adverse disease characteristics such as lymphovascular invasion or WHO grade 2 proliferative index should prompt consideration of completion right hemicolectomy.

Follow-up is not routinely recommended for patients in whom a curative resection of a small appendiceal NEN without adverse features has been accomplished by means of appendicectomy. Similarly, no follow-up is advised for patients whose treatment was by right hemicolectomy and in whom resection was complete and without lymph node metastases.

Suitable follow-up regimes for other groups are less clear. For patients with lymph node invasion or those in whom there were adverse tumour characteristics (tumour >2 cm, subserosal invasion, >WHO grade 1, lymphovascular invasion, etc.), long-term follow-up with cross-sectional imaging seems prudent though there are no data showing improved outcomes with such a strategy. ENETS guidelines suggest minimising the exposure to ionising radiation by utilising biomarker monitoring and alternative imaging such as ultrasound or MR [17].

## Colorectal Neuroendocrine Neoplasms

### *Overview*

Colorectal NENs are another group of tumours whose incidence is rising due to the expanding use of GI endoscopy, not least in the context of population-based screening programmes. These neoplasms appear to represent two distinct clinical entities. Rectal NENs are typically small, well differentiated and of low proliferative index (WHO grades 1–2), whereas colonic NENs are more commonly poorly differentiated, of higher grade and more advanced stage at diagnosis. Rectal NENs are often diagnosed following endoscopic resection performed as part of routine colonoscopy [18, 19].

### *Disease Classification, Staging and Treatment*

As for other gastroenteropancreatic (GEP) NENs, treatment is dependent on accurate risk stratification. Tumour size, stage and grade are the most important predictors of behaviour. For small (<10 mm) rectal NENs, local staging is performed using EUS and early stage (T1/T2) tumours resected endoscopically or by means of transanal endoscopic microsurgery (TEMS). For tumours between 10 and 20 mm, cross-sectional imaging (pelvic MRI) may be employed to augment EUS staging prior to local resection. Larger (>20 mm), locally advanced (T3) or high-grade (WHO grade 3) are fully staged using cross-sectional and functional imaging to exclude metastatic disease prior to resection [19, 20].

## Pancreatic Neuroendocrine Neoplasms

### *Overview*

This group of neuroendocrine neoplasms can be divided into those associated with a syndrome resulting from the secretion of bioactive peptides—functional pancreatic neuroendocrine tumours (F-p-NETs)—and those without such clinical manifestations, non-functional pancreatic neuroendocrine tumours (NF-p-NETS). The commonest F-p-NETs are gastrinomas and insulinomas, whilst there are a disparate group of rare tumours known to secrete other bioactive peptides, which are further sub-classified as rare functional tumours (RFTs). F-p-NETs are frequently associated with MEN-1 (20–30% of gastrinomas, <5% insulinomas and RFTs) [21–23].

Whilst F-p-NETs typically present with symptoms attributable to the action of their secreted peptides, NF-p-NETs are more commonly found incidentally or else present following the development of locally advanced or metastatic disease. The incidental diagnosis of NF-p-NETs is an increasingly common event owing to the expanding use and improving performance of cross-sectional imaging techniques.

## *Disease Classification and Staging*

As well as biochemical studies to measure the circulating levels of F-p-NET related peptides, staging of p-NETs is performed using CT, MRI and EUS (± guided fine-needle aspiration). $^{68}$Ga-labelled somatostatin analogue PET-CT is both sensitive and specific for p-NETs and is therefore recommended for use to improve the accuracy of staging and tumour localisation prior to surgery. This modality is less useful in imaging insulinomas however. In patients whose symptoms are poorly controlled and in whom surgery is warranted, tumour localisation can be achieved using functional imaging techniques which utilise radiolabelled glucagon-like peptide-1 (GLP-1) or selective intra-arterial calcium injection and hepatic venous insulin gradients [24, 25].

## *Treatment*

In the absence of MEN-1, metastatic disease or patient-related contraindications, surgical exploration with a view to tumour resection and lymph node dissection is recommended for F-p-NETs. In those patients thought not to be suitable surgical candidates, techniques such as radiofrequency ablation are thought to be effective alternatives.

The role for a surgical approach in NF-p-NETs is not routinely recommended unless there are adverse tumour characteristics (size >20 mm, higher grade, etc.)

## *Medical Treatment of Gastrinomas and Zollinger-Ellison Syndrome (ZES)*

The development of effective anti-secretory agents, notably the proton-pump inhibitors (PPIs), has greatly improved the outlook for patients with ZES and form the cornerstone of medical treatment. When used in sufficiently high dosage, adequate control of acid secretion is achieved in almost all patients. The gastrin antagonist netazepide may be of benefit in refractory cases, but this is not yet commercially available. In a substantial proportion of patients thought to have had all gastrinomas surgically resected, acid hypersecretion can persist for several years, and so caution should be exercised in the withdrawal of PPIs following surgery [26, 27].

### *Medical Treatment of Insulinomas*

Prior to surgical resection or in patients not suitable for surgery, the treatment of insulinoma-related hypoglycaemia is with regular meals and administration of the potassium channel activator diazoxide [28].

## Metastatic Neuroendocrine Tumour Disease

### *Overview*

A substantial proportion of NENs (particularly those arising in the small intestine, right colon and pancreas) are found to have metastasised at the time of diagnosis with the liver the predominant site for distant metastatic disease. The rate of metastasis is unsurprisingly greater in tumours of higher grade (WHO grade 3) than in those of lower grade, and carcinoid syndrome is a common feature in metastatic disease arising from small intestinal primaries [29, 30].

### *Liver-Targeted Treatment*

Therapies directed at liver-predominant disease should be considered early in the management of unresectable, metastatic NENs. Care must be exercised in the setting of functional tumour disease where prior treatment with somatostatin analogues is recommended to avoid the precipitation of carcinoid crises following treatment [30]. There are no large trials comparing the use of the varied methods of liver-targeted therapy with one another or with systemic treatment, and—to some degree—the treatment selected is dependent on local expertise and resource availability.

Debulking liver surgery might be considered in patients with functional tumours refractory to systemic treatment or in those whose symptoms are related to bulky liver disease [31]. Loco-regional or ablative treatments such as bland embolisation, chemoembolisation and radiofrequency ablation are considered in patients whose liver-predominant disease is unsuitable for surgical debulking or in whom surgery is contraindicated. These techniques can be used repeatedly in recurrent or progressive disease [30].

### *Somatostatin Analogues*

Somatostatin analogues (SSAs) are used as first-line treatment in patients with symptoms of carcinoid syndrome and/or as a cytostatic treatment in midgut or p-NENs and where somatostatin receptor positivity is demonstrated by means of functional imaging.

There are two commercially available long-acting agents—lanreotide autogel (60–120 mg subcutaneous injection monthly) and octreotide LAR (10–30 mg intramuscular injection monthly). They are equally efficacious in the treatment of carcinoid syndrome with a symptomatic response rate of approximately 65–70%. Refractory symptoms can be managed by dose escalation and/or increased frequency of administration without intolerable side effects [32].

SSAs are employed for their antiproliferative effects in both midgut and pancreatic NENs with Ki67 indices of ≤10%. Two large RCTs have provided evidence of significantly extended progression-free survival with SSAs. Both agents are used in the treatment of intestinal NETs, whilst lanreotide is recommended for the treatment of p-NEN. The decision to commence SSA treatment in non-functional NENs is usually predicated on the presence of extensive disease volume or after disease progression is observed though some expert advocate treatment initiation at the time of diagnosis [33, 34].

## *Interferon*

Interferon-alpha (IFN-α) may be used for treatment of carcinoid syndrome in addition to SSAs when monotherapy has not brought about complete symptom control and where the combination may have a synergistic effect. IFN is less efficacious for the treatment of carcinoid syndrome when used alone and its use is further limited by the high incidence of adverse effects such as fever, lethargy and myelosuppression [35, 36].

## *Telotristat*

Telotristat is an oral serotonin synthesis inhibitor which has been shown to improve symptomatic control in carcinoid syndrome when added to SSA. It is also posited that its direct effect on circulating 5HIAA levels may reduce the development of carcinoid heart disease [37].

## *Molecular Targeted Therapies*

Everolimus and sunitinib are novel targeted agents whose use has been evaluated in several recent phase III trials.

Everolimus is an oral mTOR inhibitor shown to increase median progression-free survival (PFS) in WHO grades 1–2 p-NENS and si-NENs compared with placebo. Unfortunately, side effects prompting withdrawal of treatment is reported in 12–19% of trial subjects with diarrhoea and stomatitis among the symptoms commonly reported [38–40].

Sunitinib is a tyrosine kinase inhibitor acting to inhibit angiogenesis and proliferative activity via vascular endothelial growth factor (VEGF) and platelet-derived growth factor (PDGF). In a recent phase III randomised controlled trial, PFS was significantly increased in patients with progressive p-NENs when compared with placebo [41].

The role of combining these novel drugs with SSAs for tumour control and carcinoid syndrome treatment is not yet supported by robust data.

### *Peptide Receptor Radionuclide Therapy (PRRT)*

Targeted therapy with radionuclide is considered second-line therapy for SSTR-positive NEN disease following progression or symptoms refractory to treatment with SSAs. SSA labelled with a radioactive isotope is administered with the intention of establishing radiation-induced tumour DNA damage. The recent NETTER-1 trial compared 177Lu-Dotatate to octreotide LAR for the treatment of progressive midgut NENs and showed markedly increased PFS and response rate in the PRRT group. PRRT is limited to provision in specialist centres [42, 43].

### *Cytotoxic Chemotherapy*

Systemic chemotherapy is usually reserved for the treatment of progressive pNET or high-grade NEN. Other indications for treatment include large-volume disease, refractory symptoms and rapid tumour progression. The treatment of non-pancreatic NENs with chemotherapy is not usually recommended unless the tumours are of high grade (Ki67 >15%), rapidly growing or if functional imaging demonstrates paucity of tracer avidity suggesting SSTR-negative disease. Combination therapy with streptozotocin (STZ) and fluorouracil (5-FU) has been shown to be superior to STZ monotherapy.

Chemotherapy treatment for neuroendocrine carcinomas (NECs) is well established and is typically inclusive of platinum-based drugs with etoposide [30, 44].

## Resection

Resection remains the only curative option for neuroendocrine liver metastases (NLMs). Complete resection (R0/1) of NLM can offer a 5-year survival of 60–80% [31, 45–47], as compared to around 30% 5-year survival for the non-resected group [48]. There are two main indications in offering resection in NLM, namely, curative intent with R0/1 resection and debulking resection for symptomatic control. Few elements have to be factored in before the consideration of liver resection for this group of patient. These elements are histological grade of the NLM, distribution of the liver metastases, presence of extra-hepatic metastases, status and resectability of the primary tumour and functionality of the neuroendocrine tumour.

Liver resection is generally only offered in well-differentiated neuroendocrine tumour (NET) (G1/G2), with only very few exception in solitary high-grade NLM. For liver resection with "curative intent", absence of extra-hepatic metastases and resectability of the primary tumour must be confirmed by high-resolution contrast computer tomography and functional imaging such as SPECT/CT or much more sensitive Gallium-68 PET/CT prior to surgical intervention.

Technical resectability for NLM is dependent on the distribution of liver lesions, which can be broadly categorised into three main types: (1) simple pattern (unilobar or limited), (2) complex pattern (bilobar) and (3) diffuse pattern. Liver resection is associated with low mortality rate of less than 5% and an overall morbidity of around 30% [49]. For simple pattern NLM, minor resection (less than 3 or more segments) or non-anatomical resections are normally sufficient to achieve a R0 resection margin. When surgery is contraindicated, curative therapy in the form microwave or radiofrequency ablation can be offered.

For complex pattern distribution, it is normally associated with bilobar disease or tumour location involving main intrahepatic vasculature requiring major hepatectomy in combination with or without intraoperative ablation technique. When the estimated future liver remnant after major hepatectomy is less than 30%, a two-step liver resection with ipsilateral inflow occlusion prior to resection can be employed to augment the remnant liver volume. A two-stage ALPPS approach has also been suggested to improve the feasibility of resecting borderline NLM [50]. When surgery is contraindicated, liver-only metastases can be managed by chemoembolisation or selective internal radiation therapy [51]. Surgical option is generally limited for diffuse pattern disease. Other treatment in the form of systemic therapy is normally required. These treatment pathways are summarised in Fig. 20.1.

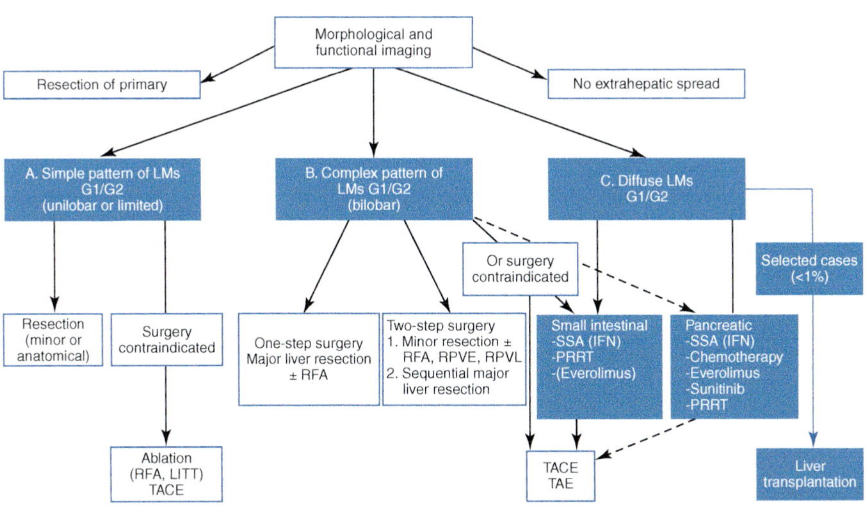


**Fig. 20.1** Treatment approach to neuroendocrine liver metastases without extra-hepatic spread (*Need approval from ENET consensus guideline* [11])

The other indication for liver resection (debulking procedure) is for symptomatic control secondary to functioning tumours. Debulking procedures involve hepatectomies, primary tumour resection and lymphadenectomy, with or without ablative therapies aiming to remove >90% of tumour burden [52, 53]. Although debulking procedure is mainly for palliative setting, studies have demonstrated an improvement in quality of life in patients' refractory to medical treatment [46, 53]. However, it is debatable regarding the extent of tumour burden that should be resected in debulking procedure.

## Liver Transplantation

With limited evidence on the long-term outcome of liver transplantation in NLM, transplantation is currently not indicated in the UK. The benefit for liver transplantation has to be weighted out against the peri-operative morbidities and mortalities, the long-term immunosuppression for an underlying malignant condition and the ethical distribution of already scarce liver graft. In addition to the criteria for resection above, ENET consensus guideline has also suggested a limited age of 50 years old and a low Ki-67 level to be included as part of the criteria for liver transplantation [30]. Nonetheless, the small percentage of tumour-free patients after 5 years in liver transplantation would be more realistically a palliation rather than a curative goal.

## References

1. Niederle MB, Hackl M, Kaserer K, Niederle B. Gastroenteropancreatic neuroendocrine tumours: the current incidence and staging based on the WHO and European Neuroendocrine Tumour Society classification: an analysis based on prospectively collected parameters. Endocr Relat Cancer. 2010;17(4):909–18.
2. Rindi G, Klöppel G, Couvelard A, Komminoth P, Körner M, Lopes JM, et al. TNM staging of midgut and hindgut (neuro) endocrine tumors: a consensus proposal including a grading system. Virchows Arch. 2007;451(4):757–62.
3. La Rosa S, Inzani F, Vanoli A, Klersy C, Dainese L, Rindi G, et al. Histologic characterization and improved prognostic evaluation of 209 gastric neuroendocrine neoplasms. Hum Pathol. 2011;42(10):1373–84.
4. Burkitt MD, Pritchard DM. Review article: pathogenesis and management of gastric carcinoid tumours. Aliment Pharmacol Ther. 2006;24(9):1305–20.
5. Cavallaro A, Zanghì A, Cavallaro M, Menzo EL, Carlo ID, Vita MD, et al. The role of 68-Ga-DOTATOC CT-PET in surgical tactic for gastric neuroendocrine tumors treatment: our experience: a case report. Int J Surg. 2014;12:S225–31.
6. Thomas D, Tsolakis AV, Grozinsky-Glasberg S, Fraenkel M, Alexandraki K, Sougioultzis S, et al. Long-term follow-up of a large series of patients with type 1 gastric carcinoid tumors: data from a multicenter study. Eur J Endocrinol. 2013;168(2):185–93.
7. Rindi G, Azzoni C, Rosa SL, Klersy C, Paolotti D, Rappel S, et al. ECL cell tumor and poorly differentiated endocrine carcinoma of the stomach: prognostic evaluation by pathological analysis. Gastroenterology. 1999;116(3):532–42.

8. Campana D, Nori F, Pezzilli R, Piscitelli L, Santini D, Brocchi E, et al. Gastric endocrine tumors type I: treatment with long-acting somatostatin analogs. Endocr Relat Cancer. 2008;15(1):337–42.
9. Murugesan SV, Steele IA, Dimaline R, Poston GJ, Shrotri M, Campbell F, et al. Correlation between a short-term intravenous octreotide suppression test and response to antrectomy in patients with type-1 gastric neuroendocrine tumours. Eur J Gastroenterol Hepatol. 2013;25(4):474–81.
10. Moore AR, Boyce M, Steele IA, Campbell F, Varro A, Pritchard DM. Netazepide, a gastrin receptor antagonist, normalises tumour biomarkers and causes regression of Type 1 gastric neuroendocrine tumours in a nonrandomised trial of patients with chronic atrophic gastritis. PLoS One. 2013;8(10):e76462.
11. Moore AR, Varro A, Pritchard DM. Zollinger-Ellison syndrome. Gastrointest Nurs. 2012;10(5):44–9.
12. Jensen RT, Niederle B, Mitry E, Ramage JK, Steinmüller T, Lewington V, et al. Gastrinoma (duodenal and pancreatic) ENETS guidelines. Neuroendocrinology. 2006;84(3):173–82.
13. Delle Fave G, Kwekkeboom DJ, Van Cutsem E, Rindi G, Kos-Kudla B, Knigge U, et al. ENETS consensus guidelines for the management of patients with gastroduodenal neoplasms. Neuroendocrinology. 2012;95(2):74–87.
14. Sato Y, Hashimoto S, Mizuno K, Takeuchi M, Terai S. Management of gastric and duodenal neuroendocrine tumors. World J Gastroenterol. 2016;22(30):6817–28.
15. Jann H, Roll S, Couvelard A, Hentic O, Pavel M, Müller-Nordhorn J, et al. Neuroendocrine tumors of midgut and hindgut origin: tumor-node-metastasis classification determines clinical outcome. Cancer. 2011;117(15):3332–41.
16. Pape UF, Perren A, Niederle B, Gross D, Gress T, Costa F, et al. ENETS consensus guidelines for the management of patients with neuroendocrine neoplasms from the jejuno-ileum and the appendix including goblet cell carcinomas—abstract. Neuroendocrinology. 2012;95(2):135–56.
17. Pape U-F, Niederle B, Costa F, Gross D, Kelestimur F, Kianmanesh R, et al. ENETS consensus guidelines for neuroendocrine neoplasms of the appendix (excluding goblet cell carcinomas). Neuroendocrinology. 2016;103(2):144–52.
18. Jung YS, Yun KE, Chang Y, Ryu S, Park JH, Kim HJ, et al. Risk factors associated with rectal neuroendocrine tumors: a cross-sectional study. Cancer Epidemiol Prev Biomark. 2014;23(7):1406–13.
19. Ramage JK, Herder WWD, Fave GD, Ferolla P, Ferone D, Ito T, et al. ENETS consensus guidelines update for colorectal neuroendocrine neoplasms. Neuroendocrinology. 2016;103(2):139–43.
20. Shen C, Yin Y, Chen H, Tang S, Yin X, Zhou Z, et al. Neuroendocrine tumors of colon and rectum: validation of clinical and prognostic values of the World Health Organization 2010 grading classifications and European Neuroendocrine Tumor Society staging systems. Oncotarget. 2016;8(13):22123–34.
21. Niina Y, Fujimori N, Nakamura T, Igarashi H, Oono T, Nakamura K, et al. The current strategy for managing pancreatic neuroendocrine tumors in multiple endocrine neoplasia type 1. Gut Liver. 2012;6(3):287–94.
22. Thakker RV, Newey PJ, Walls GV, Bilezikian J, Dralle H, Ebeling PR, et al. Clinical practice guidelines for multiple endocrine neoplasia type 1 (MEN1). J Clin Endocrinol Metab. 2012;97(9):2990–3011.
23. Brandi ML, Gagel RF, Angeli A, Bilezikian JP, Beck-Peccoz P, Bordi C, et al. Consensus: guidelines for diagnosis and therapy of MEN type 1 and type 2. J Clin Endocrinol Metab. 2001;86(12):5658–71.
24. Sharma J, Duque M, Saif MW. Emerging therapies and latest development in the treatment of unresectable pancreatic neuroendocrine tumors: an update for clinicians. Ther Adv Gastroenterol. 2013;6(6):474–90.
25. McKenna LR, Edil BH. Update on pancreatic neuroendocrine tumors. Gland Surg. 2014;3(4):258–75.

26. Wilcox CM, Seay T, Arcury JT, Mohnen J, Hirschowitz BI. Zollinger–Ellison syndrome: presentation, response to therapy, and outcome. Dig Liver Dis. 2011;43(6):439–43.
27. Boyce M, Dowen S, Turnbull G, van den Berg F, Zhao C-M, Chen D, et al. Effect of netazepide, a gastrin/CCK2 receptor antagonist, on gastric acid secretion and rabeprazole-induced hypergastrinaemia in healthy subjects. Br J Clin Pharmacol. 2015;79(5):744–55.
28. Kittah NE, Vella A. Management of endocrine disease: pathogenesis and management of hypoglycemia. Eur J Endocrinol. 2017;177(1):R37–47.
29. Yao JC, Hassan M, Phan A, Dagohoy C, Leary C, Mares JE, et al. One hundred years after "carcinoid": epidemiology of and prognostic factors for neuroendocrine tumors in 35,825 cases in the United States. J Clin Oncol. 2008;26(18):3063–72.
30. Pavel M, O'Toole D, Costa F, Capdevila J, Gross D, Kianmanesh R, et al. ENETS consensus guidelines update for the management of distant metastatic disease of intestinal, pancreatic, bronchial neuroendocrine neoplasms (NEN) and NEN of unknown primary site. Neuroendocrinology. 2016;103(2):172–85.
31. Sarmiento JM, Heywood G, Rubin J, Ilstrup DM, Nagorney DM, Que FG. Surgical treatment of neuroendocrine metastases to the liver: a plea for resection to increase survival. J Am Coll Surg. 2003;197(1):29–37.
32. O'Toole D, Ducreux M, Bommelaer G, Wemeau JL, Bouché O, Catus F, et al. Treatment of carcinoid syndrome: a prospective crossover evaluation of lanreotide versus octreotide in terms of efficacy, patient acceptability, and tolerance. Cancer. 2000;88(4):770–6.
33. Rinke A, Muller H-H, Schade-Brittinger C, Klose K-J, Barth P, Wied M, et al. Placebo-controlled, double-blind, prospective, randomized study on the effect of octreotide lar in the control of tumor growth in patients with metastatic neuroendocrine midgut tumors: a report from the PROMID study group. J Clin Oncol. 2009;27(28):4656–63.
34. Caplin ME, Pavel M, Ćwikła JB, Phan AT, Raderer M, Sedláčková E, et al. Lanreotide in metastatic enteropancreatic neuroendocrine tumors. N Engl J Med. 2014;371(3):224–33.
35. Faiss S, Pape U-F, Böhmig M, Dörffel Y, Mansmann U, Golder W, et al. Prospective, randomized, multicenter trial on the antiproliferative effect of lanreotide, interferon alfa, and their combination for therapy of metastatic neuroendocrine gastroenteropancreatic tumors—The International Lanreotide and Interferon Alfa study group. J Clin Oncol. 2003;21(14):2689–96.
36. Arnold R, Rinke A, Klose K-J, Müller H-H, Wied M, Zamzow K, et al. Octreotide versus octreotide plus interferon-alpha in endocrine gastroenteropancreatic tumors: a randomized trial. Clin Gastroenterol Hepatol. 2005;3(8):761–71.
37. Pavel M, Hörsch D, Caplin M, Ramage J, Seufferlein T, Valle J, et al. Telotristat etiprate for carcinoid syndrome: a single-arm, multicenter trial. J Clin Endocrinol Metab. 2015;100(4):1511–9.
38. Pavel ME, Hainsworth JD, Baudin E, Peeters M, Hörsch D, Winkler RE, et al. Everolimus plus octreotide long-acting repeatable for the treatment of advanced neuroendocrine tumours associated with carcinoid syndrome (RADIANT-2): a randomised, placebo-controlled, phase 3 study. Lancet. 2011;378(9808):2005–12.
39. Yao JC, Shah MH, Ito T, Bohas CL, Wolin EM, Van Cutsem E, et al. Everolimus for advanced pancreatic neuroendocrine tumors. N Engl J Med. 2011;364(6):514–23.
40. Yao JC, Fazio N, Singh S, Buzzoni R, Carnaghi C, Wolin E, et al. Everolimus for the treatment of advanced, non-functional neuroendocrine tumours of the lung or gastrointestinal tract (RADIANT-4): a randomised, placebo-controlled, phase 3 study. Lancet Lond Engl. 2016;387(10022):968–77.
41. Faivre S, Sablin M-P, Dreyer C, Raymond E. Novel anticancer agents in clinical trials for well-differentiated neuroendocrine tumors. Endocrinol Metab Clin N Am. 2010;39(4):811–26.
42. Strosberg J, El-Haddad G, Wolin E, Hendifar A, Yao J, Chasen B, et al. Phase 3 trial of 177Lu-Dotatate for midgut neuroendocrine tumors. N Engl J Med. 2017;376(2):125–35.
43. Cives M, Strosberg J. Radionuclide therapy for neuroendocrine tumors. Curr Oncol Rep. 2017;19(2):9.

44. Alexandraki KI, Karapanagioti A, Karoumpalis I, Boutzios G, Kaltsas GA. Advances and current concepts in the medical management of gastroenteropancreatic neuroendocrine neoplasms. Biomed Res Int. 2017;2017:9856140.
45. Chamberlain RS, Canes D, Brown KT, Saltz L, Jarnagin W, Fong Y, et al. Hepatic neuroendocrine metastases: does intervention alter outcomes? J Am Coll Surg. 2000;190(4):432–45.
46. Chen H, Hardacre JM, Uzar A, Cameron JL, Choti MA. Isolated liver metastases from neuroendocrine tumors: does resection prolong survival? J Am Coll Surg. 1998;187(1):88–92. discussion-3
47. Elias D, Lasser P, Ducreux M, Duvillard P, Ouellet JF, Dromain C, et al. Liver resection (and associated extrahepatic resections) for metastatic well-differentiated endocrine tumors: a 15-year single center prospective study. Surgery. 2003;133(4):375–82.
48. Kianmanesh R, O'Toole D, Sauvanet A, Ruszniewski P, Belghiti J. Surgical treatment of gastric, enteric pancreatic endocrine tumors. Part 2. Treatment of hepatic metastases. J Chir (Paris). 2005;142(4):208–19.
49. Glazer ES, Tseng JF, Al-Refaie W, Solorzano CC, Liu P, Willborn KA, et al. Long-term survival after surgical management of neuroendocrine hepatic metastases. HPB (Oxford). 2010;12(6):427–33.
50. Alvarez FA, Ardiles V, de Santibanes M, Pekolj J, de Santibanes E. Associating liver partition and portal vein ligation for staged hepatectomy offers high oncological feasibility with adequate patient safety: a prospective study at a single center. Ann Surg. 2015;261(4):723–32.
51. Grozinsky-Glasberg S, Kaltsas G, Kaltsatou M, Lev-Cohain N, Klimov A, Vergadis V, et al. Hepatic intra-arterial therapies in metastatic neuroendocrine tumors: lessons from clinical practice. Endocrine. 2018;60(3):499–509.
52. Ahlman H, Wangberg B, Jansson S, Friman S, Olausson M, Tylen U, et al. Interventional treatment of gastrointestinal neuroendocrine tumours. Digestion. 2000;62(Suppl 1):59–68.
53. Sarmiento JM, Que FG. Hepatic surgery for metastases from neuroendocrine tumors. Surg Oncol Clin N Am. 2003;12(1):231–42.

# Part IV
# Colo-Rectal Metastases and Benign Liver Tumours

# Chapter 21
# Colorectal Liver Metastasis

Rafael Diaz-Nieto and Graeme J. Poston

**Key Learning Points**
1. Up to 60% of patients with colorectal cancer will develop colorectal liver metastases.
2. Irrespective of the extension of the disease, all patients with colorectal liver metastases must be discussed in a specialized multidisciplinary committee.
3. Intervention for liver metastases can provide long-term survival benefit.
4. Surgical resection remains the best curative intent treatment.
5. Combination of systemic chemotherapy and locoregional therapies to the liver can offer survival benefits even in the palliative settings.

## Introduction

Colorectal cancer (CRC) is the third most common cause of cancer in both men and women and the third cause of cancer-related deaths in the United States [1]. Twenty-five percent of patients diagnosed with CRC present with synchronous liver metastasis (LM), and up to 60% of patients will develop liver metastases at some point in their course of their disease [2]. Metastases identified at the time of the diagnosis of the primary tumour are defined as synchronous, and those identified after the diagnosis of the original colorectal cancer are considered to be metachronous.

R. Diaz-Nieto (✉) · G. J. Poston
Hepatobiliary Surgery, Digestive Diseases Unit, Aintree University Hospital, Liverpool, UK
e-mail: Rafael.Diaz-Nieto@aintree.nhs.uk; graemeposton@blueyonder.co.uk



T. Cross, D. H. Palmer (eds.), *Liver Cancers*,
https://doi.org/10.1007/978-3-319-92216-4_21

The liver is a very common site for metastases, not only from colorectal cancer but also from many other tumours including pancreatic cancer, breast cancer and gastric cancer. Intuitively, the tumour cells reach the liver microcirculation via the portal circulation and then seed into the hepatic parenchyma. However, most of these cells fail in metastasizing successfully. Factors determining the progression of these stem cells into new tumours include adhesion, angiogenesis and final cell survival [3]. Carcinogenesis and progression of CRC involve multiple genetic and epigenetic changes in many genes. Recent investigations have demonstrated that at least 46 genes are significantly related to the liver metastasis process of CRC: KRAS, p53, APC, B-catenin and AXIN being the most common [4]. However, the whole underlying process remains poorly understood.

## Tumour Biology

The understanding of tumour biology is evolving but is now being introduced into clinical practice based on the molecular and genetic analysis of the different tumours. The recent research on these genetic markers has introduced a deeper understanding of molecular variations between tumours, so bringing tumour biology further into clinical practice. Advances in the knowledge of KRAS, NRAS, BRAF and PIK3CA mutations have shown the importance of their roles as prognostic factors following surgery [5]. Our group, for example, has added KRAS mutation into the traditional clinical risk score for prediction of survival for colorectal liver metastasis, resulting in a modified clinical score that stratifies patients overall survival with disease-free survival [6].

A good example of how tumour biology impacts on clinical practice is KRAS mutational status. KRAS status (wild- vs mutant-type) implies sensitivity or resistance to treatment using anti-epidermal growth factor receptor (EGFR) monoclonal antibodies (such as cetuximab and panitumumab) and is also associated with poorer overall survival (OS) and disease-free survival (DFS) and worse pattern of unresectable extrahepatic recurrence [7]. Additionally mutation of KRAS and BRAF predicts poorer survival outcomes after surgical resections [8, 9]. However this is even more complex as, based on a recent analysis, there is no 100% concordance in KRAS mutation between the primary tumour and the metastases [10].

## Management

Management of colorectal liver metastasis is now an extremely complex multidisciplinary process. There is now strong evidence suggesting that despite being previously considered incurable metastatic disease, interventions to colorectal liver metastases can achieve long-term survival benefit and high rates of cure [11].

The complexity of patient management now relies on more detailed diagnoses, careful preoperative assessment and multidisciplinary approaches with combinations of systemic treatments and locoregional treatments to the liver, all in combination with the already complex management of the primary tumour.

## Diagnosis

Clinical diagnosis remains the mainstay in managing the primary colorectal cancer. However liver metastasis can be completely asymptomatic. Imaging modalities are therefore essential in the diagnosis of colorectal liver metastasis, irrespective of the lack of clinical suspicion. These modalities are also of extreme importance not only for the diagnosis itself but also in the context of planning liver surgery. Assessment of the quality of the background liver, evaluation of resectability, estimation of liver volumes prior to surgery and assessment of response to systemic therapies are additional requirements for the appropriate management of colorectal liver metastasis. Figure 21.1 illustrates the most common modalities used for the diagnosis of colorectal liver metastasis.

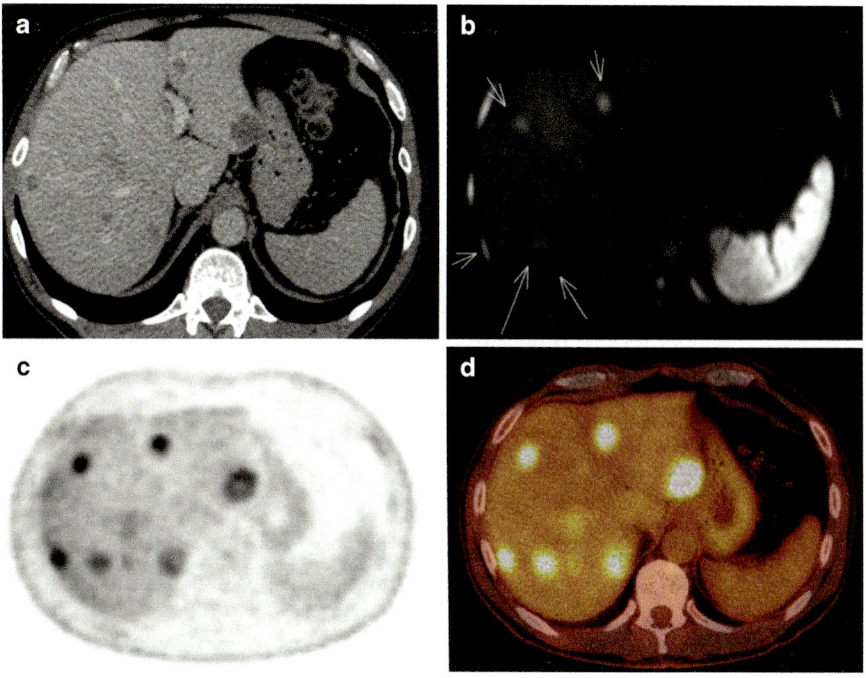


**Fig. 21.1** Comparison between different diagnostic modalities for colorectal liver metastasis. Clinical scenario of bilateral liver metastasis from colorectal cancer. (**a**) Contrast-enhanced computer tomography (CT). (**b**) Contrast-enhanced magnetic resonance (diffusion-weighted images). Arrows pointing metastatic deposits. (**c**) Functional study with fluorodeoxiglucose positron emission tomography (FDG-PET). (**d**) Combination of FDG-PET and CT (PET-CT)

### *Ultrasound Scanning*

Ultrasound (US) is frequently used for the diagnosis of hepatobiliary diseases. Some patients with colorectal liver metastasis may present with non-specific symptoms and deranged liver function test, and therefore US may be the front-line investigation. However, US itself is not adequate to differentiate between colorectal liver metastasis and other solid liver tumours. It is helpful when characterizing cystic liver lesions, and it is of paramount importance as an intraoperative technique at the time of liver resections, both for diagnosis and location of tumours, but also for planning the anatomy of the liver resection [12].

Additionally, the current use of contrast-enhanced US (CEUS) can be helpful when the diagnosis is unclear, and it is becoming a very important tool for the surgeon in the operative management of disappearing metastasis (lesions that are not further visible after a course of chemotherapy). CEUS improves US sensitivity from 67.4–71.6% to 93.4–95.8%. On a lesion-by-lesion analysis, CEUS improves the sensitivity of US from 60.9–64.9% to 85.3–92.8% and increased its specificity from 50–60% to 76.7–83.3% [13]. CEUS can be therefore an adequate alternative to MRI or CT in cases of contra-indication [14].

### *Computed Tomography*

Computed tomography (CT) is the gold standard for staging colorectal cancer. Contrast-enhanced CT is the standard technique that most commonly will identify hypodense lesions both in the arterial and portal phases with a pooled sensitivity of 80.5% (67.0–89.4%) [12]. Atypical characteristics as hypervascular or cystic metastases are also possible and may require further characterization with complementary tests. Calcification can be also an atypical presentation, but is more common in patients who have received systemic chemotherapy [15].

### *Magnetic Resonance*

Magnetic resonance (MR) increases the detection of metastases within the liver, especially when adding specific hepatobiliary contrast with combination of diffusion-weighted imaging [16]. Again, with some exceptions, colorectal liver metastasis will be shown on MR as hypovascular lesions, and it has a sensitivity of 85.7% (69.7–94.0%) [17]. Not all hepatobiliary centres routinely use MR as part of staging and diagnosis of colorectal cancer, but MR increases the sensitivity and specificity of CT for smaller metastases. Another limitation of CT that MR is able to overcome is the presence of background liver disease (steatosis, fatty infiltration, cirrhosis).

### *Positron Emission Tomography*

Positron emission tomography (PET) is the only functional test applicable to colorectal liver metastasis. Identification of hypermetabolic hepatic tumours in the context of colorectal cancer can be diagnostic of metastatic disease; however PET does not have the morphological/anatomical characteristic of other imaging modalities. It has however a valuable role in the identification of widespread metastatic disease as it scans the whole body. The combination of PET and CT overcomes its limitations as simply a functional investigation. Some reports have also correlated the grade of contrast uptake on PET with long-term outcomes [18]. However, limitations include small tumours (sub-centimetre) that are not visible with this modality and atypical metastases such as mucinous tumours; hypometabolic metastasis will not necessarily be PET avid, and it may be affected by recent chemotherapy [17]. The most common modality used in PET is fluorodeoxiglucose (FDG-PET), with a pooled sensitivity of 81.3% (64.1–91.4%) for FDG-PET and 71.0% (64.3–76.9%) for FDG-PET/CT, whilst in patients who have received chemotherapy, sensitivity rates were 54.5% (46.7–62.1%) for FDG-PET and 51.7% (37.8–65.4%) for FDG-PET/CT [17].

This diagnostic modality however is not available in every centre and is not usually included in the routine diagnostic or staging algorithm for colorectal cancer. Our group however uses PET-CT in patients with colorectal liver metastasis in cases of diagnostic doubts, clarification of postoperative/post-ablation changes in the liver and especially for identification of extrahepatic and occult metastasis [19].

Alternatively the development of MR-PET may play a role in the future staging of colorectal cancer, but this modality is not currently available in most centres, and there are no data to support its routine application [20].

With all this in mind, it is important to define adequate diagnostic algorithms that are cost-effective and provide the most accurate diagnosis. In our centre, CT of the chest abdomen and pelvis is the first diagnostic test, and in liver-limited disease, it can help to determine curative intent management for around 25% of patients. Those patients who are considered for curative intent treatment (potential surgical candidates) are then further investigated with FDG-PET and liver MRI. Our experience showed that FDG-PET identified an extra 12% of patients who had extrahepatic disease missed on the initial CT, and MRI precluded surgery in an additional 4% of patients considered resectable by CT. This staged model (or so-called hybrid model) proved to be the most cost-effective and has the shortest time to decision regarding definitive liver resection [21].

## Treatment

Historically, only liver resection offered the possibility of cure for these patients; however only one third of patients with liver-limited disease are presently considered surgically resectable at the time of diagnosis [2]. Five-year survival rates following successful liver resection are around 50% and 10-year survival approaches 25% [22, 23]. On the contrary median survival from the diagnosis of patients receiving no treatment is 6–12 months, with no 5 year survival [22, 24].

Available treatments for colorectal liver metastasis include surgery, ablation, systemic chemotherapy and regional chemotherapy and radiation therapy [25]. A recently published randomized clinical trial has demonstrated the real survival benefit of ablation of such liver metastases combined with chemotherapy in comparison with chemotherapy alone, and there are extensive data from non-randomized clinical trials demonstrating that surgical resections of colorectal liver metastasis provide long-term survival benefits [23, 26, 27]. However, such good long-term survival is a result of the combination of multimodal therapies to provide the highest survival rates. Every single patient with colorectal liver metastases must be discussed in a multidisciplinary team meeting where gastroenterologists, colorectal surgeons, hepatobiliary surgeons, thoracic surgeons, oncologist, radiologists and histopathologists can determine a structured treatment plan that may combine systemic chemotherapy, surgical resections and/or locoregional interventions.

## Surgery

Surgical resection of liver metastases from colorectal cancer remains the best treatment with curative intent. Advances in liver surgery have dramatically improved outcomes for this procedure and allow more patients to benefit. The last few years have also seen the introduction of minimally invasive surgery in the field of liver resections. Awaiting stronger evidence comparing open and laparoscopic surgery, it seems that both are equally feasible and safe in terms of survival outcomes, with laparoscopic surgery offering advantages in terms of reduced postoperative morbidity and blood loss [28].

Appropriate patient selection is essential. Patient fitness is crucial, and detailed anaesthetic assessment is strongly advised prior to surgery; however nowadays there is no single factor, including age, that is considered a contraindication to surgery.

The aim of surgery should be the complete removal of all the tumours within the liver. Whilst there are recent debates around debulking surgery [29], there is still lack of evidence to support surgery which doesn't remove all of the disease. Resection margins should be free of tumour; however the acceptable width of the margin remains unclear. It is commonly accepted that 1 mm is enough and can be considered an R0 resection. However when tumours are in contact with contralateral portal pedicles, then R1 resections are acceptable and can be considered as curative intent surgery and have proven long-term survival benefit [23, 30]. Indeed, R1 resection might have less impact on long-term survival than other more recently considered prognostic factors such as KRAS mutational status [31]. However most authors consider R1 resection to be associated with decreased OS and DFS [32], and so the surgical resection should be planned for a complete resection of the tumour with at least 1 mm margin. Macroscopic presence of tumour at the resection margin (R2 resection) has definitely poorer survival outcomes when compared with R0/R1 resections [11].

The definition of resectability is a constantly evolving concept. The current definition of resectability is the removal of all tumours whilst preserving an adequate remnant (25–30%) of the viable, disease-free healthy liver. Nevertheless even in some circumstances where there is not enough future liver remnant, new strategies are currently used to increase and optimize liver volumes and hence turning initially non-resectable patients into resectable. With this objective in mind, the surgical technique can vary. From typical anatomical (resection of anatomical segments or sectors of the liver), we have now moved into more parenchymal-sparing hepatectomies where a more limited resection is performed in order to preserve more remnant liver, thus decreasing operative morbidity [33].

Some of the strategies to convert unresectable patients to resectability include two-stage hepatectomy (TSH)–clearance of the metastases in one or two sectors of the liver combined with intraoperative or postoperative ligation/embolization of the contralateral portal vein, followed by a second hepatectomy to clear the rest of the disease. Portal vein embolization (PVE)–occlusion of portal vein branches to that part of the liver to be subsequently resected aims at increasing the future liver remnant volume by leading to hypertrophy of the other side in the subsequent weeks (Fig. 21.2). A combination of both as associated liver partition and portal vein ligation for staged hepatectomy (ALLPS)–where at the time of the first stage, the transection of the liver parenchyma is combined with ligation of the contralateral portal vein. This technique is meant to reduce the cross flow of blood through the liver parenchyma to the contralateral liver, in addition to the occlusion of the portal vein flow. All these techniques aim to occlude the inflow (portal vein) to the sector of the liver that would be potentially removed, so allowing the future remnant liver to hypertrophy prior to the resection. ALLPS results in a quicker growth rate than the other techniques, which could potentially reduce the risk of disease progression between the two stages, leading to irresectability, whilst on the other hand it is associated with higher mortality and morbidity rates [34].

Median overall survival following two-stage hepatectomy is 38.9 months with a median disease-free survival of 15.7 months. However, up to 30% of patients will not reach the second stage of surgery mainly because of disease progression during the interval between embolization and resection [35]. Staged hepatectomy has a postoperative morbidity and mortality after the first stage of around 17% and 0.5%, respectively and of 40% and 3%, respectively, after the second stage [36]. Again in this setting, 20–30% of patients will not reach the second stage mainly because of tumour progression, but for those who complete both stages, R0 resection rate is of 75%, and median overall survival is 37 months (range, 24–44) months [36]. The concept of ALPPS is to reduce the interval time between stages, ideally increasing the number of patients who will reach the second stage. This shorter period of time should avoid the development of new metastases whilst carrying with it increased morbidity and mortality [34].

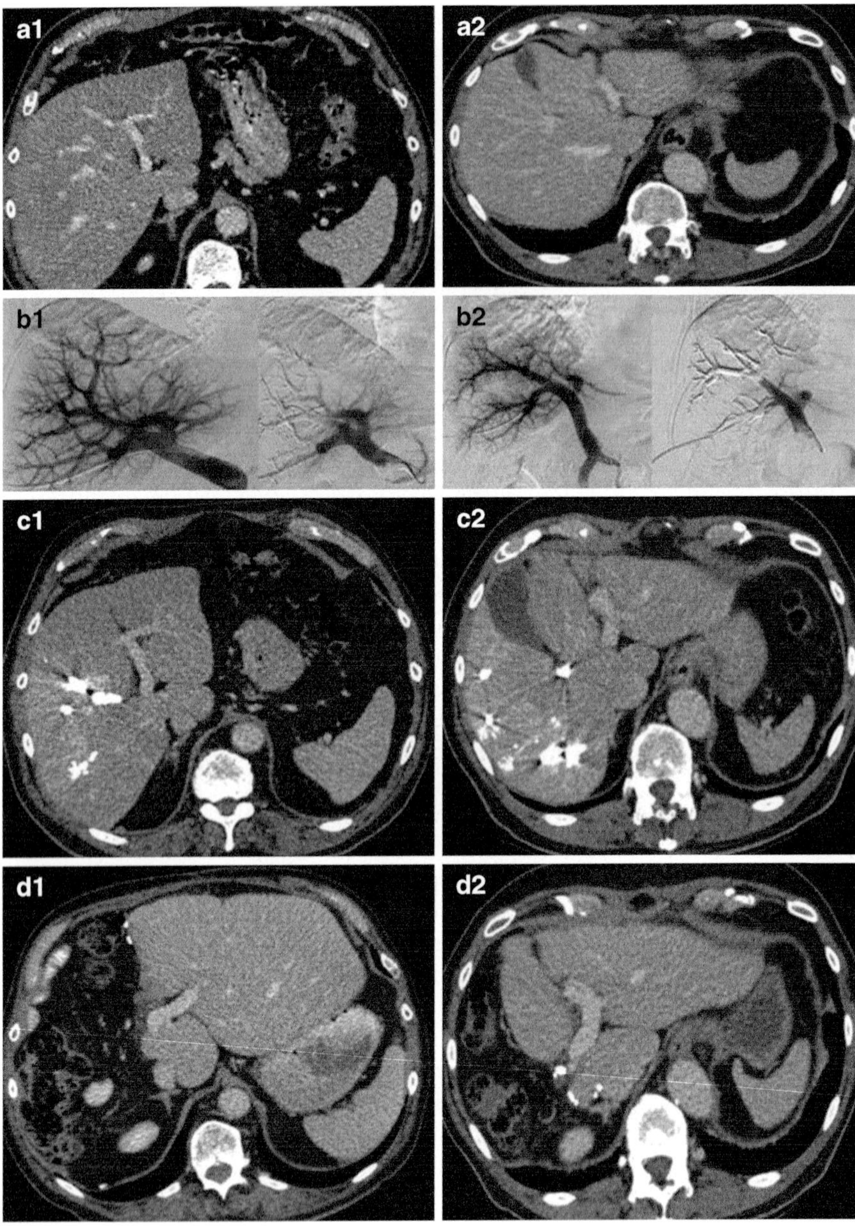


**Fig. 21.2** Examples of portal vein embolization for insufficient future liver remnant prior to liver resection. Clinical scenarios **a** and **b** of insufficient future liver remnant volume in the left hemi-liver prior to liver resection. **a1/b1**: Initial scans before intervention. **a2/b2**: Venograms before and after right-sided portal vein embolization. **c1/c2**: Post-embolizaton scans showing left-sided hypertrophy. **d1/d2**: Scans after liver resection showing final liver volume

All these strategies are in the setting of initially unresectable disease, and most protocols include the use of systemic chemotherapy (sometimes known as conversion chemotherapy) in order to reduce the bulk of the disease in the liver and subsequently proceed with surgery. An additional advantage of this approach is the treatment of micrometastases and also the selecting out of patients with more aggressive biology.

## Systemic Therapies

There is now a wide range of drugs and regimens available to treat advanced colorectal cancer. Systemic therapy has evolved from single agent fluorouracil (5-FU) to multiple combinations of antineoplastic agents in addition to anti-angiogenic drugs (bevacizumab, regorafenib and aflibercept) and anti-epidermal growth factor receptor agents (anti-EGFR), such as cetuximab and panitumumab. Most of the standard regimens include 5-FU modulated by folinic acid, oxaliplatin or irinotecan. Nomenclature is also complex, and the traditional concept of neoadjuvant chemotherapy can be confusing if the patient has undergone an earlier bowel resection with subsequent adjuvant chemotherapy which could be considered as neoadjuvant to the resection of the liver metastases. Perioperative chemotherapy includes all regimens given either before or after surgery.

The most reliable evidence supporting perioperative chemotherapy and showing survival benefit in terms of disease-free survival comes from the use of FOLFOX4 [37, 38].

Neoadjuvant systemic chemotherapy prior to liver resection for resectable liver metastases has many theoretical advantages, such as assessing tumour sensitivity, decreasing large or multiple liver lesions, increasing resectability, and treating micrometastases [39]. However there are inherit risks related to delaying the surgical resection specially the risk of disease progression (6%) and 30% of patients who don't respond to chemotherapy [40], induction of liver toxicity (steatohepatitis with irinotecan and sinusoidal congestion syndrome with oxaliplatin) and increasing postoperative morbidity [38] and mortality [41]. There is a need for stronger evidence therefore to support the routine use of systemic chemotherapy for resectable liver metastasis prior to liver resection, both in the setting of synchronous presentation and metachronous presentation.

Adjuvant chemotherapy is even more controversial. There are discrepancies between trials regarding benefits in OS and DFS; however as mentioned before, the use of perioperative chemotherapy (rather than adjuvant only chemotherapy) is justified, supported by the fact that recurrence after liver resection remains around 60% [41]. Based on the publication of the randomized clinical trial for resectable liver metastasis (EORTC 40983), perioperative administration of FOLFOX4 (six 14-day cycles of oxaliplatin 85 mg/m$^2$, folinic acid 200 mg/m$^2$

(DL form) or 100 mg/m$^2$ (L form) on days 1–2 plus bolus and fluorouracil 400 mg/m$^2$ (bolus) and 600 mg/m$^2$ (continuous 22 h infusion), before and after surgery) has become the standard regimen. This trial reported a significant DFS benefit in those patients who underwent liver resection [38] but failed to demonstrate long-term OS benefit as it was insufficiently powered [42]. A more recent meta-analysis has suggested that the routine use of adjuvant systemic chemotherapy after resection of liver metastasis improved OS rates for 23% of the patients versus surgery alone (HR, 0.77; 95% confidence interval [CI] 0.67–0.88; $p < 0.001$) and improved DFS for 29% of the patients (HR, 0.71; 95% CI 0.61–0.83; $p < 0.001$) [43].

Up to 70% of patients will have unresectable disease at the time of presentation. This is where conversion chemotherapy plays a very important role. Recently the METHEP trial reported that the FOLFIRINOX regimen (combination of folinic acid, 5-FU, oxaliplatin and irinotecan) resulted in a very good response in patients with unresectable liver-limited disease with up to 67% of the patients become resectable [44]. More recent addition of bevacizumab or other regimens including capecitabine may also increase this resection rate and offer alternatives for initial nonresponders [45, 46]. Median pooled overall survival for patients who underwent liver resection after FOLFIRINOX-Bev was 30.2 months, and median DFS was 12.4 months [47]. The addition of cetuximab to standard systemic chemotherapy significantly improves the outcomes in RAS wild-type patients with unresectable liver-limited colorectal metastases in terms of OS, DFS and also conversion to resectable and improved R0 rates after surgery [48]. However postoperative administration of FOLIRI after R0 resection of liver metastases did not show any benefit in overall survival but increased the rate of chemotherapy-related toxicity [41, 44].

In the palliative setting, chemotherapy remains the basis of management for the majority of patients with stage 4 colorectal cancer. Surgery has traditionally only played a role in these patients for the treatment of symptoms related to the primary tumour [49]. Administration of the chemotherapy regimens discussed above provides a survival benefit to patients of 24 months OS [49]. Further results from randomized clinical trials suggest that, when possible, liver-targeted interventions for the liver metastases (mainly ablation techniques) offer a survival benefit when compared to chemotherapy alone [26]. Alternative therapies for patients with liver-limited disease when systemic treatment (following one or more treatment lines) has failed to control the disease, include regional treatment to the liver such as hepatic artery infusional (HAI) chemotherapy and radioembolization (yttrium-90 (Y90)) [50, 51]. However current evidence to support such treatment strategies is limited. Drug-eluting beads with irinotecan (DEBIRI) may offer equivalent effect with potentially reduced side effects. Its use as neoadjuvant treatment has recently proved to be as effective as systemic chemotherapy for resectable liver metastases [52].

## Thermal Ablation

Thermal ablation (TA) technologies destroy neoplastic tissue by coagulative necrosis. Radiofrequency ablation (RFA) and microwave ablation (MWA) use extremely high temperatures (>60 °C), whilst cryotherapy (CA) uses liquid nitrogen to disrupt the tissue by freezing [53, 54].

A recent systematic review compared these three techniques, and in accordance with most of the available literature, it seems that CA has the highest local recurrence rates (12–39%), RFA local recurrence rates ranged between 10 and 31%, and MWA had the lowest (5–13%) [55–57]. More recently, the use of irreversible electroporation (IRE) has reported similar outcomes [58], but there remains a need for well-designed trials to compare these different techniques. However, IRE seems to be beneficial for tumours very close to the main portal pedicles and major hepatic veins, where others types of thermal ablations are considered unsafe [58].

The advantage of TA over liver resection (LR) is lower morbidity/mortality [59, 60]; however there are limitations relating to tumour location and size and number of metastases [61]. A recent consensus concluded that less than five tumours, all smaller than 3 cm, are acceptable for percutaneous ablation, if more than a 5 mm ablation margin can be achieved [62].

Despite the lack of strong evidence and the heterogeneity of clinical trials, it seems that liver resection, when feasible, is superior to TA in achieving local control [63]. Recent reports suggest that LR was superior to RFA in the treatment of patients, irrespective of solitary or multiple metastases and the size of the tumours [64–67]. However, in the setting of the multidisciplinary team and complementary to surgery and chemotherapy, TA has a very important role in the management of colorectal liver metastasis, both for curative intent treatment and palliative management [61].

## Liver Transplantation

Liver transplantation is, in concept, an alternative treatment to colorectal liver metastasis. It was actually one of the initial indications for transplantation; however poor outcomes and early recurrence made centres abandon these techniques for liver malignancies, and only hepatocellular carcinoma remains as a standard indication for liver transplantation [25]. The lack of donor organs for transplantation to treat end-stage chronic liver diseases precluded for the indications of transplantation for malignancies. Some centres however have explored this field and innovations in some immune-modulating agents, rather than immunosuppressive drugs may change this indication [25]. Despite remaining a unique outcome, Hagness et al. reported a 1-, 3- and 5-year OS of 95%, 68% and 60%, respectively, following orthotopic liver transplantation for patients with unresectable liver-limited colorectal liver metastases [68].

## Recurrence After Treatment

In the lack of strong evidence, most commonly used follow-up protocols after curative intended liver resection for colorectal liver metastases include regular CTs of the chest abdomen and pelvis every 6 months to a year for a minimum of 5 years. In addition, CEA has proven to be an adequate tumour marker to monitor recurrence.

If the disease recurs in the liver, then all of the therapies discussed above can be reconsidered. Surgery remains the ideal treatment option despite the limitations of a previous liver resection. In this setting, if technically possible then repeated hepatectomies have proven to be as effective in survival outcomes as the first hepatectomy, despite the surgical limitations of adhesions from previous surgeries [69]. There is no limit to the number of hepatectomies that can be performed, with large series reporting long-term survival benefits after repeated hepatectomies [70]. The limitation is related however to the future liver remnant that would be progressively compromised. Alternatively, thermal ablation can be considered. However our recent experience shows that despite being feasible, ablation has a poorer outcome when compared to surgery for recurrent colorectal liver metastases [71].

## Presence of Extrahepatic Disease

Although the liver is the most common site for metastatic colorectal cancer, up to 38% of patients will develop metastases at other sites. Lung, peritoneum and lymph nodes are the most common site for extrahepatic metastases. The complexity of management is obviously greater, but long-term survival is still possible. Extrahepatic disease is no longer an absolute contraindication, and if R0 resection is possible at all anatomical sites, then treatment strategies to achieve this objective should be considered [72].

From our experience a multidisciplinary approach is of key importance. Tumours that have initially responded to chemotherapy can be re-challenged using the same chemotherapy regimen. Following a lack of response, then consideration should be given to second-line chemotherapy. Nowadays it is mandatory that every patient with colorectal liver metastases, irrespective of the extent of disease or the concomitance of disease at other sites, is discussed in a specialized liver centre where a liver surgeon can assess resectability [73]. Even more so, multidisciplinary management of patients with colorectal cancer has proven to diagnose and stage patients more accurately with a subsequent positive impact in OS [74].

## References


1. Siegel RL, Miller KD, Jemal A. Cancer statistics, 2016. CA Cancer J Clin. 2016;66(1):7–30.
2. Sag AA, Selcukbiricik F, Mandel NM. Evidence-based medical oncology and interventional radiology paradigms for liver-dominant colorectal cancer metastases. World J Gastroenterol. 2016;22(11):3127–49.
3. Rudmik LR, Magliocco AM. Molecular mechanisms of hepatic metastasis in colorectal cancer. J Surg Oncol. 2005;92(4):347–59.
4. Ki DH, Jeung HC, Park CH, Kang SH, Lee GY, Lee WS, et al. Whole genome analysis for liver metastasis gene signatures in colorectal cancer. Int J Cancer. 2007;121(9):2005–12.
5. Palomba G, Doneddu V, Cossu A, Paliogiannis P, Manca A, Casula M, et al. Prognostic impact of KRAS, NRAS, BRAF, and PIK3CA mutations in primary colorectal carcinomas: a population-based study. J Transl Med. 2016;14(1):292.
6. Brudvik KW, Jones RP, Giuliante F, Shindoh J, Passot G, Chung MH, et al. RAS mutation clinical risk score to predict survival after resection of colorectal liver metastases. Ann Surg. 2017.
7. Andreatos N, Ronnekleiv-Kelly S, Margonis GA, Sasaki K, Gani F, Amini N, et al. From bench to bedside: Clinical implications of KRAS status in patients with colorectal liver metastasis. Surg Oncol. 2016;25(3):332–8.
8. Passiglia F, Bronte G, Bazan V, Galvano A, Vincenzi B, Russo A. Can KRAS and BRAF mutations limit the benefit of liver resection in metastatic colorectal cancer patients? A systematic review and meta-analysis. Crit Rev Oncol Hematol. 2016;99:150–7.
9. Brudvik KW, Kopetz SE, Li L, Conrad C, Aloia TA, Vauthey JN. Meta-analysis of KRAS mutations and survival after resection of colorectal liver metastases. Br J Surg. 2015;102(10):1175–83.
10. Mao C, Wu XY, Yang ZY, Threapleton DE, Yuan JQ, Yu YY, et al. Concordant analysis of KRAS, BRAF, PIK3CA mutations, and PTEN expression between primary colorectal cancer and matched metastases. Sci Rep. 2015;5:8065.
11. Allard MA, Adam R, Giuliante F, Lapointe R, Hubert C, Ijzermans JNM, et al. Long-term outcomes of patients with 10 or more colorectal liver metastases. Br J Cancer. 2017;117(5):604–11.
12. Torzilli G, Procopio F. State of the art of intraoperative ultrasound in liver surgery: current use for resection-guidance. Chirurgia (Bucur). 2017;112(3):320–5.
13. Cantisani V, Ricci P, Erturk M, Pagliara E, Drudi F, Calliada F, et al. Detection of hepatic metastases from colorectal cancer: prospective evaluation of gray scale US versus SonoVue(R) low mechanical index real time-enhanced US as compared with multidetector-CT or Gd-BOPTA-MRI. Ultraschall Med. 2010;31(5):500–5.
14. Cantisani V, Grazhdani H, Fioravanti C, Rosignuolo M, Calliada F, Messineo D, et al. Liver metastases: contrast-enhanced ultrasound compared with computed tomography and magnetic resonance. World J Gastroenterol. 2014;20(29):9998–10007.
15. Hale HL, Husband JE, Gossios K, Norman AR, Cunningham D. CT of calcified liver metastases in colorectal carcinoma. Clin Radiol. 1998;53(10):735–41.
16. Zech CJ, Herrmann KA, Reiser MF, Schoenberg SO. MR imaging in patients with suspected liver metastases: value of liver-specific contrast agent Gd-EOB-DTPA. Magn Reson Med Sci. 2007;6(1):43–52.
17. van Kessel CS, Buckens CF, van den Bosch MA, van Leeuwen MS, van Hillegersberg R, Verkooijen HM. Preoperative imaging of colorectal liver metastases after neoadjuvant chemotherapy: a meta-analysis. Ann Surg Oncol. 2012;19(9):2805–13.
18. Xia Q, Liu J, Wu C, Song S, Tong L, Huang G, et al. Prognostic significance of (18)FDG PET/CT in colorectal cancer patients with liver metastases: a meta-analysis. Cancer Imaging. 2015;15:19.

19. Yip VS, Poston GJ, Fenwick SW, Wieshmann H, Athwal T, Malik HZ. FDG-PET-CT is effective in selecting patients with poor long term survivals for colorectal liver metastases. Eur J Surg Oncol. 2014;40(8):995–9.
20. Lee DH, Lee JM. Whole-body PET/MRI for colorectal cancer staging: is it the way forward? J Magn Reson Imaging. 2017;45(1):21–35.
21. Yip VS, Collins B, Dunne DF, Koay MY, Tang JM, Wieshmann H, et al. Optimal imaging sequence for staging in colorectal liver metastases: analysis of three hypothetical imaging strategies. Eur J Cancer. 2014;50(5):937–43.
22. Wilson SM, Adson MA. Surgical treatment of hepatic metastases from colorectal cancers. Arch Surg. 1976;111(4):330–4.
23. Hosokawa I, Allard MA, Gelli M, Ciacio O, Vibert E, Cherqui D, et al. Long-term survival benefit and potential for cure after R1 resection for colorectal liver metastases. Ann Surg Oncol. 2016;23(6):1897–905.
24. Scheele J, Stangl R, Altendorf-Hofmann A, Gall FP. Indicators of prognosis after hepatic resection for colorectal secondaries. Surgery. 1991;110(1):13–29.
25. Moris D, Tsilimigras DI, Chakedis J, Beal EW, Felekouras E, Vernadakis S, et al. Liver transplantation for unresectable colorectal liver metastases: a systematic review. J Surg Oncol. 2017;116(3):288–97.
26. Ruers T, Punt C, Van Coevorden F, Pierie JP, Borel-Rinkes I, Ledermann JA, et al. Radiofrequency ablation combined with systemic treatment versus systemic treatment alone in patients with non-resectable colorectal liver metastases: a randomized EORTC Intergroup phase II study (EORTC 40004). Ann Oncol. 2012;23(10):2619–26.
27. Ruers T, Punt CJA, Van Coevorden F, Pierie JPEN, Borel-Rinkes I, Ledermann JA, Poston G, et al. Long-term survival results of a randomised phase II study of the EORTC-NCRI CCSG-ALM intergroup 40004 (CLOCC). J Clin Oncol. 2015;33(Suppl).
28. Hallet J, Beyfuss K, Memeo R, Karanicolas PJ, Marescaux J, Pessaux P. Short and long-term outcomes of laparoscopic compared to open liver resection for colorectal liver metastases. Hepatobiliary Surg Nutr. 2016;5(4):300–10.
29. Tanaka K, Murakami T, Yabushita Y, Hiroshima Y, Matsuo K, Endo I, et al. Maximal debulking liver resection as a beneficial treatment strategy for advanced and aggressive colorectal liver metastases. Anticancer Res. 2014;34(10):5547–54.
30. de Haas RJ, Wicherts DA, Flores E, Azoulay D, Castaing D, Adam R. R1 resection by necessity for colorectal liver metastases: is it still a contraindication to surgery? Ann Surg. 2008;248(4):626–37.
31. Truant S, Sequier C, Leteurtre E, Boleslawski E, Elamrani M, Huet G, et al. Tumour biology of colorectal liver metastasis is a more important factor in survival than surgical margin clearance in the era of modern chemotherapy regimens. HPB (Oxford). 2015;17(2):176–84.
32. Tranchart H, Chirica M, Faron M, Balladur P, Lefevre LB, Svrcek M, et al. Prognostic impact of positive surgical margins after resection of colorectal cancer liver metastases: reappraisal in the era of modern chemotherapy. World J Surg. 2013;37(11):2647–54.
33. Alvarez FA, Sanchez Claria R, Oggero S, de Santibanes E. Parenchymal-sparing liver surgery in patients with colorectal carcinoma liver metastases. World J Gastrointest Surg. 2016;8(6):407–23.
34. Moris D, Ronnekleiv-Kelly S, Kostakis ID, Tsilimigras DI, Beal EW, Papalampros A, et al. Operative results and oncologic outcomes of Associating Liver Partition and Portal Vein Ligation for Staged Hepatectomy (ALPPS) versus Two-Stage Hepatectomy (TSH) in patients with unresectable colorectal liver metastases: a systematic review and meta-analysis. World J Surg. 2017.
35. Ironside N, Bell R, Bartlett A, McCall J, Powell J, Pandanaboyana S. Systematic review of perioperative and survival outcomes of liver resections with and without preoperative portal vein embolization for colorectal metastases. HPB (Oxford). 2017;19(7):559–66.

36. Lam VW, Laurence JM, Johnston E, Hollands MJ, Pleass HC, Richardson AJ. A systematic review of two-stage hepatectomy in patients with initially unresectable colorectal liver metastases. HPB (Oxford). 2013;15(7):483–91.
37. de Gramont A, Figer A, Seymour M, Homerin M, Hmissi A, Cassidy J, et al. Leucovorin and fluorouracil with or without oxaliplatin as first-line treatment in advanced colorectal cancer. J Clin Oncol. 2000;18(16):2938–47.
38. Nordlinger B, Sorbye H, Glimelius B, Poston GJ, Schlag PM, Rougier P, et al. Perioperative chemotherapy with FOLFOX4 and surgery versus surgery alone for resectable liver metastases from colorectal cancer (EORTC Intergroup trial 40983): a randomised controlled trial. Lancet. 2008;371(9617):1007–16.
39. Nordlinger B, Benoist S. Benefits and risks of neoadjuvant therapy for liver metastases. J Clin Oncol. 2006;24(31):4954–5.
40. Masi G, Loupakis F, Pollina L, Vasile E, Cupini S, Ricci S, et al. Long-term outcome of initially unresectable metastatic colorectal cancer patients treated with 5-fluorouracil/leucovorin, oxaliplatin, and irinotecan (FOLFOXIRI) followed by radical surgery of metastases. Ann Surg. 2009;249(3):420–5.
41. Fiorentini G, Sarti D, Aliberti C, Carandina R, Mambrini A, Guadagni S. Multidisciplinary approach of colorectal cancer liver metastases. World J Clin Oncol. 2017;8(3):190–202.
42. Nordlinger B, Sorbye H, Glimelius B, Poston GJ, Schlag PM, Rougier P, et al. Perioperative FOLFOX4 chemotherapy and surgery versus surgery alone for resectable liver metastases from colorectal cancer (EORTC 40983): long-term results of a randomised, controlled, phase 3 trial. Lancet Oncol. 2013;14(12):1208–15.
43. Araujo RL, Gonen M, Herman P. Chemotherapy for patients with colorectal liver metastases who underwent curative resection improves long-term outcomes: systematic review and meta-analysis. Ann Surg Oncol. 2015;22(9):3070–8.
44. Ychou M, Hohenberger W, Thezenas S, Navarro M, Maurel J, Bokemeyer C, et al. A randomized phase III study comparing adjuvant 5-fluorouracil/folinic acid with FOLFIRI in patients following complete resection of liver metastases from colorectal cancer. Ann Oncol. 2009;20(12):1964–70.
45. Okines A, Puerto OD, Cunningham D, Chau I, Van Cutsem E, Saltz L, et al. Surgery with curative-intent in patients treated with first-line chemotherapy plus bevacizumab for metastatic colorectal cancer First BEAT and the randomised phase-III NO16966 trial. Br J Cancer. 2009;101(7):1033–8.
46. Wong R, Cunningham D, Barbachano Y, Saffery C, Valle J, Hickish T, et al. A multicentre study of capecitabine, oxaliplatin plus bevacizumab as perioperative treatment of patients with poor-risk colorectal liver-only metastases not selected for upfront resection. Ann Oncol. 2011;22(9):2042–8.
47. Tomasello G, Petrelli F, Ghidini M, Russo A, Passalacqua R, Barni S. FOLFOXIRI plus bevacizumab as conversion therapy for patients with initially unresectable metastatic colorectal cancer: a systematic review and pooled analysis. JAMA Oncol. 2017;3(7):e170278.
48. Lv W, Zhang GQ, Jiao A, Zhao BC, Shi Y, Chen BM, et al. Chemotherapy plus cetuximab versus chemotherapy alone for patients with KRAS wild type unresectable liver-confined metastases colorectal cancer: an updated meta-analysis of RCTs. Gastroenterol Res Pract. 2017;2017:8464905.
49. Costi R, Leonardi F, Zanoni D, Violi V, Roncoroni L. Palliative care and end-stage colorectal cancer management: the surgeon meets the oncologist. World J Gastroenterol. 2014;20(24):7602–21.
50. Cercek A, Gendel V, Jabbour S, Moore D, Chen C, Nosher J, et al. A comparison of Yttrium-90 microsphere radioembolization to hepatic arterial infusional chemotherapy for patients with chemo-refractory hepatic colorectal metastases. Curr Treat Options in Oncol. 2017;18(7):42.
51. Bhutiani N, Martin RC 2nd. Transarterial therapy for colorectal liver metastases. Surg Clin North Am. 2016;96(2):369–91.

52. Jones RP, Malik HZ, Fenwick SW, Terlizzo M, O'Grady E, Stremitzer S, et al. PARAGON II—a single arm multicentre phase II study of neoadjuvant therapy using irinotecan bead in patients with resectable liver metastases from colorectal cancer. Eur J Surg Oncol. 2016;42(12):1866–72.
53. Wu ZB, Si ZM, Qian S, Liu LX, Qu XD, Zhou B, et al. Percutaneous microwave ablation combined with synchronous transcatheter arterial chemoembolization for the treatment of colorectal liver metastases: results from a follow-up cohort. Onco Targets Ther. 2016;9:3783–9.
54. Poston G. Cryosurgery for colorectal liver metastases. Hepato-Gastroenterology. 2001;48(38):323–4.
55. Pathak S, Jones R, Tang JM, Parmar C, Fenwick S, Malik H, et al. Ablative therapies for colorectal liver metastases: a systematic review. Color Dis. 2011;13(9):e252–65.
56. Correa-Gallego C, Fong Y, Gonen M, D'Angelica MI, Allen PJ, DeMatteo RP, et al. A retrospective comparison of microwave ablation vs. radiofrequency ablation for colorectal cancer hepatic metastases. Ann Surg Oncol. 2014;21(13):4278–83.
57. Martin RC, Scoggins CR, McMasters KM. Safety and efficacy of microwave ablation of hepatic tumors: a prospective review of a 5-year experience. Ann Surg Oncol. 2010;17(1):171–8.
58. Scheffer HJ, Melenhorst MC, Echenique AM, Nielsen K, van Tilborg AA, van den Bos W, et al. Irreversible electroporation for colorectal liver metastases. Tech Vasc Interv Radiol. 2015;18(3):159–69.
59. Hammill CW, Billingsley KG, Cassera MA, Wolf RF, Ujiki MB, Hansen PD. Outcome after laparoscopic radiofrequency ablation of technically resectable colorectal liver metastases. Ann Surg Oncol. 2011;18(7):1947–54.
60. Jakobs TF, Hoffmann RT, Trumm C, Reiser MF, Helmberger TK. Radiofrequency ablation of colorectal liver metastases: mid-term results in 68 patients. Anticancer Res. 2006;26(1B):671–80.
61. Diaz-Nieto R, Fenwick S, Malik H, Poston G. Defining the optimal use of ablation for metastatic colorectal cancer to the liver without high-level evidence. Curr Treat Options in Oncol. 2017;18(2):8.
62. Gillams A, Goldberg N, Ahmed M, Bale R, Breen D, Callstrom M, et al. Thermal ablation of colorectal liver metastases: a position paper by an international panel of ablation experts, The Interventional Oncology Sans Frontieres meeting 2013. Eur Radiol. 2015;25(12):3438–54.
63. de Meijer VE, Verhoef C, Kuiper JW, Alwayn IP, Kazemier G, Ijzermans JN. Radiofrequency ablation in patients with primary and secondary hepatic malignancies. J Gastrointest Surg. 2006;10(7):960–73.
64. Wu YZ, Li B, Wang T, Wang SJ, Zhou YM. Radiofrequency ablation vs hepatic resection for solitary colorectal liver metastasis: a meta-analysis. World J Gastroenterol. 2011;17(36):4143–8.
65. Abdalla EK, Vauthey JN, Ellis LM, Ellis V, Pollock R, Broglio KR, et al. Recurrence and outcomes following hepatic resection, radiofrequency ablation, and combined resection/ablation for colorectal liver metastases. Ann Surg. 2004;239(6):818–25. discussion 25-7
66. Lee KH, Kim HO, Yoo CH, Son BH, Park YL, Cho YK, et al. Comparison of radiofrequency ablation and resection for hepatic metastasis from colorectal cancer. Korean J Gastroenterol. 2012;59(3):218–23.
67. Lee H, Heo JS, Cho YB, Yun SH, Kim HC, Lee WY, et al. Hepatectomy vs radiofrequency ablation for colorectal liver metastasis: a propensity score analysis. World J Gastroenterol. 2015;21(11):3300–7.
68. Hagness M, Foss A, Line PD, Scholz T, Jorgensen PF, Fosby B, et al. Liver transplantation for nonresectable liver metastases from colorectal cancer. Ann Surg. 2013;257(5):800–6.
69. Wurster EF, Tenckhoff S, Probst P, Jensen K, Dolger E, Knebel P, et al. A systematic review and meta-analysis of the utility of repeated versus single hepatic resection for colorectal cancer liver metastases. HPB (Oxford). 2017;19(6):491–7.
70. Adam R, Pascal G, Azoulay D, Tanaka K, Castaing D, Bismuth H. Liver resection for colorectal metastases: the third hepatectomy. Ann Surg. 2003;238(6):871–83. discussion 83-4

71. Dupre A, Jones R, Diaz-Nieto R, Fenwick S, Poston G, Malik H. Curative-intent treatment of recurrent colorectal liver metastases: a comparison between ablation and resection. Eur J Surg Oncol. 2017;43(10):1901–7.
72. Hadden WJ, de Reuver PR, Brown K, Mittal A, Samra JS, Hugh TJ. Resection of colorectal liver metastases and extra-hepatic disease: a systematic review and proportional meta-analysis of survival outcomes. HPB (Oxford). 2016;18(3):209–20.
73. Jones RP, Vauthey JN, Adam R, Rees M, Berry D, Jackson R, et al. Effect of specialist decision-making on treatment strategies for colorectal liver metastases. Br J Surg. 2012;99(9):1263–9.
74. Ye YJ, Shen ZL, Sun XT, Wang ZF, Shen DH, Liu HJ, et al. Impact of multidisciplinary team working on the management of colorectal cancer. Chin Med J. 2012;125(2):172–7.

# Chapter 22
# Benign Liver Tumours

**James Pape and Charles Imber**

> **Key Learning Points**
> 1. Benign liver lesions can offer challenging dilemmas for clinicians.
> 2. Hepatic adenomas have the potential for malignant change determined by size and patient gender.
> 3. The mechanism and classification of hepatic adenomas are increasingly understood.
> 4. Haemangiomas, FNH and cysts are often asymptomatic but may cause problems due to pressure effects.
> 5. Surgical intervention must weigh up the risks to the patient and the potential benefits.
> 6. Liver transplantation may be indicated in a small number of polycystic liver disease cases, where patients are very symptomatic and the quality of life poor.

## Hepatocellular Adenoma

Hepatocellular adenoma (HCA) is a rare benign liver tumour derived from the proliferation of mature hepatocytes, with an incidence of 1 case for 1,000,000 people [1]: the incidence increases to 1–3 cases for 100,000 in females which use or have used an oral contraceptive long term.

J. Pape (✉) · C. Imber
Centre For HPB Surgery and Liver Transplantation, Royal Free Hospital, London, UK
e-mail: james.pape@nhs.net; charles.imber@nhs.net



T. Cross, D. H. Palmer (eds.), *Liver Cancers*,
https://doi.org/10.1007/978-3-319-92216-4_22

## Presentation and Clinical Features

More than 50% of adenomas are asymptomatic and identified incidentally; large lesions (6–30 cm) can cause right upper quadrant discomfort or pain due to expansion of the liver capsule. A potentially acute and life-threatening presentation occurs if a large peripheral or exophytic tumour breaks and bleeds into the abdominal cavity.

The main risk factor for HCA development is oestrogen exposure, explaining the predominance of female cases and the association with oral contraception. Also some congenital diseases such as glycogen storage diseases, as well as some metabolic syndrome manifestations such as diabetes mellitus, insulin resistance, dyslipidaemia and obesity, are considered as risk factors for the development and progression of HCA.

Men with metabolic syndrome are at a much higher risk (ten times more likely than females) for malignant degeneration of liver adenomas (anyway rare, <5%). Other risk factors for degeneration are androgen use, large tumours (>5 cm) and histological subtype (β-catenin-mutated).

## Pathophysiology

HCAs usually are solitary, well-delineated and, occasionally, pedunculated tumours with parenchyma composed of plates of hepatocytes separated by sinusoids without portal tract elements or bile ductules, a key feature in the histological distinction of HCA from focal nodular hyperplasia (FNH).

With regard to the morphomolecular aspects of the disease, the great leap forward was the discovery that hepatocellular adenoma was not a single entity and that at least three different subtypes exist, with specific underlying gene mutations [2]. These mutations affect the *HNF1A* gene, several genes leading to JAK/STAT3 pathway activation and the *CTNNB1* gene. All of them are associated with more or less specific histopathological characteristics and can be recognised using immunohistochemistry either with specific antibodies or with surrogate markers.

## Diagnostic Workup

Confronted with a potentially benign liver tumour, the first key clinical point is to perform a precise and unambiguous diagnosis. Abnormal liver function tests may occur in patients with large HCA tumours including increased γ-glutamyl transferase levels, alkaline phosphatase secondary to cholestasis or an increase in transaminase levels as a result of hepatic steatosis. Serum biomarkers of inflammation including fibrinogen and C-reactive protein were increased in 90% of patients with inflammatory HCA and returned to normal after surgical resection of the tumour.

Imaging is useful to rule out focal nodular hyperplasia (FNH) and hepatic haemangioma. Most HCAs are diagnosed on contrast-enhanced, multiphase computed tomography (CT) or magnetic resonance imaging (MRI). Multiphase dynamic contrast-enhanced MRI is considered the modality of choice in the diagnosis of HCA and its subtypes [3]. Histological analysis after percutaneous image-driven biopsy remains the gold standard of HCA diagnosis and can also help to rule out differential diagnoses, such as hepatocellular carcinoma (HCC) or FNH.

## *Management and Complications*

Classically, HCAs have been considered an indication for surgical resection due to their potential for both bleeding and malignant transformation. Yet, growing knowledge of this condition has showed that bleeding and malignant transformation were mainly observed in lesions >5 cm and rarely in lesions less than this size. It has also been shown that malignant transformation is ten times more frequent in males, especially in the presence of steroid intake. These features have led to the management of hepatic adenomas based on size and gender, with resection of HCAs >5 cm in females and of all HCAs in males. The surgical approach does not require a wide resection margin or a regional lymphadenectomy even in the case of suspected malignancy owing to the minimal risk of vascular invasion or lymph node involvement, and a laparoscopic approach may be considered for a non-haemorrhagic HCA. Intraoperative ultrasound is useful because HCA tumours often are soft and non-palpable with ill-defined margins between the tumour and the adjacent steatotic hepatic parenchyma.

Recent molecular subtyping of adenomas has revolutionised the field and further refined indications for resection of HCAs [4]. In several reference centres, it has revived the use of preoperative biopsies for more personalised management. Thus, liver surgeons must be fully educated on the molecular subtypes of hepatic adenomas. HCA molecular subtypes drive the prognosis and natural history of these lesions, have a good correlation with imaging; and can be studied on biopsy specimens using specific immunochemistry. Obesity is a risk factor for inflammatory HCA and ‘sonic hedgehog’ HCA, which also has a high risk of bleeding. Hepatocyte nuclear factor 1 alpha HCA has a low potential for malignant transformation, while b-catenin-activated HCA has a high potential for progressing to malignancy. Less than 10% of HCAs are not characterised by imaging or immunohistochemistry. All are precipitated by oral contraceptives in females and the size and gender rule (higher risk of bleeding and malignancy in lesions >5 cm and of malignancy in males) remains valid in all subtypes. These findings are summarised in Table 22.1.

**Table 22.1** Classification and significance of different subtypes of hepatic adenoma

| Bordeaux group risk prediction tool for adenoma | | | | |
|---|---|---|---|---|
| Tumour subtype | Prevalence | HCC association | Bleeding risk | Immunohistochemical markers |
| Hepatocyte nuclear factor 1α | 30–50% | Rare | N/A | Liver fatty acid-binding protein |
| β-Catenin activated | 10–15% | 46% association | N/A | β-Catenin |
| Inflammatory | 35% | None | N/A | Serum amyloid A |
| Sonic hedgehog | 4% | Rare | High | GLI1 activation |
| Unclassified | 5–10% | N/A | N/A | None |

### *Prognosis*

Most patients are asymptomatic, and small lesions in women have an excellent prognosis. In men or women with larger tumours, histological subtyping and/or consideration of resection is necessary.

## Haemangioma

### *Presentation and Clinical Features*

Hepatic haemangiomas account for up to 70% of benign liver lesions. Estimated prevalence varies from 0.4 to 20%, making them the most common liver lesion. Most are discovered incidentally during laparotomy or imaging for an unrelated indication.

Haemangiomas are typically asymptomatic, but larger lesions may cause symptoms which are most commonly right upper quadrant pain or fullness. Nausea, loss of appetite and early satiety are less common and may occur due to compression of adjacent structures. If there is thrombosis or bleeding within the tumour, sudden severe abdominal pain may result, associated with liver function derangement and fever. Rarely, rupture into the biliary tree leads to haemobilia.

In children, giant haemangiomas have been associated with high-output cardiac failure.

Generally physical examination is unremarkable, but occasionally a liver mass is palpable.

Haemangiomas of the liver may be associated with haemangiomas of other organs, focal nodular hyperplasia and bile duct hamartomas.

## *Pathophysiology*

Haemangiomas range in size from a few millimetres to more than 20 cm diameter. They are often solitary but may be multiple in up to 40% of patients [5]. Lesions larger than 5 cm are referred to as giant haemangiomas and are more likely to grow or cause symptoms.

The tumour is made up of different sizes of cavernous vascular spaces lined with a single layer of endothelium and filled with blood which may thrombose. This thrombosis may lead to the development of a collagenous scar or fibrous nodule. Lesions are surrounded by a thin capsule.

Sex hormones may influence tumour growth as haemangiomas enlarge in pregnancy and during administration of oestrogen or progesterone. The lesions often regress after withdrawal of the therapy. However, oestrogen receptors have not been found in all haemangiomas, and tumour growth has been reported in the absence of oestrogen therapy and in postmenopausal women, and so the association is not yet entirely defined.

## *Diagnostic Workup*

In the absence of compressive effects, liver function tests are normal unless there is acute bleeding or thrombosis within the haemangioma. Alpha-fetoprotein (AFP) is normal.

Ultrasound usually strongly suggests haemangioma, but other modalities are added to confirm the diagnosis if the patient has a history of malignancy or chronic liver disease, as malignant tumours have similar patterns on ultrasound. Smaller lesions are usually easier to identify, but the thrombosis and fibrosis in larger lesions make confident diagnosis more challenging. Contrast agents used in conjunction with ultrasound improve the detection rate [6].

CT scanning with contrast and a portal venous phase shows initial peripheral enhancement of the lesion and the centre filling in thereafter. Larger lesions may opacify atypically due to differing sizes of vascular spaces, scar tissue and the presence of cystic spaces.

MRI is highly accurate and may be further enhanced when combined with liver-specific IV contrast.

Technetium-99 m pertechnetate-labelled red blood cells are highly specific, but sensitivity is affected by the presence of fibrosis and thrombosis. Single-photon emission CT (SPECT) has an accuracy close to that of MRI.

Angiography is rarely used for diagnosis but may assist for atypical tumours that elude definitive diagnosis after non-invasive imaging.

Percutaneous needle biopsy has been associated with fatal haemorrhage, and as the diagnostic yield is low its value is debatable and use is best avoided.

## *Management*

Patients with asymptomatic small lesions may be reassured and observed. Lesions <5 cm are often not followed up provided there is diagnostic certainty. Larger lesions are more likely to grow and should have repeat imaging in 6–12 months. Prophylactic resection cannot be justified as the risk of bleeding is low.

There is controversy as to whether patients with haemangiomas should be advised against pregnancy. Oral contraceptives and pregnancy seem associated with haemangioma development and growth, but there is insufficient evidence to make a conclusive link.

Indications for treatment include failure to exclude malignancy radiologically, incapacitating symptoms or complications including rupture and intraperitoneal bleeding. The management of asymptomatic lesions that are large or growing is controversial, as complications of observing these remain mild and do not outweigh the risk of surgery [7].

Where the indication is pain, other causes should be ruled out beforehand as a number of patients have persistent pain after haemangioma treatment.

Surgical treatment options are resection, enucleation, hepatic artery ligation and transplantation.

Non-surgical treatments include arterial embolisation, radiotherapy and interferon alpha-2a.

Arterial embolisation may be used for acute bleeding control and treatment, or to reduce the size of lesions preoperatively.

Radiotherapy is used occasionally for the treatment of childhood haemangiomas but is rarely a first-line therapy due to risks of secondary malignancy and effects on growth [8].

Interferon alpha-2a is used for treatment of infants with life-threatening extrahepatic haemangiomas but with limited success, and it has not been well studied for hepatic haemangiomas [9].

## *Natural History and Complications*

The natural history of hepatic haemangioma is not completely understood, with variable results reported in available studies. This makes it challenging to determine what proportion of the lesions will progress. Spontaneous rupture is a rare but serious complication and occurs usually in large haemangiomas that are located peripherally. Rupture following abdominal trauma is also possible but uncommon.

## *Prognosis*

Most patients are asymptomatic, and the lesions have an excellent prognosis.

# Focal Nodular Hyperplasia

Focal nodular hyperplasia (FNH) is a generally benign liver lesion that usually occurs in a normal liver and only occasionally becomes symptomatic. It can be challenging to differentiate radiologically from some more sinister liver pathology.

## *Presentation and Clinical Features*

The incidence of FNH is estimated at 0.3% [10]. It occurs most commonly in adults, especially women of childbearing age. It is more common in females with reported ratios varying from 8 to 15:1 [11, 12]. Lesions in men are often smaller and more likely to be atypical.

FNH accounts for approximately 8% of primary liver tumours and is between three and ten times more common than hepatocellular adenoma.

Most FNH are found incidentally in patients without symptoms. 12–13% are discovered when abnormal liver function tests are investigated.

Symptoms are rare but include abdominal pain, a palpable mass (2–4%) or hepatomegaly.

Differential diagnosis is challenging, especially with other hypervascular entities such as hepatocellular adenoma, hepatocellular carcinoma and hypervascular metastases, which appear similar on imaging. MRI and CT can lead to diagnosis when typical features are demonstrated, but these are not always present [11].

## *Pathogenesis*

FNH probably develops secondary to local hemodynamic instability in the liver. An arterial malformation leads to hyperperfusion of an area of the liver causing a regenerative response. At present the pathophysiology remains unclear, but FNH is accepted to be truly benign and is not expected to bleed spontaneously or undergo malignant transformation [10, 13].

FNH has been associated with hepatic haemangiomas and various vascular malformations, leading to the hypothesis that it may result from a congenital vascular abnormality [11].

Oral contraceptives do not cause FNH, but established FNH may further develop in response to oestrogens. Patients taking oral contraceptives tend to have larger more vascular tumours. The reports of haemorrhage and rupture of FNH that have occurred have all been in patients taking oral contraceptives. FNH are well-differentiated lesions without a capsule and contain scar tissue. Fibrous stroma divides the lesion into small hepatocellular nodules. The stroma is prominent and forms a central stellate scar. There is disruption of the central veins and portal tracts of the normal hepatic lobule and large dystrophic arteries.

Arteries drain into adjacent hepatic veins producing a 'spoke and wheel' pattern that is seen on angiography. FNH can be differentiated from hepatocellular adenoma by the presence of sinusoids and Kupffer cells [11].

## *Diagnostic Workup*

Laboratory testing is often unremarkable, but mild disruption of hepatic enzymes may occur. Alpha-fetoprotein is normal [11].

Ultrasound often incidentally detects FNH, but its appearance varies greatly. Lesions may appear hypo- or isoechoic and rarely as hyperechoic. The central scar is only seen in about 20% of cases, and it may be difficult to distinguish FNH from adenoma or malignant lesions. Ultrasound becomes more informative when combined with IV contrast, which may show arterial phase enhancement of the central stellate arteries. Emerging research suggests that the ability of contrast-enhanced ultrasound to differentiate solid liver tumours is comparable with MRI.

CT is often suggestive of the diagnosis and should be performed without contrast and then with hepatic arterial and portal venous phases. The lesion is iso- or hypodense before contrast and then hyperdense with contrast. The central scar often enhances prominently. CT has been shown to have a sensitivity of 75% and specificity of 92% [14].

MRI is considered highly accurate in diagnosis of FNH and useful when other imaging techniques are inadequate for diagnosis. The use of IV contrast allows for definitive diagnosis if typical behaviour is present [13].

In FNH behaving atypically, differentiation can be difficult. Gadolinium-based hepato-specific contrast agents may assist—these are taken up by the liver and excreted in the biliary system. Since adenomas and metastases do not contain bile ducts, they can be distinguished from FNH.

Angiography may reveal the diagnostic 'spoked wheel' but is rarely indicated [14].

If doubt still exists, image-guided biopsy may be undertaken, but existing data shows a poor correlation between a biopsy diagnosis of FNH and the histology of subsequently resected specimens [15].

## *Management*

Management remains controversial due to the lack of randomised trials comparing elective resection with conservative management. However the absence of malignant transformation and the relative rarity of complications support a conservative approach if sufficient diagnostic certainty can be achieved. This is especially true for small asymptomatic lesions that do not enlarge at follow-up [15].

Suggested indications for resection include diagnostic doubt, tumour enlargement (3–5 cm/year) and symptomatic lesions, although no randomised controlled trials have studied the benefit of elective surgery [13]. Surgery for FNH has been demonstrated to be safe. Moreover, it is associated with both a low morbidity and in providing long-term relief from symptoms [13, 15].

Angio-embolisation has been described and may be considered when symptomatic lesions are not resectable.

### *Prognosis*

FNH generally runs a benign course and has a very good prognosis.

## Hepatic Cysts

Hepatobiliary cystic lesions are more common than previously thought. With advances in modern cross-sectional imaging, the prevalence of hepatobiliary cystic lesions has increased from a presumed 2–3% historically to 18%. The differential diagnosis of hepatobiliary cystic lesions is broad, and it ranges from benign, asymptomatic lesions to infectious lesions and aggressive malignancies.

### *Presentation and Clinical Features*

In many cases, hepatobiliary cysts are asymptomatic and are found incidentally on imaging for other reasons. This is especially true for simple hepatic cysts, although large simple cysts may produce abdominal pain, vague discomfort or fullness, early satiety, palpable mass or abdominal distention. In the setting of polycystic liver disease (PCLD), patients often present with a protuberant abdomen from massive hepatomegaly with or without associated autosomal dominant polycystic kidney disease.

Infectious hepatic cysts, including parasitic, amoebic and pyogenic abscesses, often present with fever, malaise, right upper quadrant pain and even sepsis. Additionally, there is often a history of antecedent intra-abdominal infection or biliary tract manipulation. Pyogenic liver abscesses can result from haematogenous seeding from extra-abdominal infections, especially in immunosuppressed individuals. Parasitic liver abscesses are most commonly due to echinococcal infection (hydatid disease), which is endemic in the Middle East, Asia, Australia, New Zealand and South America.

Neoplastic hepatic cysts which include cystadenoma, cystadenocarcinoma and intraductal papillary mucinous neoplasm of biliary origin (IPMN-B) are rare and are thought to account for <1% of all cystic lesions. Diagnosis is typically delayed for these lesions because symptoms are indolent and nonspecific. They include abdominal pain or discomfort, abdominal swelling and jaundice.

## *Diagnostic Workup*

Blood tests will normally be unrevealing in this situation. Patients with infectious cysts may have leukocytosis and elevated alkaline phosphatase, gamma-glutamyl transferase and transaminases. Erythrocyte sedimentation rate and C-reactive protein are also frequently elevated. The armamentarium for diagnosis and characterisation of hepatobiliary cystic neoplasms includes ultrasound, cross-sectional imaging (CT and MRI), magnetic resonance cholangiopancreatography (MRCP) and endoscopic retrograde cholangiopancreatography (ERCP).

Cyst fluid is typically acellular and is not helpful in distinguishing simple cysts from other cysts, including neoplastic cysts. Multiple recent studies have demonstrated that cyst and serum concentrations of CEA and CA 19-9 in patients with simple cysts and cystadenoma are comparable [16].

## *Management*

Asymptomatic simple cysts do not require intervention. If symptomatic the primary treatment modalities for simple hepatic cysts include sclerotherapy and laparoscopic or open fenestration. Aspiration is not recommended as definitive therapy due to a nearly 100 percent recurrence rate.

In symptomatic patients with polycystic liver disease, the goal of therapy is to reduce liver volume to the greatest extent possible. In this setting, cyst recurrence is the rule. Medical therapies include octreotide, lanreotide and sirolimus, all of which have been shown to achieve modest reductions in liver volume by inhibiting cyst fluid secretion and are of limited value. Additional options include aspiration and sclerotherapy, cyst fenestration or liver resection in cases where one area of the liver is predominantly affected, and there is little to no functional parenchyma in that area. Liver transplant is rarely indicated for PCLD as the uninvolved liver parenchyma functions normally, but for quality of life improvement if extremely symptomatic, it can be considered. If the patient is losing weight and muscle mass, this may lend weight to the indication or if combined liver kidney transplant is required because of worsening renal function due to coexistent polycystic kidney disease.

In patients presenting with pyogenic liver abscess, blood cultures should be obtained immediately, and broad-spectrum IV antibiotics should be administered as soon as possible. If the abscess is secondary to an intra-abdominal infection, the source should be addressed (i.e. appendicitis, diverticulitis, cholangitis, etc.). As with any abscess, the key to successful treatment is drainage. Ultrasound-guided percutaneous drainage can be achieved by simple aspiration or catheter drainage and is generally recommended as the first therapeutic approach. Aspiration is well-suited for multiple small abscesses, whereas catheter drainage is recommended for large abscesses with loculation. If percutaneous drainage fails, surgical drainage is required and can be performed via a laparoscopic or open approach.

Recommended treatment for hydatid cysts includes chemotherapy combined with surgery or percutaneous aspiration, injection and re-aspiration (PAIR).

Neoplastic hepatic cysts include biliary cystadenoma, cystadenocarcinoma and the more recently recognised IPMN-B. There is as of yet no way to distinguish between cystadenoma, a premalignant lesion, and cystadenocarcinoma in the absence of metastatic disease. Regardless, both lesions should be treated with complete resection by enucleation, partial hepatectomy or bile duct resection with bilio-enteric reconstruction for extrahepatic lesions [15]. Partial resection and drainage are inadequate due to high recurrence rates.

## *Prognosis*

Hepatobiliary cystic lesions encompass a range of benign and malignant conditions. Clinical presentation, laboratory investigations and imaging can often lead to a diagnosis prior to surgical intervention. In more complex cases, patients should be presented and discussed in a multidisciplinary setting.

# Conclusion

Benign liver tumours are not infrequently seen, and a robust diagnostic approach is necessary to avoid missing malignancies and also to prevent harm being done from unnecessary medical interventions. The natural history of hepatic adenomas and their underlying pathophysiology are being increasingly understood. Haemangiomas, FNH and cysts often require no intervention, but should the patient become symptomatic, the harms and benefits must be carefully considered and fully discussed with the patient prior to any intervention. Treatment, including surgery and embolic procedures, should only be offered in centres with experience in managing these patients. Table 22.2 summarises the key differences between the most commonly seen benign liver tumours.

**Table 22.2** Summary of clinical features of the common benign liver tumours

| Features of benign liver tumours | | | | |
|---|---|---|---|---|
| | Adenoma | Haemangioma | FNH | Simple liver cyst |
| Prevalence | Very rare | Common | Infrequent | Common |
| Presentation | >50% asymptomatic | Asymptomatic | Mostly incidental | Simple cysts generally asymptomatic. Infective cysts with features of inflammation |
| Pathology | Plates of hepatocytes<br>3 morphological subtypes | Cavernous vascular spaces with single layer of endothelium. Thrombosis may lead to collagenous scar | Fibrous central stellate scar | Variety of pathologies—simple, infective, neoplastic |
| Laboratory tests | Large lesions may cause cholestasis<br>Increased fibrinogen and CRP | Normal unless compressive effects | Occasional mild hepatic enzyme disruption | Usually normal, infective cysts with appropriately raised makers. |
| Radiological and other investigations | Variable per subtypes<br>No capsule<br>Consider biopsy for molecular subtyping | Homogenous. Peripheral enhancement with contrast followed by central filling. No capsule | Hypodense becoming hyperdense with contrast, with visible central scar | Fluid-filled lesion with distinct capsule |
| Management | Surgical resection (males, or >5 cm lesion in females) due to risk of bleeding and malignant transformation | Conservative if asymptomatic | Conservative—resect if large or symptomatic | Conservative, or sclerotherapy or fenestration if symptomatic |

# References


1. Rooks JB, Ory HW, Ishak KG, et al. Epidemiology of hepatocellular adenoma. The role of oral contraceptive use. JAMA. 1979;242:644–8.
2. Bioulac-Sage P, Rebouissou S, Thomas C, et al. Hepatocellular adenoma subtype classification using molecular markers and immunohistochemistry. Hepatology. 2007;46:740–8.
3. Ronot M, Bahrami S, Calderaro J, et al. Hepatocellular adenomas: accuracy of magnetic resonance imaging and liver biopsy in subtype classification. Hepatology. 2011;53:1182–91.
4. Bioulac-Sage P, Laumonier H, Couchy G, et al. Hepatocellular adenoma management and phenotypic classification: the Bordeaux experience. Hepatology. 2009;50:481–9.
5. Tait N, Richardson AJ, Muguti G, Little JM. Hepatic cavernous haemangioma: a 10 year review. Aust N Z J Surg. 1992;62(7):521–4. http://www.ncbi.nlm.nih.gov/pubmed/1610320. [cited 2018 Jan 14]

6. Leifer DM, Middleton WD, Teefey SA, Menias CO, Leahy JR. Follow-up of patients at low risk for hepatic malignancy with a characteristic hemangioma at US. Radiology. 2000;214(1):167–72. http://pubs.rsna.org/doi/10.1148/radiology.214.1.r00ja09167. [cited 2018 Jan 14]
7. Miura JT, Amini A, Schmocker R, Nichols S, Sukato D, Winslow ER, et al. Surgical management of hepatic hemangiomas: a multi-institutional experience. HPB. 2014;16(10):924–8. http://www.ncbi.nlm.nih.gov/pubmed/24946109. [cited 2018 Jan 14]
8. Gaspar L, Mascarenhas F, da Costa MS, Dias JS, Afonso JG, Silvestre ME. Radiation therapy in the unresectable cavernous hemangioma of the liver. Radiother Oncol. 1993;29(1):45–50. http://www.ncbi.nlm.nih.gov/pubmed/8295987. [cited 2018 Jan 14]
9. Ezekowitz RAB, Mulliken JB, Folkman J. Interferon Alfa-2a therapy for life-threatening hemangiomas of infancy. N Engl J Med. 1992;326(22):1456–63. http://www.ncbi.nlm.nih.gov/pubmed/1489383. [cited 2018 Jan 14]
10. Wanless IR, Mawdsley C, Adams R. On the pathogenesis of focal nodular hyperplasia of the liver. Hepatology. 1985;5(6):1194–200. http://www.ncbi.nlm.nih.gov/pubmed/4065824. [cited 2018 Jan 4]
11. Nguyen BN, Fléjou JF, Terris B, Belghiti J, Degott C. Focal nodular hyperplasia of the liver: a comprehensive pathologic study of 305 lesions and recognition of new histologic forms. Am J Surg Pathol. 1999;23(12):1441–54. http://www.ncbi.nlm.nih.gov/pubmed/10584697. [cited 2018 Jan 5]
12. Luciani A, Kobeiter H, Maison P, Cherqui D, Zafrani E-S, Dhumeaux D, et al. Focal nodular hyperplasia of the liver in men: is presentation the same in men and women? Gut. 2002;50(6):877–80. http://www.ncbi.nlm.nih.gov/pubmed/12010893. [cited 2018 Jan 5]
13. Cristiano A, Dietrich A, Spina JC, Ardiles V, de Santibañes E. Focal nodular hyperplasia and hepatic adenoma: current diagnosis and management. Updates Surg. 2014;66(1):9–21. http://www.ncbi.nlm.nih.gov/pubmed/23807711. [cited 2018 Jan 3]
14. Rogers JV, Mack LA, Freeny PC, Johnson ML, Sones PJ. Hepatic focal nodular hyperplasia: angiography, CT, sonography, and scintigraphy. AJR Am J Roentgenol. 1981;137(5):983–90. http://www.ajronline.org/doi/10.2214/ajr.137.5.983. [cited 2018 Jan 6]
15. Vogt DP, Henderson JM, Chmielewski E. Cystadenoma and cystadenocarcinoma of the liver: a single center experience. J Am Coll Surg. 2005;200:727–33.
16. Seo JK, Kim SH, Lee SH, et al. Appropriate diagnosis of biliary cystic tumors: comparison with atypical hepatic simple cysts. Eur J Gastroenterol Hepatol. 2010;22:989–96.

# Appendix

## New Directions in the Management of Hepatocellular Carcinoma

The majority of patients with HCC present with non-curative disease, i.e. BCLC stage B–D disease [1]. As mentioned in earlier chapters, there has been an expansion in the treatments available from ablation therapies (microwave, radio frequency, cryoablation and irreversible electroporation (IRE) for early-stage disease patients not fit for surgery) to embolic therapies (transarterial embolization (TAE), transarterial chemoembolization (TACE) and selective internal radiation therapy (SIRT)) for patients with intermediate-stage disease through to the introduction of sorafenib [2] and the new generation of systemic therapies for first-line (lenvatinib [3]) or second-line therapies (regorafinib [4]). Yet, the only way a clinician can assess response is to give treatment and follow the patient up. Surely, it would be better if the clinician knew beforehand that the treatment being offered was very likely to be successful. The 'holy grail' for much of medicine and not just peculiar to oncology is the development of personalized medicine.

The historical reluctance to biopsy liver tumours due to the overstated risk of tumour seeding and bleeding has, in retrospect, hindered our understanding of this malignancy and in the process allowed potential targets for treatment to remain elusive. In the future, particularly when cure with resection or liver transplantation is not considered possible, it may become standard practice to biopsy dominant liver lesions and perform DNA sequencing to identify targets best suited to treat and individualize care based on those findings. With refinements in technique, it may be possible to identify circulating markers and DNA accurately from peripheral blood. This in turn may lead to the identification of new biomarkers that permit earlier detection of the disease to improve the quality and sensitivity of surveillance and also provide a further way to assess response to treatment (provided that the test is cheap, effective and readily available in a target population).



T. Cross, D. H. Palmer (eds.), *Liver Cancers*,
https://doi.org/10.1007/978-3-319-92216-4

Patients with intermediate-stage disease who progress on treatments such as TACE have few options for liver-confined disease. Some centres use alternative chemotherapeutic against or bland embolizations, but these are not proven to be superior and data is lacking. For lesions too large for ablation or unresponsive to TACE/TAE and where TARE, as in the UK, is not universally available, the options for patients and clinicians are limited. Unlike other forms of malignancy, the role of radiotherapy had taken a back seat and was not considered a viable or relevant treatment option. But the development of stereotactic body radiotherapy (SBRT) is changing this perception. At present, this technique does not fit in anywhere among the algorithms applied by BCLC or AASLD guidelines although it has been proposed that SBRT could be applied across the HCC spectrum of disease from very early to very advanced stages [5]. This treatment requires careful staging and planning on how to deliver multiple beams of radiation to be delivered in a highly targeted and focussed way. It is thought that radiation may have a directly ablative effect on the tumour as well as have direct effects on the endothelium (fuKs). A further intriguing mechanism is whether radiation induces a tumour antigen-specific immune response that enhances the effectiveness of tumour cell death [6].

This degree of accuracy was not previously possible, and the concern was that excessive toxicity and local tissue damage might be incurred. Several observational studies from around the world have suggested this technique may be a further tool to be added to the armamentarium directed against HCC. Sanuki and colleagues assessed outcomes in a retrospective series of 185 patients. Dose of radiation was 35 Gy for patients with Childs-Pugh B disease or 40 Gy if the patient had Childs-Pugh A disease, in five fractions. In short, the 3-year local control rate and overall survival were 91% and 70%, respectively. Equivalent outcomes were observed regardless of the dose of radiation administered [7]. A similar study was done by Wahl and colleagues when outcomes were compared between radio-frequency ablation or SBRT for small inoperable HCC. Two hundred patients were identified of which 161 (249 tumours) underwent RFA and 63 had SBRT (83 tumours). The rates of freedom from local progression at 1 and 2 years was 83.6% and 80.2% for RFA and 97.4 and 83.8% for SBRT. The overall survival at 1 and 2 years was 70% and 53% for RFA versus 74% and 46% after SBRT [8].

In the UK, several centres have been involved in a service evaluation of the role of HCC in selected cases. A trial is planned in the future, and it is likely that SBRT may be compared against lesions that fail to respond to TACE. A study in South Korea showed that patients with an incomplete response to TACE had similar survival outcomes after SBRT to those patients who had an initial good response to TACE, suggesting this approach might be an alternative for patients not having an initial response to chemoembolization [9]. There is also emerging evidence that SBRT might have an emerging role in treating patients with portal vein tumour thrombosis related to HCC [10]. The procedure does require multiple visits to the hospital, but it does obviate the need for a hospital admission. Unfortunately, in the UK, the centres in England are predominantly in the south of the country, and there is only one centre in the North of England in Leeds.

Thus, many patients are some distance from these centres, and this might be disadvantageous, particularly as one of the highest UK prevalences of HCC is in North West of England.

The development of immune therapies has revolutionized the outcome for patients diagnosed with lung cancer, malignant melanoma and renal cell carcinoma. Given the historically poor outcomes in these patients, it is not too optimistic to expect that similar outcomes could be delivered in HCC or its cousin in young adults, fibrolamellar HCC, when surgical resection is not possible. The future management of patients with or at risk of HCC is likely to include better targeting of patients who will benefit from surveillance; the introduction of better biomarkers to help diagnose, assess tumour biology and acquire a more rapid assessment of treatment response, with a further understanding of the tumour, liver and patient characteristics, that better select treatment regimens with scientifically selected targets. Like other forms of malignancy, tumour cells in the liver cause subversion of the immune system that ultimately leads to full-blown HCC. The place of immune checkpoints, including programmed cell death protein 1, programmed cell death ligand 1 and cytotoxic T lymphocyte antigen 4, is increasingly being recognised as targets for treatments and to modify the disease process [11]. For patients with incurable disease, this could offer improved patient survival, and the additional prospect of regenerative medicine and methods to downstage liver scarring (fibrosis) could further reduce the likelihood of cancer development in the future.

In the past, the diagnosis of hepatocellular carcinoma was met with a sense of nihilism, but in the future, rather than being one of despair, we can look ahead with cautious optimism.

## References

1. European Association for the Study of the L, European Organisation for R, Treatment of C. Clinical practice guidelines: EASL–EORTC clinical practice guidelines: management of hepatocellular carcinoma. J Hepatol. 2012;56:908–43.
2. Llovet JM, Ricci S, Mazzaferro V, Hilgard P, Gane E, Blanc JF, et al. Sorafenib in advanced hepatocellular carcinoma. N Engl J Med. 2008;359(4):378–90.
3. Cheng A-L, Finn RS, Qin S, Han K-H, Ikeda K, Piscaglia F, et al. Phase III trial of lenvatinib (LEN) vs sorafenib (SOR) in first-line treatment of patients (pts) with unresectable hepatocellular carcinoma (uHCC). J Clin Oncol. 2017;35(15_Suppl):4001.
4. Bruix J, Qin S, Merle P, Granito A, Huang YH, et al. Regorafenib for patients with hepatocellular carcinoma who progressed on sorafenib treatment (RESORCE): a randomised, double-blind, placebo-controlled, phase 3 trial. Lancet. 2017;389(10064):56–66.
5. Dawson LA. Overview: where does radiation therapy fit in the spectrum of cancer loco-regional therapies? Semin Radiat Oncol. 2011;21(4):241–6.
6. Finkelstein SE, Timmerman R, McBride WH, Schaue D, Hoffe SE, et al. The confluence of sterotactic ablative radiotherapy and tumour immunology. Clin Dev Immunol. 2011.; ID 439752
7. Sanuki N, Takeda A, Oku Y, Mizuno T, Aoki Y, et al. Stereotactic body radiotherapy for small hepatocellular carcinoma: a retrospective outcome analysis in 185 patients. Acta Oncol. 2014;53(3):399–404.

8. Wahl DR, Stenmark MH, Tao Y, Pollom EL, Caoili EM, et al. Outcomes after stereotactic body radiotherapy or radiofrequency ablation for hepatocellular carcinoma. J Clin Oncol. 2016;34(5):452–9.
9. Paik EK, Kim MS, Jang WI, Seo YS, Cho CK, et al. Benefits of stereotactic ablative radiotherapy combined with incomplete transcatheter arterial chemoembolization in hepatocellular carcinoma. Radiat Oncol. 2016;11:22.
10. Yu JI, Park HC, Lim DH, Park W, Yoo BC, Paik SW, Koh KC, Lee JH. Prognostic index for portal vein tumor thrombosis in patients with hepatocellular carcinoma treated with radiation therapy. J Korean Med Sci. 2011;26(8):1014–22.
11. Elsegood CL, Tirnitz-Parker JE, Olynuy JK, Yeoh GCT. Immune checkpoint inhibition: prospects for prevention and therapy of hepatocellular carcinoma. Clin Transl Immunol. 2017;6(11):e161.

Printed by Printforce, the Netherlands